Atlas of Diagnosis and Management of Breast Diseases

This atlas focuses on the principles of diagnosis and management of breast diseases with a target audience of trainees and junior consultants in gynaecology, together with SAS grade doctors, advanced care practitioners, and specialist nurses.

Key Features:

- Provides an expert guide to the range of breast problems presenting for the gynaecologist
- Offers a reliable summary of the possible diagnoses and follow-up management procedures involved
- Guides the front-line clinician with the information to manage and advise patients with confidence

Atlas of Diagnosis and Management of Breast Diseases

Edited by

John R. Benson, DM (Oxon), MD (Cantab), FRCS
Cambridge Breast Unit, Cambridge University Hospitals NHS Foundation Trust, and School of Medicine, Anglia Ruskin University, Cambridge, UK

Ismail Jatoi, MD, PhD, FACS
Division of Surgical Oncology, Dale H. Dorn Chair in Surgery, University of Texas Health Science Center, San Antonio, Texas, USA

Dorin Dumitru, MD
Breast Unit, Castlehill Hospital and Hull York Medical School, Hull, UK

CRC Press
Taylor & Francis Group
Boca Raton London New York

CRC Press is an imprint of the Taylor & Francis Group, an **informa** business

Designed cover image: Getty Images

First edition published 2025

by CRC Press
2385 NW Executive Center Drive, Suite 320, Boca Raton FL 33431

and by CRC Press
4 Park Square, Milton Park, Abingdon, Oxon, OX14 4RN

CRC Press is an imprint of Taylor & Francis Group, LLC

ISBN: 9781032496368 (hbk)
ISBN: 9781032485690 (pbk)
ISBN: 9781003394785 (ebk)

DOI: 10.1201/9781003394785

Typeset in Palatino
by Apex CoVantage, LLC

Contents

Contributors

Christian M. Asher
Norfolk and Norwich University Hospitals NHS Foundation Trust, Norwich, UK

Susanne Cruickshank
Royal Marsden NHS Foundation Trust, London, UK

Sue Down
University of East Anglia, Norwich, UK, and James Paget University Hospital Trust, Great Yarmouth, UK

Sarah Downey
University of East Anglia, Norwich, UK

Rasheed Elayyan
University of East Anglia, Norwich, UK

E. R. Gatfield
Addenbrooke's Hospital, Cambridge, UK

Fiona Gilbert
University of Cambridge, Cambridge, UK

Victoria Harmer
Imperial College Healthcare NHS Trust, London, UK

Nuala Healy
Cambridge University Hospitals Foundation Trust, Cambridge, UK

Jonathan J. James
Nottingham Breast Institute, Nottingham, UK

Natasha E. Jiwa
Imperial College London, UK

Fleur Kilburn-Toppin
St. John's College, Cambridge University, Cambridge, UK

Sam Leinster
Norwich Medical School, University of East Anglia, Norwich, UK

Charles M. Malata
Cambridge Breast Unit at Addenbrooke's Hospital, Cambridge; University Hospitals NHS Foundation Trust, Cambridge and Anglia; Ruskin University School of Medicine, Cambridge and Chelmsford, UK

Falak Masood
Cambridge University Hospitals Foundation Trust, Cambridge, UK

M. B. Mukesh
Colchester Hospital, East Suffolk & North Essex NHS Trust, Colchester, UK

Francesca Muscara
Cambridge University Hospitals Foundation Trust, Cambridge, UK

Elena Provenzano
Addenbrooke's Hospital, Cambridge, UK

Ahsan Rao
Anglia Ruskin University and Mid and South Essex University NHS Trust, Cambridge, UK

Nisha Sharma
Leeds Teaching Hospitals, Leeds, UK

Matthew G. Wedlich
Addenbrooke's Hospital, Cambridge University Hospitals NHS Foundation Trust, Cambridge, UK

1

Anatomy and Physiology of the Breast

Ahsan Rao

1.1 Embryology and Development

The human breast is a unique and complex organ that undergoes significant changes throughout an individual's life stages. Understanding the development and embryology of the breast is essential for healthcare professionals as it provides insights into congenital and acquired breast disorders, their diagnosis, and their treatment.

1.1.1 Breast Bud Formation

The development of the human breast begins during embryonic life, around the fourth week of gestation.[1] The mammary gland, an epidermal appendage derived from the apocrine glands, initiates its development from the ectoderm layer of the embryo.[1] This process starts with the formation of mammary ridges or milk lines, which are parallel bands of thickened ectoderm that extend from the axillary region to the inguinal area.[1] The milk lines eventually give rise to the breast buds, which are the primordial structures of the mammary gland.

1.1.2 Mammary Gland Development

Mammary gland development comprises several stages, orchestrated by complex epithelial-mesenchymal interactions and regulated by systemic hormones.[2] The primary sprout of the mammary gland emerges from the breast bud, forming a solid epithelial cord that invades the underlying mesenchyme.[2] This cord subsequently branches and canalises, giving rise to the primitive ductal system of the mammary gland.[2] The terminal end buds (TEBs) are responsible for the elongation and branching of the ducts, and they play a crucial role in shaping the structure of the mammary gland.[2]

1.1.3 Role of Hormones and Growth Factors

Hormones and growth factors play a significant role in the development of the mammary gland. Oestrogen, progesterone, and prolactin are the primary hormones involved in breast development, while insulin-like growth factors (IGFs) and epidermal growth factors (EGFs) contribute to the regulation of mammary gland growth and differentiation.[3] The intricate interplay between these hormonal and growth factor signalling pathways ensures the proper development of the mammary gland and its associated structures

1.1.4 Pubertal Development of the Breast

1.1.4.1 Lobule Formation

The main spurt of breast growth occurs during puberty, with the formation of lobules.[4] Lobules are the functional units of the mammary gland, responsible for milk production during lactation.[4,5]

1.1.4.1.1 Tanner Stages

The development of the breast during puberty can be categorised into five stages, known as the Tanner stages.[6] These stages are:

1. **Prepubertal stage:**

   No glandular tissue is present, and the nipple is slightly raised.

2. **Breast budding stage:**

   The nipple and areola enlarge, and a small amount of glandular tissue is formed.

3. **Continued breast growth:**

   The breast and areola enlarge further, and more glandular tissue is formed.

4. **Areolar mound stage:**

   The areola forms a secondary mound on the breast.

5. **Mature breast stage:**

   The breast reaches its adult size and shape, with the areola and nipple forming a single contour.

DOI: 10.1201/9781003394785-1

It is important to note that individual variations exist in the timing and progression of these stages, influenced by genetic, hormonal, and environmental factors.

1.1.5 Hormonal Influences on Breast Development

1.1.5.1 Oestrogen and Progesterone

Oestrogen and progesterone are the primary hormones involved in the regulation of breast development. Oestrogen promotes ductal growth and branching, while progesterone stimulates the formation of lobules and alveoli.[7] These hormones act in a coordinated manner to regulate the growth and differentiation of the mammary gland throughout various life stages, including puberty, pregnancy, lactation, and menopause.[8]

1.1.5.2 Prolactin

Prolactin is another hormone that plays a crucial role in breast development, particularly during pregnancy and lactation. It stimulates the growth and differentiation of mammary gland epithelial cells and promotes milk production.[9] Additionally, prolactin acts in a paracrine manner to regulate the function of mammary stem cells, contributing to the maintenance and expansion of the mammary gland during pregnancy.[10]

1.2 Anatomy

1.2.1 Structure of the Breasts

The human breast is a complex and essential part of the body, playing a vital role in the female reproductive system as well as a source of nourishment for newborns.

The breasts are paired structures located on the anterior thoracic wall, in the pectoral region. They are present in both males and females, but more prominent in females following puberty. In females, the breast organ is an accessory gland of the reproductive system and are key structures involved in lactation.[4,5]

1.2.2 Surface Anatomy

The breast is located on the anterior thoracic wall, extending horizontally from the lateral border of the sternum to the mid-axillary line. Vertically, it spans between the second and sixth costal cartilages, lying superficially to the pectoralis major and serratus anterior muscles.

The superficial structures of the breast are thought to consist of two different regions:

- **Circular body:** The most prominent and largest part of the breast
- **Axillary tail:** It is the small part of the breast that lies along the bottom edge of the pectoralis major and runs towards the axillary fossa.

At the centre of the breast is the nipple, composed mostly of smooth muscle fibres. Surrounding the nipple is a pigmented area of skin called the areola.

1.2.3 External Anatomy

The external anatomy of the breast consists of the nipple, areola, and surrounding skin. The nipple is the central protrusion of the breast, which contains multiple openings for milk secretion during lactation. The areola is the pigmented circular area surrounding the nipple, which contains sebaceous glands that aid in lubrication and protection of the nipple during breastfeeding.

1.2.3.1 Nipples and Areola

The central prominence on the circular region of the breast is known as the nipple. Each nipple consists of 9–10 milk ducts.[11]

The nipple is surrounded by an annulus of skin that is darker in colour. Montgomery's glands excrete an oily substance that serves to protect the nipple and surrounding skin from friction while nursing.[12]

1.2.4 Internal Anatomy

The internal anatomy of the breast is composed of glandular tissue, adipose tissue, connective tissue, and various supporting structures. The glandular tissue is responsible for milk production and secretion and comprises numerous lobules, which contain clusters of milk-producing alveoli. These lobules are connected to a network of ducts that transport milk to the nipple.

Adipose tissue, or fat, gives the breast its size and shape, and its distribution varies among individuals. Connective tissue, including ligaments and fascia, provides support and maintains the structural integrity of the breast.

- Lobes
- Mammary gland (lobules)
- Lactiferous ducts
- Connective tissue stroma

- Pectoral fascia and retro-mammary space
- Nipples and areola

The anatomy of the breast is illustrated schematically in Figure 1.1.

1.2.4.1 Lobes

There are 15 to 20 sections (lobes) surrounding the nipple in a spiral wheel shape in each breast.[10]

1.2.4.2 Mammary Gland (Lobules)

The mammary glands are modified sweat glands consisting of a series of ducts and secretory lobules (15–20). Each lobule consists of many alveoli drained by a single lactiferous duct. These ducts converge at the nipple like spokes of a wheel.[13] The system of each end lobule connected to its main duct is called the terminal ductal lobular unit.[13]

The mammary glands are composed of two types of tissue:

- **Endocrine tissue:** This is responsible for making hormones that stimulate breast development and maturation.
- **Exocrine tissue:** This is responsible for the production of milk.

1.2.4.3 Lactiferous Ducts

Small tubes carry milk from the exocrine tissue of the mammary gland to the nipples, which are also known as milk ducts.[14]

1.2.4.4 Connective Tissue Stroma

The connective tissue within the breasts is known as the stroma. This structure supports and strengthens the breast, divides the mammary gland tissue into separate sections, and contains nerves and blood vessels.[15] It has both a fibrous and a fatty component.

The **fibrous stroma** condenses to form suspensory ligaments (of Astley Cooper). These ligaments have two main functions:

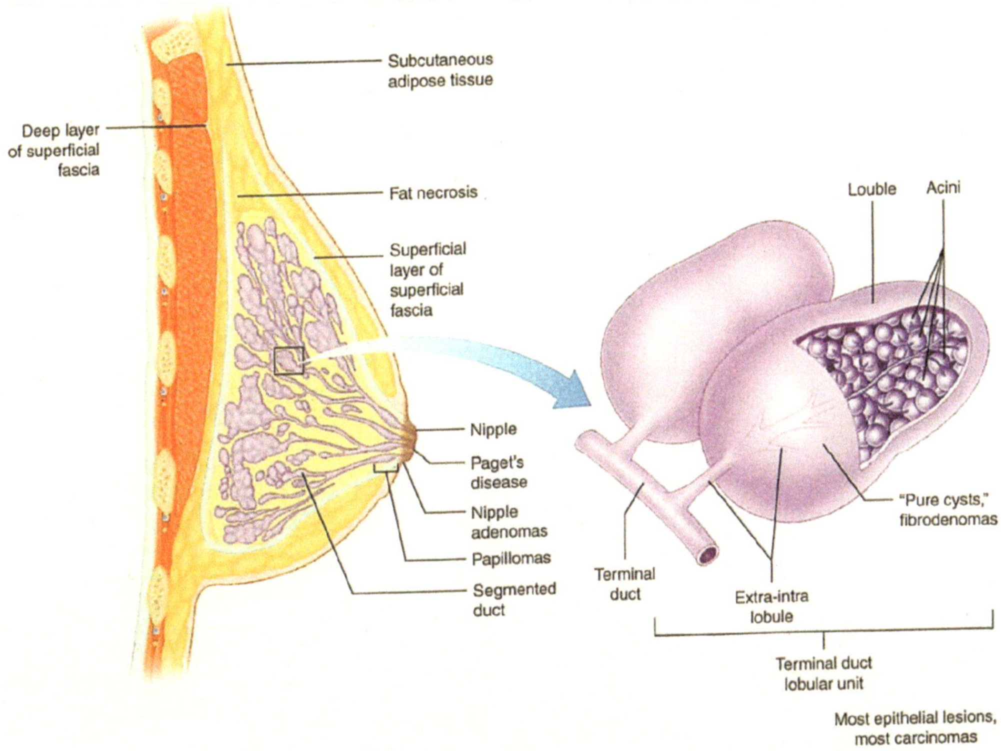

FIGURE 1.1
Schematic diagram showing arrangement of the ducts and lobules within the human breast and illustrating the basic functional unit—the terminal duct lobular unit. The latter drains into a sub-segmental and then larger segmental duct with several of these larger ducts intertwined within any single lobe.

Source: **Jatoi I, Benson J, Sbitany H, 'Anatomy of the breast', in *Atlas of Breast Surgery*, second edition, Springer, 2020, with permission.**

- Attach and secure the breast to the dermis and underlying pectoral fascia.
- Separate the secretory lobules of the breast.

1.2.4.5 Pectoral Fascia

The pectoral fascia is a sheet of connective material located just under the surface of the skin. It stretches from one side of the chest to the other, covering the chest wall and extending over the area of the nipple.[16] The base of the breast lies on the pectoral fascia—a flat sheet of connective tissue associated with the pectoralis major muscle. It acts as an attachment point for the suspensory ligaments.

1.2.4.6 Retro-Mammary Space

There is a layer of loose connective tissue between the breast and the pectoral fascia, known as the retromammary space. This potential space is often used in reconstructive plastic surgery.[17]

The retromammary region is made up of a thin sheet of soft connective tissue that lies between the pectoral fascia and the breast tissue. Muscles and ligaments in the chest wall help to expand the space when we breathe in. The breast contains extra nerves and blood vessels that make up this space.[18]

1.2.5 Inframammary Fold

The inframammary fold is a crucial anatomical feature that defines the shape and structure of the breast, particularly in women. It is located between the fifth and sixth ribs and is thought to be where the ligaments or fascia are attached to the ribs.

1.2.5.1 Vasculature

The mammary gland in the human body is abundantly supplied with blood vessels, which supply blood to each lobe as well as to the nipple area.[19]

The lobes and ducts are linked up by means of blood vessels. The blood supply for the lobes comes from the lateral thoracic artery (a branch of the thoraco-acromial artery), perforator branches of internal mammary artery medially, and perforator branches of intercostal vessels inferiorly. The blood supply to the ducts is mostly by mammary branches that come off the lateral mammary arteries and end in the ducts (Figure 1.2).[20]

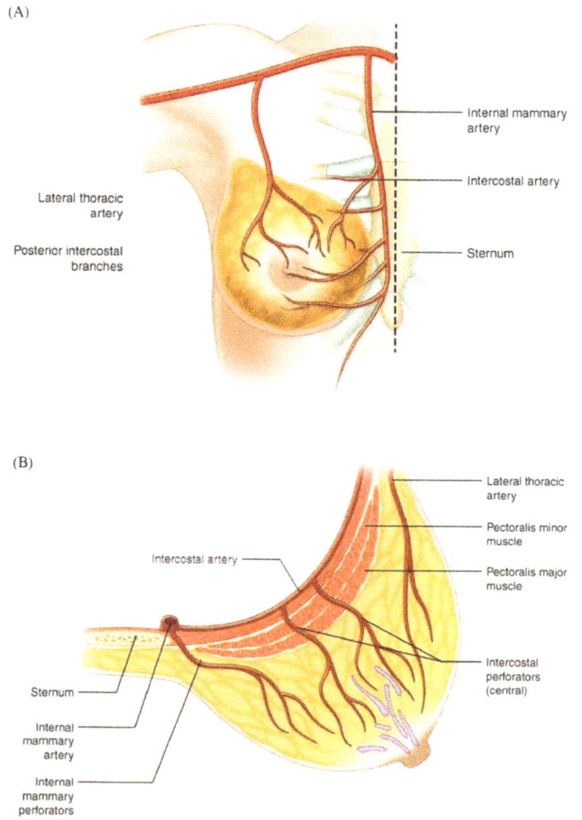

FIGURE 1.2
(A, B) The blood supply to the breast comes predominantly from the lateral thoracic and internal mammary arteries. Perforating branches from the internal mammary artery penetrate the intercostal spaces (second, third, and fourth) to pass through the pectoralis major muscle to supply the medial and deep parts of the breast. The blood supply enters the breast from superolateral and inferomedial directions with a rich network of anastomoses within the parenchyma.

Source: **Jatoi I, Benson J, Sbitany H, 'Anatomy of the breast', in *Atlas of Breast Surgery*, second edition, Springer, 2020, with permission.**

1.2.5.2 Branches of the Axillary Artery

The axillary artery gives off branches that supply the lateral thoracic, superior thoracic, subscapular, and thoracoacromial regions.[21] They travel through the brachial plexus and gives rise to the lateral thoracoacromial arteries.

1.2.5.3 Internal Thoracic Branches

These branches are located on the front of the chest just below the clavicle. They arise from the internal mammary artery and these branches supply the medial part of the breast (Figure 1.2(B)).[22]

Branches of Intercostal Arteries:

> The pectoral branches of the second, third, and fourth intercostal arteries supply the entire breast.[23]

1.2.6 Venous Drainage

There are many breast veins that follow the corresponding arteries in order to drain into the axillary, internal thoracic, and second-fourth intercostal veins.[24]

1.2.6.1 Chest Wall Musculature

The chest wall muscles can be broadly categorised into three groups: extrinsic, intrinsic, and accessory muscles. Each group serves a specific purpose and contributes to the overall function of the chest wall (Figure 1.3).

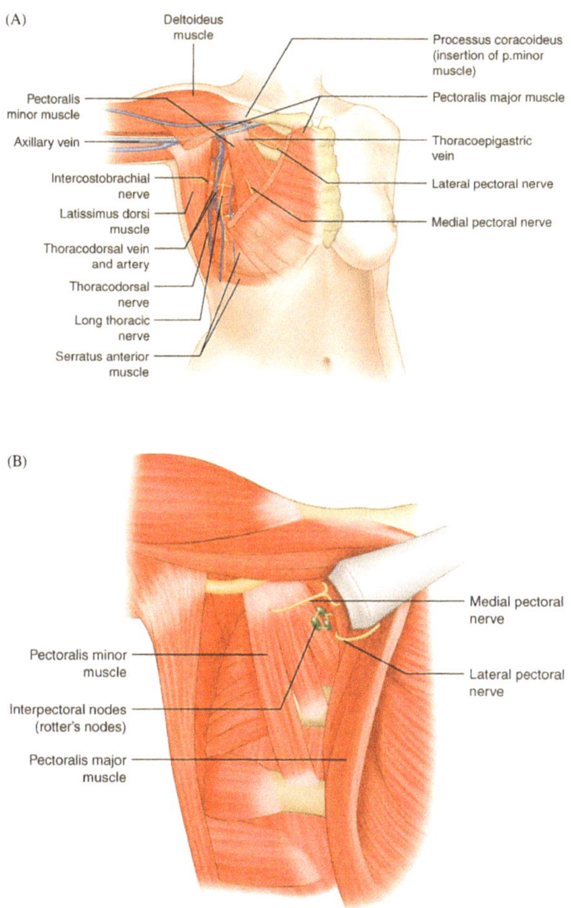

FIGURE 1.3
(A, B) Schematic illustration of the chest wall musculature including extrinsic muscles, intrinsic muscles, and accessory muscles (see text). The long thoracic and thoracodorsal nerves are important motor nerves that supply the serratus anterior and latissimus dorsi muscles, respectively, and can be damaged during breast surgery. The intercostobrachial nerve is purely sensory and derives from T1 and T2 nerve roots.

Source: **Jatoi I, Benson J, Sbitany H, 'Anatomy of the breast', in** ***Atlas of Breast Surgery,*** **second edition, Springer, 2020, with permission.**

1.2.6.2 Extrinsic Muscles

Extrinsic muscles are primarily responsible for moving the upper extremities and stabilising the shoulder girdle. These include the latissimus dorsi, pectoralis major, and pectoralis minor muscles.

1.2.6.3 Intrinsic Muscles

Intrinsic muscles are responsible for the movement of the rib cage and play a significant role in respiration. These muscles include the intercostal muscles (external, internal, and innermost), subcostal muscles, and the transversus thoracis muscles.

1.2.6.4 Accessory Muscles

Accessory muscles assist in respiration by stabilising the chest wall and aiding in the expansion and contraction of the thoracic cavity. These muscles include the serratus anterior, serratus posterior superior, and serratus posterior inferior muscles.

1.2.6.5 Latissimus Dorsi

The latissimus dorsi is the most frequently used muscle for lateral and anterior chest wall defects due to its large size, robust blood supply, and wide arc of rotation. It is supplied by the thoracodorsal neurovascular bundle and receives blood supply from branches supplying the serratus anterior. Excellent musculocutaneous collaterals allow for significant skin to be taken with the muscle during surgical procedures.

1.2.6.5.1 *Origin and Insertion*

The latissimus dorsi originates from the spinous processes of the thoracic vertebrae T6 to T12, as well as the lumbar and sacral vertebrae, and inserts into the intertubercular groove of the humerus.

1.2.6.5.2 *Function*

The primary functions of the latissimus dorsi are to extend, adduct, and medially rotate the shoulder joint. It also plays a role in assisting with respiration, particularly during forceful exhalation.

1.2.6.6 Pectoralis Major and Pectoralis Minor

The pectoralis major and minor muscles are essential for the movement and stabilisation of the shoulder joint. They also play a crucial role in chest wall reconstruction for various types of defects.[21]

1.2.6.6.1 Origin and Insertion

The pectoralis major originates from the clavicle, sternum, and costal cartilages of the first six ribs, and inserts into the lateral lip of the intertubercular groove of the humerus. The pectoralis minor originates from the third, fourth, and fifth ribs and inserts into the coracoid process of the scapula.

1.2.6.6.2 Function

The pectoralis major functions to flex, adduct, and medially rotate the shoulder joint. The pectoralis minor assists in stabilising the scapula by drawing it inferiorly and anteriorly against the thoracic wall.

1.2.6.7 Intercostal Muscles

The intercostal muscles are intrinsic muscles that play a vital role in respiration. They are located between the ribs and can be divided into three layers: external, internal, and innermost intercostal muscles.

1.2.6.7.1 Origin and Insertion

The external intercostal muscles originate from the lower border of the rib above and insert into the upper border of the rib below. The internal intercostal muscles originate from the upper border of the rib below and insert into the lower border of the rib above. The innermost intercostal muscles have a similar origin and insertion to the internal intercostal muscles but are located deeper within the chest wall.

1.2.6.7.2 Function

The external intercostal muscles function to elevate the ribs during inspiration, while the internal and innermost intercostal muscles function to depress the ribs during expiration.[23]

1.2.6.8 Subcostal and Transversus Thoracis Muscles

The subcostal and transversus thoracis muscles are intrinsic muscles that aid in respiration by assisting in the movement of the ribcage.

1.2.6.8.1 Origin and Insertion

The subcostal muscles originate from the inner surface of the lower ribs and insert into the inner surface of the second or third rib below. The transversus thoracis muscles originate from the posterior surface of the lower sternum and insert into the inner surface of the second to sixth costal cartilages.

1.2.6.8.2 Function

Both the subcostal and transversus thoracis muscles function to depress the ribs during expiration.

1.2.6.9 Serratus Anterior and Posterior Muscles

The serratus muscles are accessory muscles that play a critical role in stabilising the chest wall and assisting with respiration.

1.2.6.9.1 Origin and Insertion

The serratus anterior originates from the outer surface of the first eight or nine ribs and inserts into the medial border of the scapula. The serratus posterior superior originates from the spinous processes of the cervical and upper thoracic vertebrae and inserts into the upper borders of the second to fifth ribs. The serratus posterior inferior originates from the spinous processes of the lower thoracic and upper lumbar vertebrae and inserts into the lower borders of the eighth to twelfth ribs.[24–26]

1.2.6.9.2 Function

The serratus anterior functions to stabilise and rotate the scapula, while the serratus posterior superior and inferior muscles aid in respiration by elevating and depressing the ribs, respectively.

1.2.6.10 Nerve Supply

The breast is innervated by anterior and lateral cutaneous branches of the fourth to sixth intercostal nerves. These nerves contain both sensory and autonomic nerve fibres (the autonomic fibres regulate smooth muscle and blood vessel tone). It should be noted that these nerves do not control the production and secretion of milk. This is regulated by the hormones prolactin and oxytocin, which are secreted from the pituitary gland.

The nerves that supply the breast are the anterior and lateral cutaneous branches of the fourth to sixth intercostal nerves, containing both sensory and autonomic nerve endings.[27]

The sensory innervation to the breast originates as branches of the intercostal nerves T3–T5.[28] The lower cervical plexus provides sensory innervation to the nipple. This sensation is derived from the lateral cutaneous branch of T4 as shown in Figure 1.3.

1.2.6.11 Lymphatic System

The lymphatic drainage of the breast is of great clinical importance due to its role in the metastasis of breast cancer cells. Breast tissue is drained by lymph nodes; there are three sets of lymph nodes:

1. **Axillary lymph nodes:**

   These nodes drain 75% of the lymph from breast tissue. The lymph vessels in the breast lobes and in the nipple and areola areas (lateral quadrants mostly) are collected into the

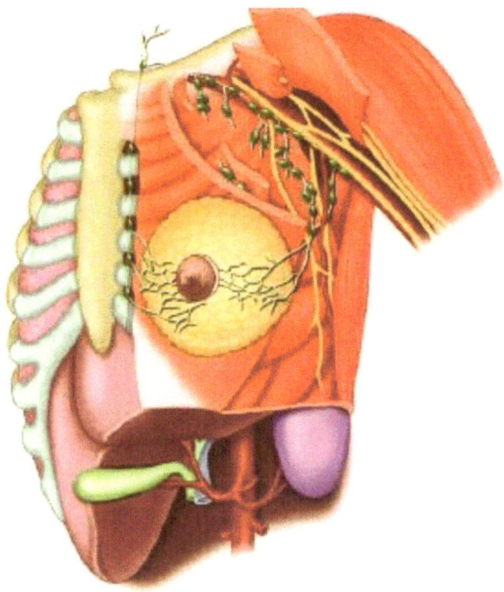

FIGURE 1.4
Lymphatic drainage of the female breast showing predominant nodal groupings in the axilla and internal mammary chain. The majority of the breast lymphatics drain to the axillary nodes.

Source: **Bland KI, Copeland EM,** ***The Breast: Comprehensive Management of Benign and Malignant Diseases*****, Elsevier, 1988, with permission.**

subareolar lymphatic plexus (of Sappey).[28] From here the lymph is drained into pectoral lymph nodes which drain into the axillary lymph nodes.

2. **Parasternal nodes:**

   These drain about 20% of the lymph from the rest of the breast tissue.[29] The parasternal lymph nodes drain into the lymphatic trunks.

3. **Posterior intercostal nodes**

   Besides axillary and parasternal lymph nodes, some drainage occurs through the posterior intercostal lymph nodes.[28]

The lymphatics of the breast skin envelope also have lymphatic drainage to the axillary, inferior deep cervical, and infraclavicular nodes (Figure 1.4).

1.3 Physiology of the Breast in Menstrual Cycle, Pregnancy, Lactation, and Menopause

The physiology of the breast is a complex and fascinating process that is influenced by various hormonal and environmental factors throughout a woman's life. From the menstrual cycle to pregnancy, lactation, and menopause, the breast undergoes significant changes in response to these events.[29]

1.3.1 Menstrual Cycle

1.3.1.1 Hormonal Influences

Breast tissue is highly responsive to hormonal changes, particularly during the menstrual cycle. The menstrual cycle is characterised by cyclical variations in hormone levels, primarily oestrogen and progesterone, which are responsible for the growth and development of the breast. These hormones play a crucial role in determining breast morphology and function.

1.3.1.2 Breast Physiology During the Menstrual Cycle

Breast morphology is profoundly affected by cyclical variations in hormonal levels during the normal menstrual cycle. Histological changes have been reported in both stroma and epithelium, reflecting the influence of oestrogen and progesterone on breast tissue.[30] These changes include an increase in ductal branching and the growth of glandular tissue, as well as alterations in the structure and composition of the breast stroma.

1.3.2 Pregnancy

1.3.3 Anatomic Changes and Mammogenesis

Mammogenesis is the process of growth and development of the mammary gland in preparation for milk production. This process begins when the mammary gland is exposed to oestrogen at puberty and is completed during the third trimester of pregnancy. Under the influence of uninterrupted and rising concentrations of oestrogen, progesterone, and prolactin during pregnancy, the water, electrolyte, and fat content of the breast increases. The resultant increase in volume is accompanied by a marked increase in the vascular supply to the breast, with the dilated subcutaneous mammary veins becoming prominent, and the blood flow increasing twofold.[31] The size and pigmentation of the nipples also increase under the influence of rising oestrogen concentrations.

1.3.3.1 Hormonal Effects

Total oestrogen excretion increases from 20 mg to 20,000 mg per 24 hours between early and late pregnancy, reflecting the rising plasma oestrogen levels that stimulate the ductal arborisation begun at puberty and the differentiation of epithelial cells into ductal, acinar, and myoepithelial elements. As the acinar-ductal system expands, it replaces much of the fatty tissue of the breast and is organised into mature, functional, lobular-alveolar-ductal units surrounded by hypertrophied myoepithelial elements.[13]

Progesterone secretion increases from 3 mg to 300 mg per day as pregnancy progresses. In the presence of oestrogen and prolactin, progesterone stimulates acinar proliferation and inhibits lactose synthesis. The high plasma concentrations of oestrogen and progesterone present before delivery inhibit the active secretory effects of prolactin on mammary alveolar epithelium.

1.3.4 Lactation

1.3.4.1 Lactogenesis

The mammary epithelium remains a presecretory tissue until the abrupt diminution in plasma oestrogen and progesterone concentration that occurs at the time of delivery. Without the inhibitory influence of progesterone on mammary epithelium, prolactin, and the other hormones active in the initiation of milk production can exert their effects on acinar cells. The initiation of milk production (lactogenesis) requires 2–5 days.

Prolactin and cortisol are essential for lactogenesis. Growth hormone, insulin, and thyroxin have facultative roles. Prolactin, a peptide hormone with a molecular weight of 23,500, is produced by the lactotrophs of the pituitary gland. Prolactin specifically binds to a receptor on the surface of the alveolar epithelium, stimulating synthesis of messenger RNA (mRNA) molecules that are necessary for the production of milk proteins and other required enzymes.

The only other specific hormone required for lactogenesis is oxytocin. Oxytocin is an octapeptide produced in the supraoptic and paraventricular nuclei of the hypothalamus and stored in the posterior lobe of the pituitary gland. It is released after suckling stimulates sensory fibres in the nipple.

1.3.4.2 Galactopoiesis

Galactopoiesis is the maintenance of milk production once it has been established by completion of lactogenesis. The single most important factor in successful galactopoiesis is regular and frequent milk removal from the mammary gland. Milk removal stimulates further milk secretion by at least three mechanisms: It promotes the secretion of prolactin and oxytocin, it triggers the release of other hormones active in milk production, and it prevents the accumulation of milk in the breast, which can lead to vascular stasis and alveolar atrophy.

1.3.4.3 Inhibition of Lactation

The success of a purposeful suppression of lactation depends on inhibiting the process of lactogenesis. Its inhibition is stimulated by rise in circulating oestrogen hormones and reduction in prolactin and oxytocin hormone due to lack of milk excretion.[32]

1.3.5 Menopause

Menopause, the cessation of menstruation, marks a significant shift in hormonal balance and breast physiology.[33] The decline in oestrogen and progesterone production during menopause leads to several changes in the breast, including:

- Decreased breast size and volume
- Reduced glandular and ductal tissue
- Loss of elastic supportive tissues
- Increased adipose tissue

These changes have implications for breast health and disease, as well as for the interpretation of breast imaging. Understanding the physiological changes that occur during menopause is essential for the proper management of breast health in post-menopausal women.[33]

1.4 Congenital Abnormalities

1.4.1 Supernumerary Breasts and Nipples

Supernumerary breasts and nipples are congenital anomalies that result from the persistence and development of the mammary ridges or milk lines. While supernumerary nipples are relatively common, affecting around 1–5% of the population, supernumerary breasts are less frequent. These anomalies may be associated with other congenital abnormalities, particularly in the renal and urogenital systems.

1.4.2 Breast Asymmetry

Breast asymmetry refers to differences in the size, shape, or position of the breasts. It is a common condition that can be caused by various factors, including hormonal imbalances, differences in the underlying chest wall, or abnormalities in the breast tissue itself. In some cases, breast asymmetry may be associated with congenital breast disorders, such as amastia (complete absence of the breast) or athelia (absence of the nipple).[33]

1.4.3 Inverted Nipples

Inverted nipples are a relatively common congenital breast condition, affecting around 2–10% of the population. This condition occurs when the nipple is retracted into the breast tissue rather than protruding outward. Inverted nipples can be classified into three grades, based on their severity and ability to be manually everted. Treatment options for inverted nipples include non-surgical interventions, such as the use of nipple shields and suction devices, as well as surgical correction.

References

1. Russo J, Russo IH. Development of the human breast. Maturitas. 2004;49(1):2–15.
2. Javed A, Lteif A. Development of the human breast. Semin Plast Surg. 2013;27(1):5–12.
3. Seltzer V. The breast: Embryology, development, and anatomy. Clin Obstet Gynecol. 1994;37(4):879–80.
4. Lemaine V, Simmons PS. The adolescent female: Breast and reproductive embryology and anatomy. Clin Anat. 2013;26(1):22–8.
5. Pandya S, Moore RG. Breast development and anatomy. Clin Obstet Gynecol. 2011;54(1):91–5.
6. Skandalakis JE. Embryology and anatomy of the breast. In: Shiffman MA, ed., Breast Augmentation: Principles and Practice. Springer, 2009:3–24.
7. Sicinski P, Donaher JL, Parker SB, et al. Cyclin D1 provides a link between development and oncogenesis in the retina and breast. Cell. 1995;82(4):621–30.
8. Howard BA, Gusterson BA. Human breast development. J Mammary Gland Biol Neoplasia. 2000;5:119–37.
9. Comsa S, Ceausu AR, Popescu R, et al. Patterns of tumor vasculogenesis on a chick embryo chorioallantoic membrane in vivo model of breast cancer. Anticancer Res. 2022;42(2):877–83.
10. Merlob P. Congenital malformations and developmental changes of the breast: A neonatological view. J Pediat Endocrinol Metabol. 2003;16(4):471–86.
11. Ramsay DT, Kent JC, Hartmann RA, et al. Anatomy of the lactating human breast redefined with ultrasound imaging. J Anat. 2005;206(6):525–34.
12. Bianchini G, Qi Y, Alvarez RH, et al. Molecular anatomy of breast cancer stroma and its prognostic value in estrogen receptor-positive and-negative cancers. J Clin Oncol. 2010;28(28):4316–23.
13. Vendrell-Torné E, Setoain-Quinquer J, Doménech-Torné FM. Study of normal mammary lymphatic drainage using radioactive isotopes. J Nucl Med. 1972;13:801.
14. Oktay K, Buyuk E, Libertella N, et al. Fertility preservation in breast cancer patients: A prospective controlled comparison of ovarian stimulation with tamoxifen and letrozole for embryo cryopreservation. J Clin Oncol. 2005;23(19):4347–53.
15. Jesinger RA. Breast anatomy for the interventionalist. Tech Vasc Interv Radiol. 2014;17(1):3–9.
16. Montagna W, Macpherson EE. Some neglected aspects of the anatomy of human breasts. J Investigat Dermatol. 1974;63(1):10–6.
17. Pandya S, Moore RG. Breast development and anatomy. Clin Obstet Gynecol. 2011;54(1):91–5.
18. Geddes DT. Inside the lactating breast: The latest anatomy research. J Midwif Women's Health. 2007;52(6):556–63.
19. de la Pared Torácica A, Mama A. Anatomy of the thoracic wall, axilla and breast. Int J Morphol. 2006;24(4):691–704.
20. Love SM, Barsky SH. Anatomy of the nipple and breast ducts revisited. Cancer. 2004;101(9):1947–57.
21. McGuire KP. Breast anatomy and physiology. In: Aydiner A, Igci A, Soran A, eds., Breast Disease: Diagnosis and Pathology. Springer, 2016:1–4.
22. Zucca-Matthes G, Urban C, Vallejo A. Anatomy of the nipple and breast ducts. Gland Surg. 2016;5(1):32.
23. Rusby JE, Brachtel EF, Michaelson JS, et al. Breast duct anatomy in the human nipple: Three-dimensional patterns and clinical implications. Breast Cancer Res Treat. 2007;106:171–9.
24. Rubino C, Mazzarello V, Farace F, et al. Ultrastructural anatomy of contracted capsules around textured implants in augmented breasts. Ann Plastic Surg. 2001;46(2):95–102.
25. Russo IH, Russo J. Mammary gland neoplasia in long-term rodent studies. Environ Health Perspect. 1996;104:938.
26. Russo J, Russo IH. Development of the human breast. In: Neville MC, Daniel CW, eds., The Mammary Gland. Plenum Press, 1987:67–93.
27. Henderson BE, Ross R, Bernstein L. Estrogens as a cause of human cancer: The Richard and Hinda Rosenthal Foundation award lecture. Cancer Res. 1988;48:246.
28. Cummings SR, Duong T, Kenyon E, et al. Serum estradiol level and risk of breast cancer during treatment with raloxifene. JAMA. 2002;287:216.
29. Rosen PP. Abnormalities of mammary growth and development. In: Rosen PP, ed., Rosen's Breast Pathology, 3rd edn. Lippincott Williams & Wilkins/Wolters Kluwer, 2009.
30. Schnitt SJ, Collins LC, eds., Biopsy Interpretation of the Breast, 3rd edn. Wolters Kluwer Health, 2018.
31. Hultborn KA, Larsson LG, Ragnhult I. The lymph drainage from the breast to the axillary and parasternal lymph nodes, studied with the aid of colloidal Au198. Acta Radiol. 1955;43:52.
32. Estourgie SH, Nieweg OE, Olmos RA, et al. Lymphatic drainage patterns from the breast. Ann Surg. 2004;239:232.
33. Byrd DR, Dunnwald LK, Mankoff DA, et al. Internal mammary lymph node drainage patterns in patients with breast cancer documented by breast lymphoscintigraphy. Ann Surg Oncol. 2001;8:234.

2

Symptomatic Triple Assessment

Francesca Muscara and John R. Benson

2.1 Epidemiology of Breast Cancer

Breast cancer is the most common malignancy worldwide with recent lifetime risk estimates of 1 in 7 for women in the United Kingdom (UK) where the annual rate has doubled in the past four decades. Breast is the primary site in one-quarter of female cancers globally and 2.3 million women worldwide were diagnosed with breast cancer in 2020 among which more than 600,000 died from their disease (breastcanceruk.org). Almost half of breast cancers are diagnosed within the screening age bracket within screened populations such as the UK where introduction of screening led to an initial surge in breast cancer. The latter is a disease predominantly of post-menopausal women and higher rates in more affluent countries has been attributed to increased usage of hormone replacement therapy (HRT). Nonetheless, use of exogenous hormones in women aged 45–69 years fell significantly after 2002 with a consequent transient reduction in breast cancer incidence amongst white American women; this decline has not been sustained despite limited contemporary usage of HRT. Breast cancer development in younger women is more likely linked to genetic factors with increasing recognition of lower penetrance genes that individually confer lower levels of risk but are collectively important. Epigenetic phenomena are frequently displayed in breast cancer and permit changes in gene expression without DNA sequence alterations and act as translators between the external environment and the genome.

Countries with historically moderate or low rates of breast cancer based on income levels are now witnessing rapid rate increases in the incidence of breast cancer that is particularly evident in China and India with a notable doubling of rates in Japan over the past 50 years. The high incidence rates in Western industrial nations have been attributed to specific lifestyles that are increasingly being adopted by women from emerging economies. These include changes in reproductive behaviour, altered dietary habits with increased consumption of polyunsaturated fats and alcohol, and a more sedentary lifestyle and physical inactivity. Breast cancer incidence could be significantly reduced by modifying these risk factors with the aim of maintaining optimum body weight, limiting alcohol intake, and engaging in regular exercise.

Mortality rates for breast cancer have fallen over the past 30 years despite a continued rise in incidence. Survival rates at 10 years for breast cancer in the UK are currently 80.4% compared with approximately 55% in the final quarter of the last century (breastcanceruk.org). Survivorship has become an important issue with an estimated 7.8 million patients around the world living with breast cancer diagnosed in the past 5 years. Survival rates will continue to improve with advances in translational research and development of tailored therapies (e.g. antibody drug conjugates) that can effectively target micrometastatic disease with acceptable levels of serious side effects—there is a balance between length and quality of life. With improved survival outcomes for breast cancer treatments, the focus has now shifted to quality-of-life issues. Although many studies have confirmed that aesthetic results of breast cancer surgery are a principal determinant of quality-of-life and patient satisfaction, functional and psychosexual outcomes are equally important and should be part of any shared decision-making process.

2.2 Clinical Breast Examination

Evaluation of breast disease is based on the principle of triple assessment, involving a combination of clinical examination, imaging, and tissue biopsy. There is much overlap in the clinical features of benign and malignant breast conditions, and physical examination alone has limited accuracy. This underscores the principle of triple assessment in which clinical examination is complemented by radiological imaging with or without some form of tissue biopsy. Triple

DOI: 10.1201/9781003394785-2

assessment has an overall accuracy exceeding 99%, and this permits the majority of patients attending 'one-stop' clinics to be reassured and discharged without further follow-up. Patients present to breast clinics with a range of symptoms but two-thirds will have either a lump or an area of lumpiness or thickening. Many breast complaints, such as pain, lumpiness, and nipple discharge, may relate to normal physiological changes taking place at different stages of reproductive life and in response to monthly cyclical hormonal changes. Benign conditions may present with lumps that fluctuate with the menstrual cycle or have decreased in size since first noticed by the patient. These include fibroadenosis and fibroadenomas and are also more likely to be associated with pain and tenderness than a malignant breast lesion. A previous history of benign breast conditions, particularly cysts or fibrocystic change can be important indicators of the likely nature of any current breast problem. Many patients ostensibly presenting with a breast lump will not have a discrete or dominant mass, but rather an area of focal nodularity; this represents a prominent area of normal glandular tissue or an abnormality of normal development and involution (ANDI). The latter is a spectrum of changes in the breast parenchyma (epithelial and stromal elements). Distinction may be evident on clinical examination, but often further evaluation with ultrasound is necessary to confirm the presence of a discrete mass (Figure 2.1). Ultrasound examination can usually distinguish between benign, malignant, and suspicious lesions and has a high sensitivity for detection of focal mass lesions (Figure 2.2). A mammogram would not normally be performed on patients under 35–40 years of age as the sensitivity of mammography is innately lower in young women with dense breast tissue and there is some risk from unnecessary radiation exposure (Figure 2.3). However, when a suspicious lesion is identified on ultrasound in a younger patient, this should be further evaluated with mammography that can provide additional information such as associated microcalcification. Clinical classification is based on a scoring system as follows:

E(P)1 = normal
E(P)2 = benign
E(P)3 = suspicious probably benign
E(P)4 = suspicious probably malignant
E(P)5 = malignant

The designation of a lesion as E3 can sometimes be problematic; the important question is whether further evaluation with needle biopsy is indicated following discussion between the clinician and radiologist.

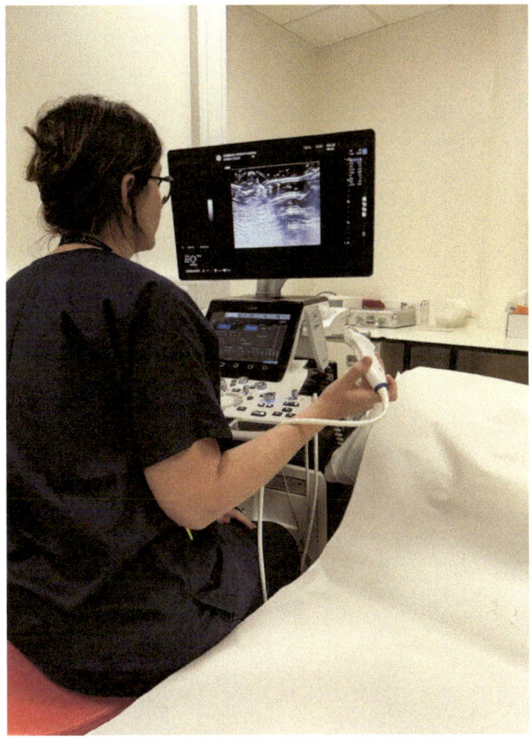

FIGURE 2.1
Modern B-mode breast ultrasound machine with a handheld probe (imaging breast or axilla).

There is evidence that performance in clinical breast examination is highly variable depending on clinical grade and experience (range 44.6–65.9%)[1] and arguably patients examined by a non-consultant grade/resident with an E3 lump and normal/benign imaging (without needle biopsy) should be re-examined by another clinician. When patients are discharged after triple assessment', it is mandatory to inform patients that if they remain worried or changes persist, they should return to their doctor for reassessment. It should be emphasised that patients do not require routine follow-up with clinical review and/or repeat ultrasound examination for benign and non-suspicious findings on triple assessment. Despite persistence and even enlargement of a lump, patients can be falsely reassured after attending a one-stop clinic and being informed that there are no suspicious findings. Hence, patients must always be instructed to seek further medical attention if a breast lump fails to regress spontaneously or increases in size.

The principle of triple assessment implies that patients are considered for some form of percutaneous biopsy, but this is not mandatory and failure to undergo biopsy does not reflect an inadequate evaluation (Figure 2.4). Usually needle biopsy is prompted when there is a palpable, discrete mass and there is a suspicious correlate on clinical or radiological assessment. Sometimes a patient will have an area of focal

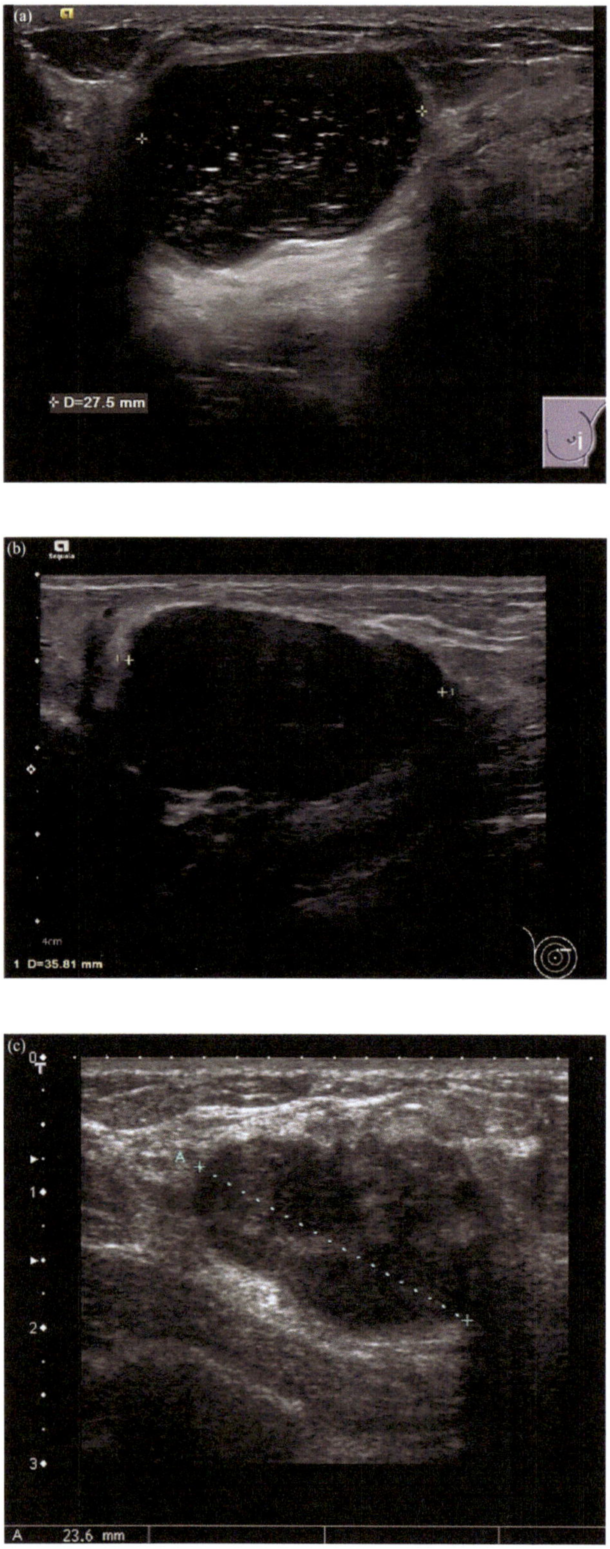

FIGURE 2.2
Ultrasound appearances of (a) breast cyst, (b) fibroadenoma, and (c) malignant tumour (see text for explanation).

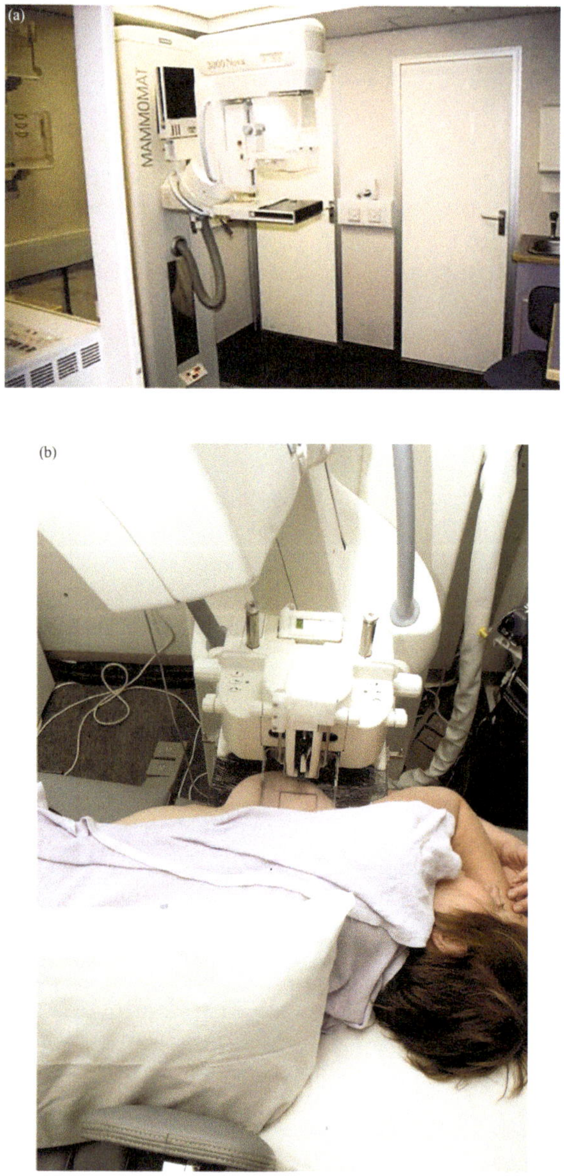

FIGURE 2.3
(a) Current generation of mammography machines; (b) breast compressed between plates of mammogram machine to capture as much of the breast tissue as possible (very posterior lesions may not be visualised).

nodularity with the impression of a dominant lesion within, but no overtly dominant mass. A localised area of focal nodularity attributable to fibrocystic changes can appear clinically suspicious but quite innocent on ultrasound with no focal abnormality that can be readily targeted for biopsy. It is important to maintain a favourable benign to malignant biopsy ratio as this is an important quality control parameter, particularly for screen-detected lesions. Fewer than 10% of cancers are radiologically occult on mammography or ultrasound (more tumours fail to be visualised on

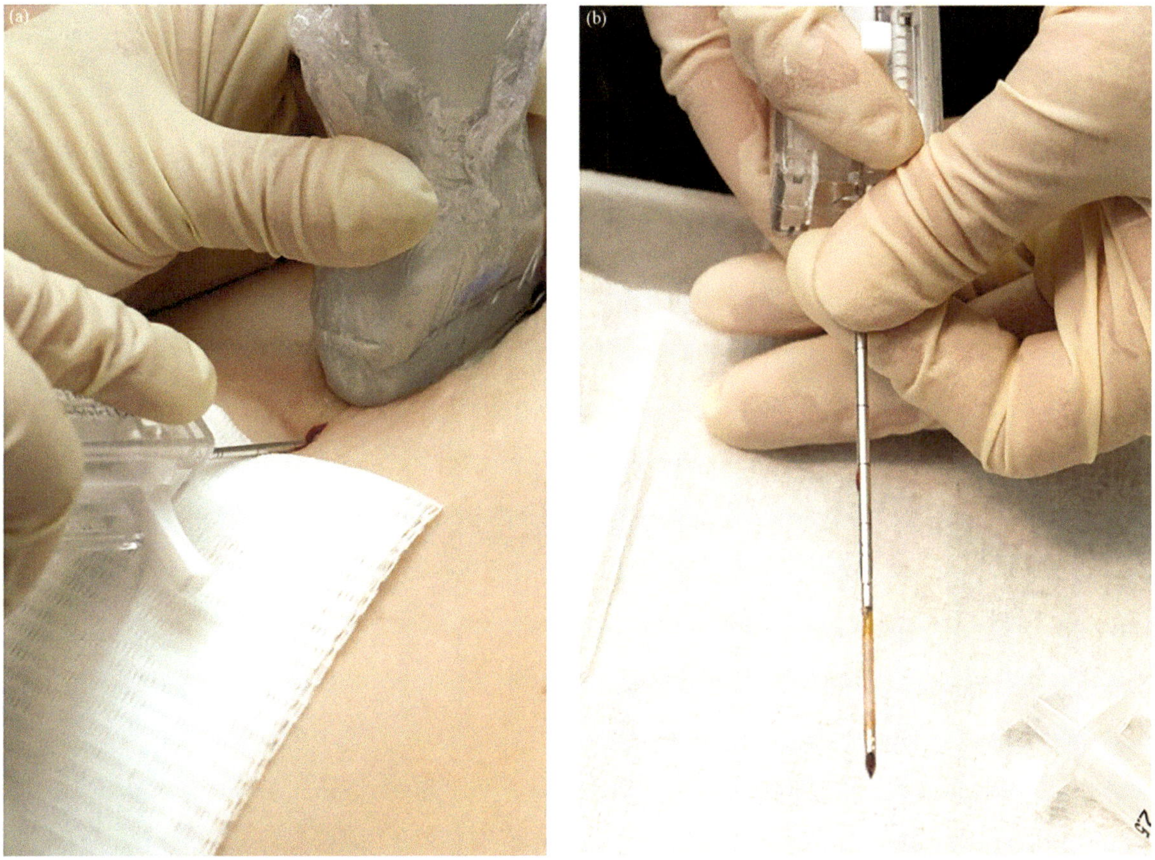

FIGURE 2.4
(a, b) Core biopsy performed under ultrasound-guidance employing a spring-loaded biopsy device.

mammography, than ultrasound examination). An innocent ultrasound assessment performed by an experienced operator can usually exclude more sinister pathology, but there is much variation in the sensitivity of clinical breast examination (CBE) between clinicians and a lesion considered suspicious (E3) by one may be rated as benign (E2) by another. The clinical classification necessarily has a subjective element in these indeterminate cases and this presents a challenge for triple assessment; an excessive proportion of 'B2 cores' should be avoided, but missed cancers minimised. Therefore, a balance must be reached based on clinical and radiological features and discussion between clinician and radiologist. An interesting study from North America found that more than 40% of doctors considered themselves to have poor clinical breast examination skills and only 50% were moderately confident with their clinical judgement in this area.

In the absence of core biopsy, a follow-up examination can be arranged after a few weeks to determine whether the area of clinical concern has regressed. Faced with an unchanged situation, a core biopsy could then be undertaken (a cancer is unlikely to have enlarged significantly during a 6-week period) or further radiological interrogation done with MRI imaging.

2.3 Imaging Studies

Mammography: Mammography is usually undertaken for all women aged ≥40 years presenting with a breast mass. Some units in the United States will routinely perform mammography over the age of 30 years, but relatively high breast density in the age group 30–40 reduces sensitivity with limitations on the accuracy and interpretation of imaging. Mammography may reveal a discrete mass that may be well/poorly circumscribed or an asymmetric density with distinction between these entities sometimes being unclear; the former is a localised lesion of homogeneous density that is round in shape with convex margins (Figure 2.5). By contrast, an asymmetric density has mixed density and concave margins (Figure 2.6). Benign lesions characteristically have well-defined

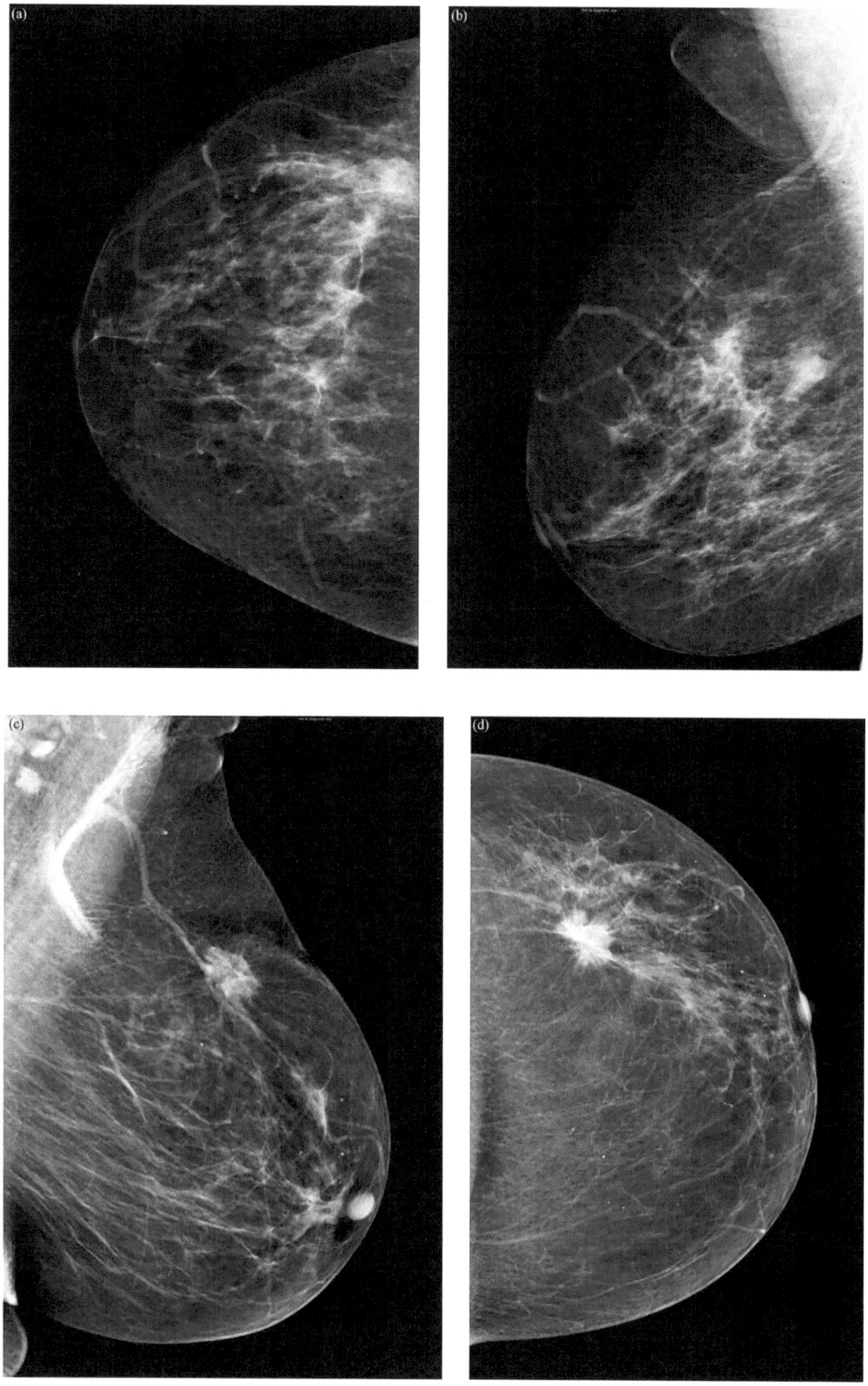

FIGURE 2.5
Discrete mass lesions within the breast may be well circumscribed (a, b) or less well-defined (c, d).

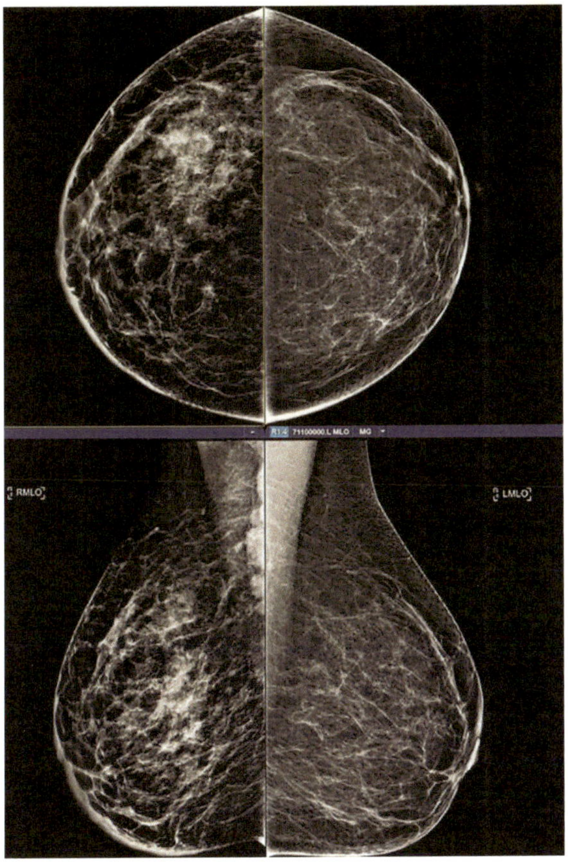

FIGURE 2.6
An asymmetric density representing an invasive carcinoma.

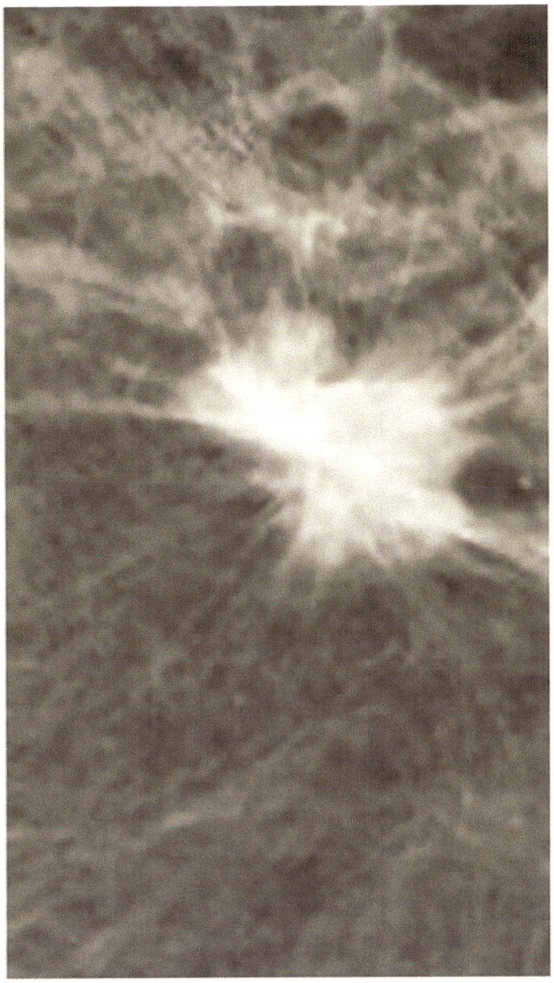

FIGURE 2.7
Spiculate mass lesion characteristic of an invasive carcinoma; the radiating spicules represent a desmoplastic reaction within the surrounding connective tissue and can provide a radiological signature for otherwise impalpable lesions.

margins, whilst the hallmark of a typical malignant lesion is an ill-defined, spiculate mass that represents a desmoplastic reaction within surrounding stromal elements (Figure 2.7). Radiological assessment of a lesion on mammography must take account of a patient's age together with the number, size, morphology, and density of lesions in addition to the presence of microcalcifications (Figure 2.8). Tomosynthesis is increasingly being employed as a supplemental investigation for breast assessment in patients with relatively dense breast tissue and those with a lesion manifest as a subtle opacity. This radiological technique serves to spread out the breast tissue and prevent a lesion being obscured against the background of normal breast parenchyma (Figure 2.9).

Ultrasound: This is complementary to mammography for assessment of a mass lesion and modern B-mode ultrasound can readily differentiate between benign and malignant lesions. Benign lesions are wider than tall, have an absent or homogeneously reduced internal echo pattern and a bright distal acoustic shadow (Figure 2.2b). By contrast, malignant lesions tend to be taller than wide, have a heterogeneously reduced internal echo pattern and distal acoustic shadowing (Figure 2.2c). Ultrasound examination is the primary radiological modality for evaluation of breast lesions in women under the age of 40 years and is used for image-guided biopsy of breast masses. Once malignancy is suspected on an initial ultrasound examination in a younger patient (confirmed on biopsy), mammography should be undertaken to determine the presence of calcification and ascertain extent of disease (MRI is usually the subsequent investigation). Modern forms of ultrasound examination are very accurate with a high negative predictive value—if the ultrasound is innocuous (U2), there is a low probability of malignancy. Nonetheless, ultrasound is very operator dependent and interpretation will vary depending on experience/skill of the individual performing the procedure.

Magnetic resonance imaging (MRI): This is helpful in a diagnostic context for clarification of tumour extent

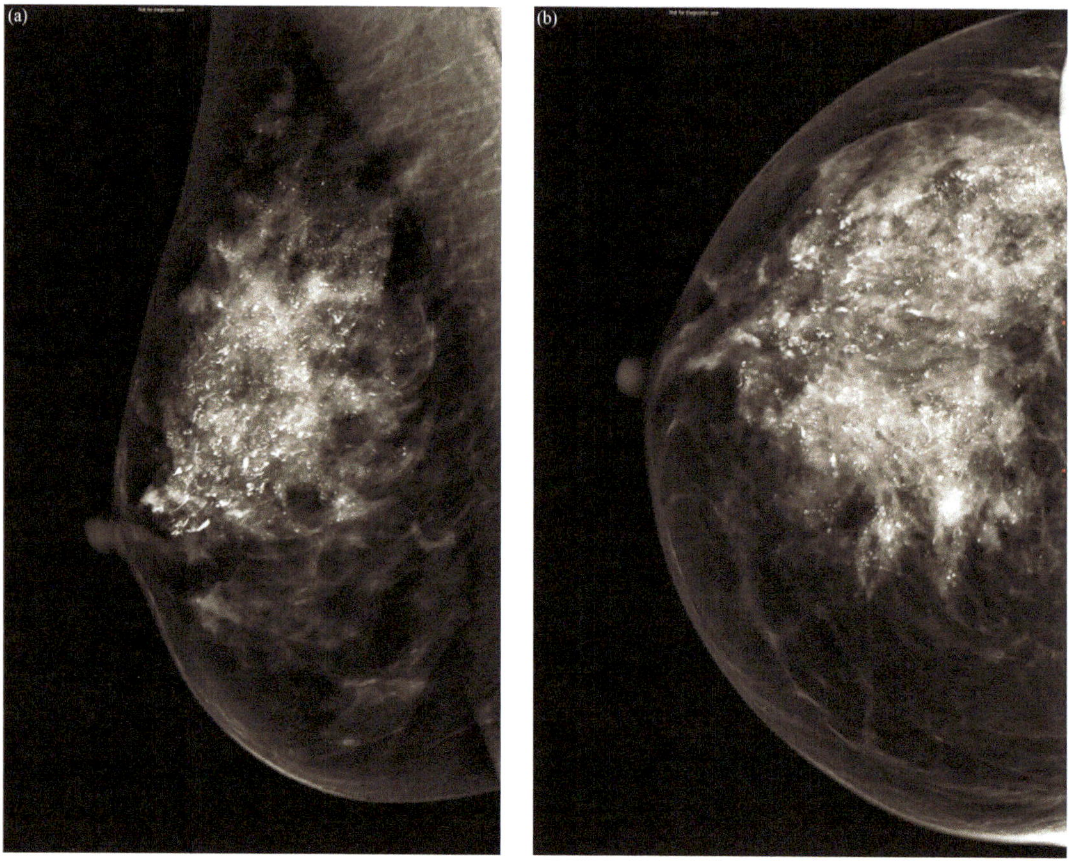

FIGURE 2.8
(a, b) Malignant mass lesion with associated pleiomorphic microcalcification.

and exclusion of multifocal lesions prior to surgery (Figure 2.10). It is important to undertake thorough local staging of disease prior to any complex oncoplastic surgical procedure and determine whether any distant ipsilateral lesions or a contralateral cancer is present at the time of diagnosis (especially for lesions with a lobular phenotype) (Figure 2.11). A principal disadvantage of MRI imaging relates to false positive results; benign lesions (such as fibroadenomas) have active blood flow and can be visualised as an enhancing lesion on MRI that may hinder distinction from malignant lesions (Figure 2.12). The pattern of dynamic contrast enhancement differs for benign and malignant lesions; the former demonstrate slow uptake (type 1 curve), whilst the latter have a rapid uptake and washout (type 3 curve). Indeterminate lesions have a type 2 curve with moderate early enhancement and will prompt a second-look ultrasound examination in the first instance (MR3, MR4). If such indeterminate lesions are sonographically occult, then MRI-guided biopsy may be necessary, especially for an MR4 lesion. MRI-guided biopsies require special equipment and highly skilled personnel, and these facilities may only be available at a geographically separate institution. Hence, organisation of these procedures can lead to significant delay, but there is no change in surgical plan for what may prove to be a unifocal cancer when additional foci of disease are not confirmed. Increasing numbers of patients present with breast problems and a prior history of breast augmentation that can render mammography either difficult or impossible (Figure 2.13). Posterior displacement techniques can be used for implants placed in the sub-pectoral plane, but for sub-glandular implants, there might still be significant shadowing which can obscure some breast parenchyma.

2.4 Percutaneous Needle Biopsy Techniques

Percutaneous needle biopsy techniques can provide a definitive diagnosis for the majority of both benign and malignant lesions and have dramatically reduced the need for open surgical biopsy. Triple assessment can provide a definitive pre-operative diagnosis in >95%

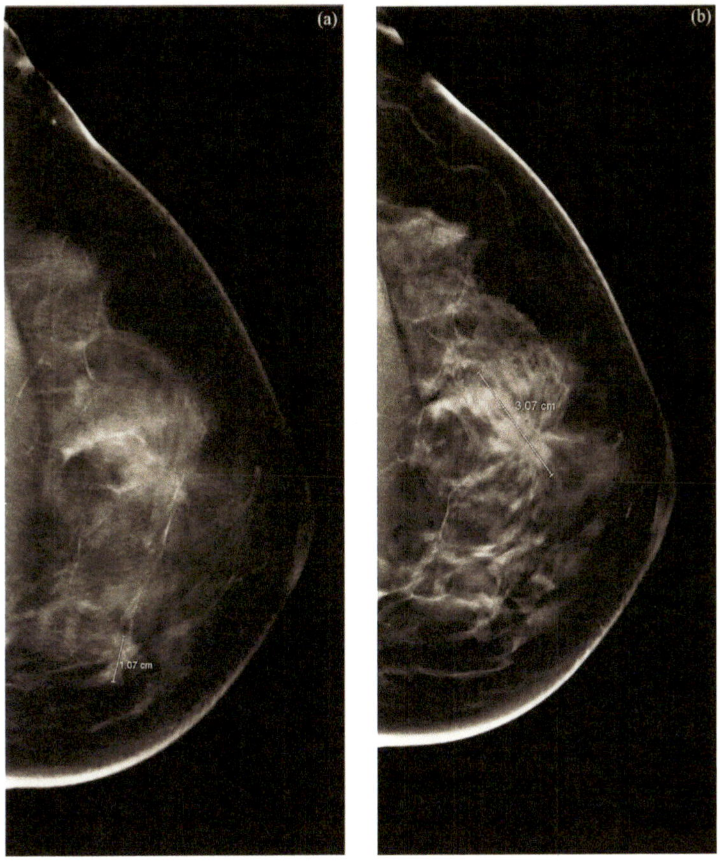

FIGURE 2.9
(a, b) Tomosynthesis images to show how tissue is imaged to prevent lesion being obscured by overlapping breast parenchymal tissue; (a) conventional mammography; (b) tomosynthesis.

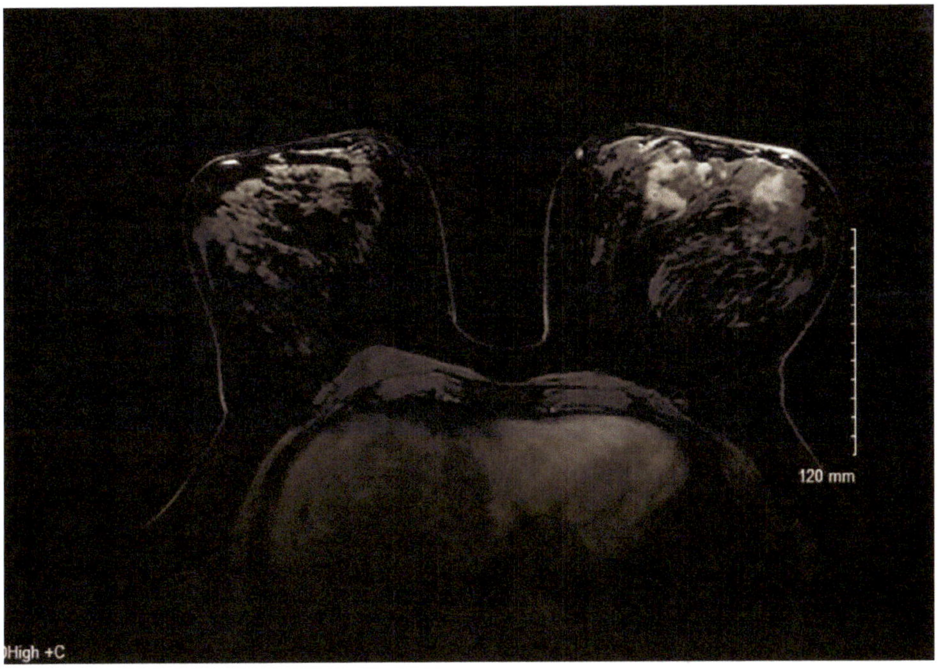

FIGURE 2.10
MRI images showing multifocal cancer in right breast. Conventional imaging had suggested a unifocal lesion only.

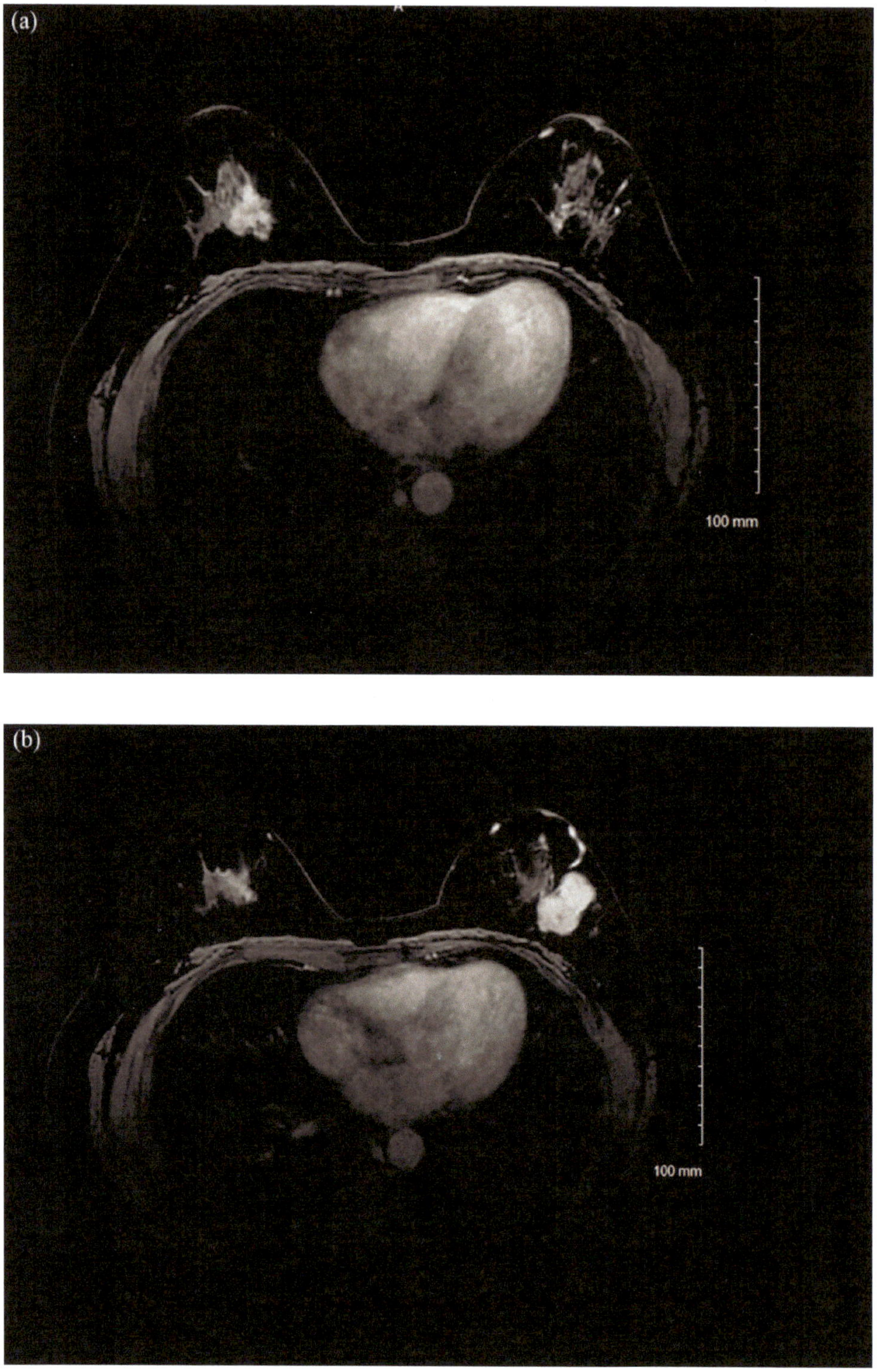

FIGURE 2.11
(a, b) MRI examination showing synchronous bilateral cancers that are more commonly found in patients with lobular cancers (an indication for routine MRI imaging).

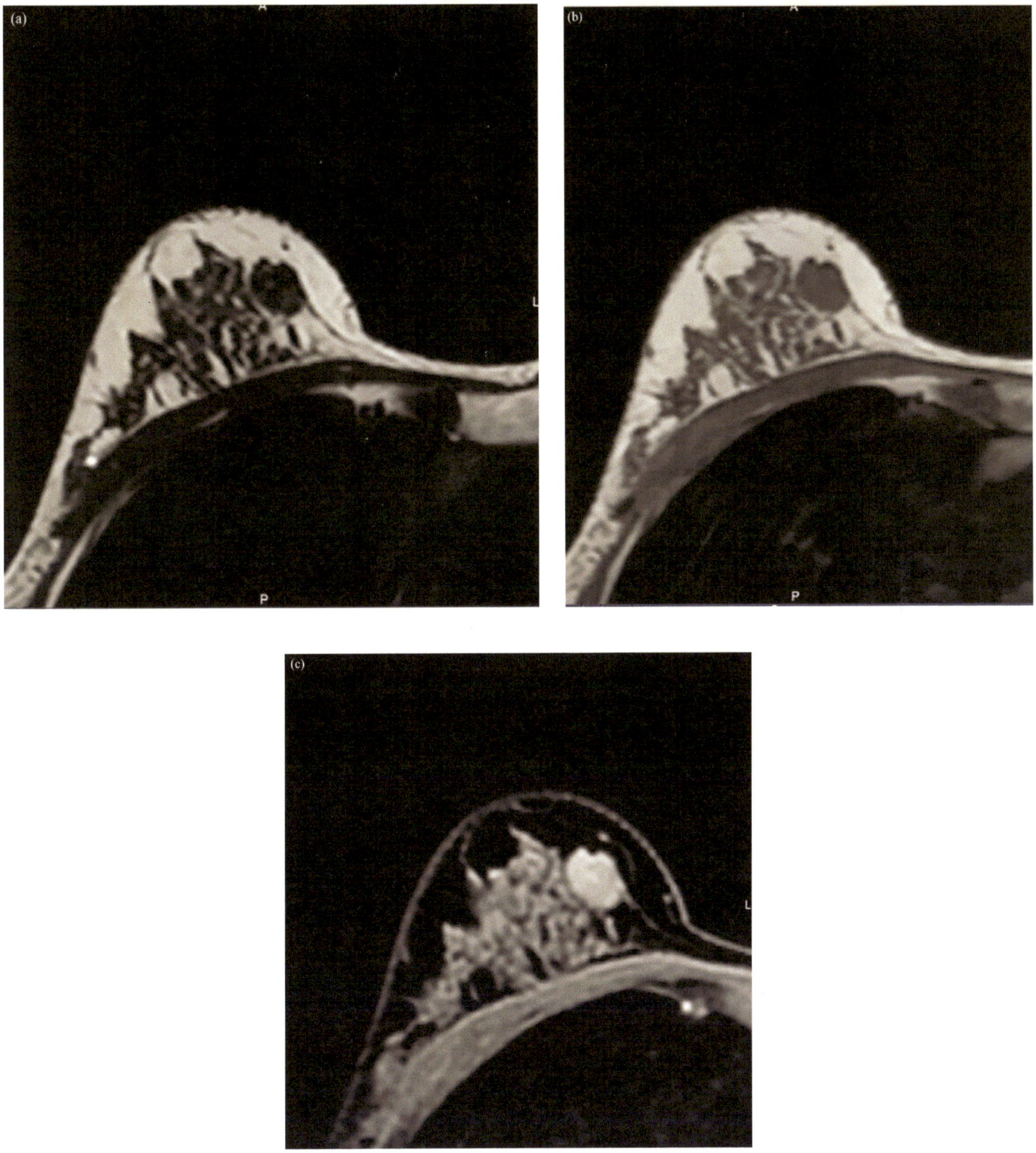

FIGURE 2.12
(a–c) Enhancement on MRI imaging is dependent on increased blood flow and therefore fibroadenomas can yield false positive results due to their rich blood supply.

of cancer cases, which allows planning of treatment with the patient and a fully informed shared decision-making process about surgical options. It is arguably unacceptable nowadays to perform a diagnostic excision biopsy without any prior image-guided needle biopsy of a breast mass. Use of ultrasound to guide needle biopsy allows accurate direction and placement of needles for either fine-needle aspiration cytology (FNAC) or core biopsy with real-time visualisation of the needle within the lesion (Figure 2.14). Both the needle and the lesion can be clearly identified during the biopsy procedure using linear ultrasound transducers of 7.5 MHz or 10 MHz. Wide bore core-needle biopsy is preferred to fine-needle aspiration and yields cores of tissue that maintain tissue architecture and in particular permit distinction between invasive

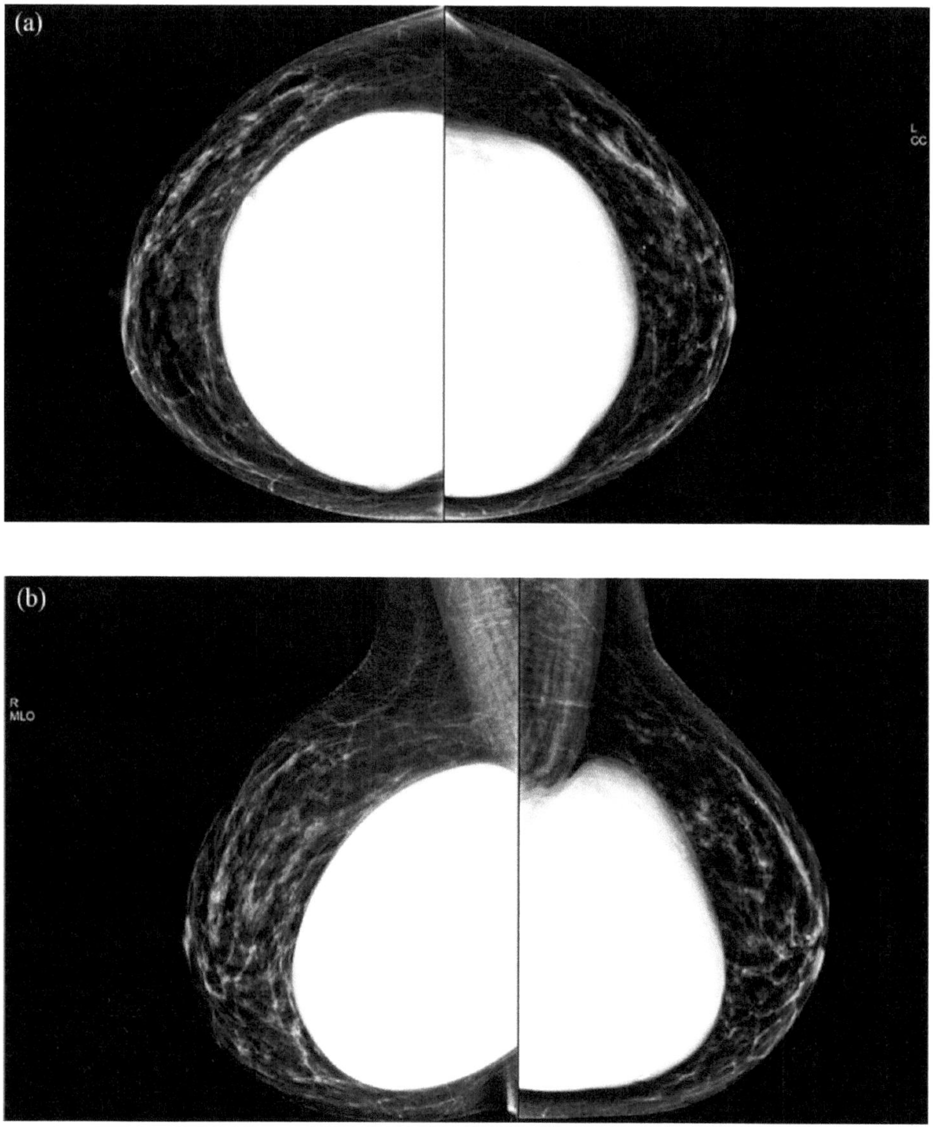

FIGURE 2.13
Mammography in a patient with implants following cosmetic breast augmentation on the (a) right and (b) left. It may be impossible to employ posterior displacement techniques during mammography, and therefore, MRI imaging may be indicated.

and noninvasive carcinoma (Figure 2.15). The standard core biopsy needle is either 14-gauge or 16-gauge but larger volumes of tissue can be obtained from vacuum-assisted core biopsy devices—most often 11-gauge (Figure 2.16). These larger needles reduce underdiagnosis and increase the chance of obtaining a definitive pre-operative cancer diagnosis. There are some units that continue to employ and have good results from FNAC of breast lesions performed either freehand or under ultrasound guidance and indeed many radiologists prefer the ease and safety of FNAC for biopsy of axillary nodes. Nonetheless, core-needle biopsy techniques are the recommended method for percutaneous needle biopsy of breast lesions and are not reliant on availability of a skilled cytopathologist. Not infrequently, FNAC will yield equivocal results that prompt subsequent core biopsy.

Fine-needle aspiration cytology: Historically, this technique underpinned the concept of a one-stop clinic in which a patient could attend for assessment and receive a definitive diagnosis during the clinic on the same day. An experienced cytopathologist can provide accurate results with sensitivity of about 95% and specificity approaching 100%. Although false positive rates are very low, FNAC cannot distinguish between invasive and noninvasive disease and a subsequent core-needle biopsy is often needed to ascertain receptor profiles (oestrogen receptor, progesterone receptor, HER2 and Ki-67). Although FNAC is a technically simple procedure and performed under local anaesthesia with a

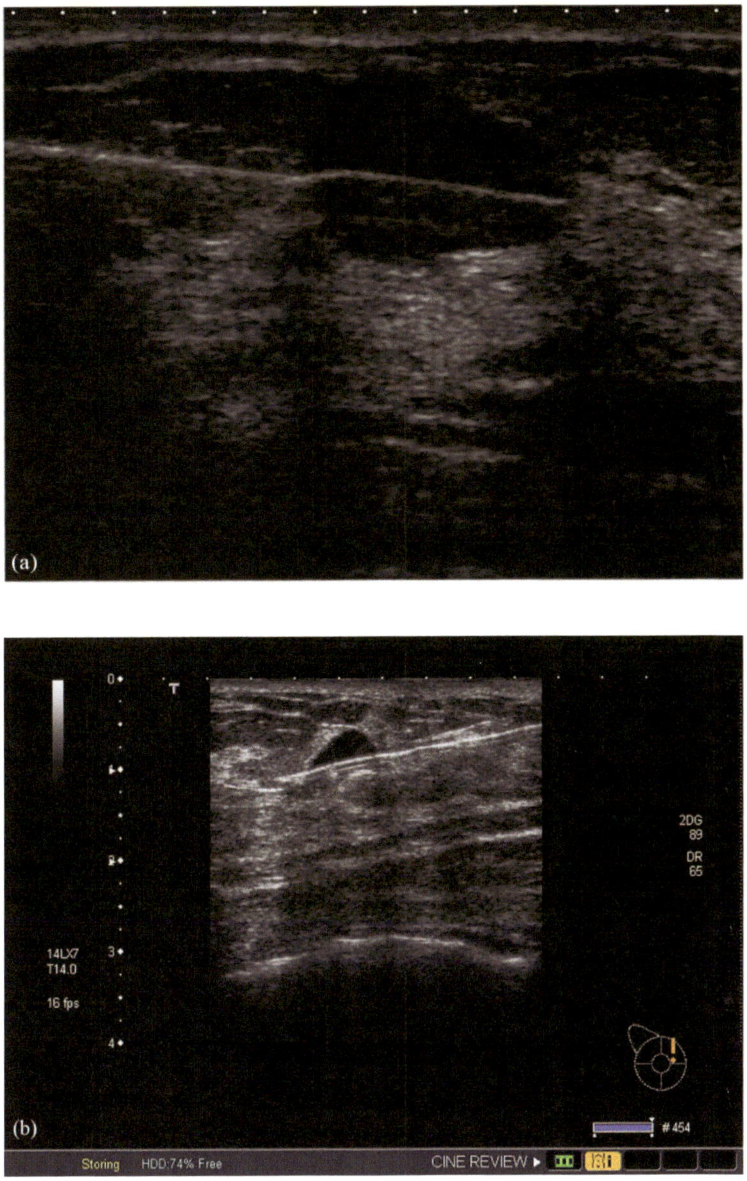

FIGURE 2.14
(a, b) US-guided percutaneous core biopsy showing needle traversing lesion (tip of wire must advance beyond lesion to obtain satisfactory sample (cf. fine-needle aspiration where tip of needle lies within centre of lesion).

21-gauge needle, it can be associated with complications such as haematoma, pneumothorax, and infection. It is important to introduce the needle at a tangent to the chest wall to avoid penetration into the pleural cavity. False negative rates for FNAC are 2–3%, which are relatively high and attributable to sampling error; in the event of a C2 diagnosis and lack of concordance between clinical, radiological, and cytological findings, either core biopsy or diagnostic excision biopsy must be undertaken (sometimes an MRI may be requested as the next investigation prior to any further biopsy).

Core-needle biopsy: There has been a shift away from FNAC to core biopsy in recent years due to inadequacy of sampling and inability to diagnose invasive cancer.[2] Core-needle biopsy provides solid pieces of breast tissue (20–25 g) that can be examined histologically as fresh or paraffin-embedded material thereby permitting assessment of both breast architecture and cellular morphology (Figure 2.17). Standard techniques for core biopsy utilise either 14-gauge or 16-gauge needles attached to disposable, automated spring-loaded devices that provide accurate sampling and good quality cores for routine histology and immunohistochemical analysis (Figure 2.18). Specimen cores are typically up to 2 cm in length corresponding to the throw of the needle. Techniques for core-needle biopsy can be applied to either palpable or impalpable lesions with image-guided practices now

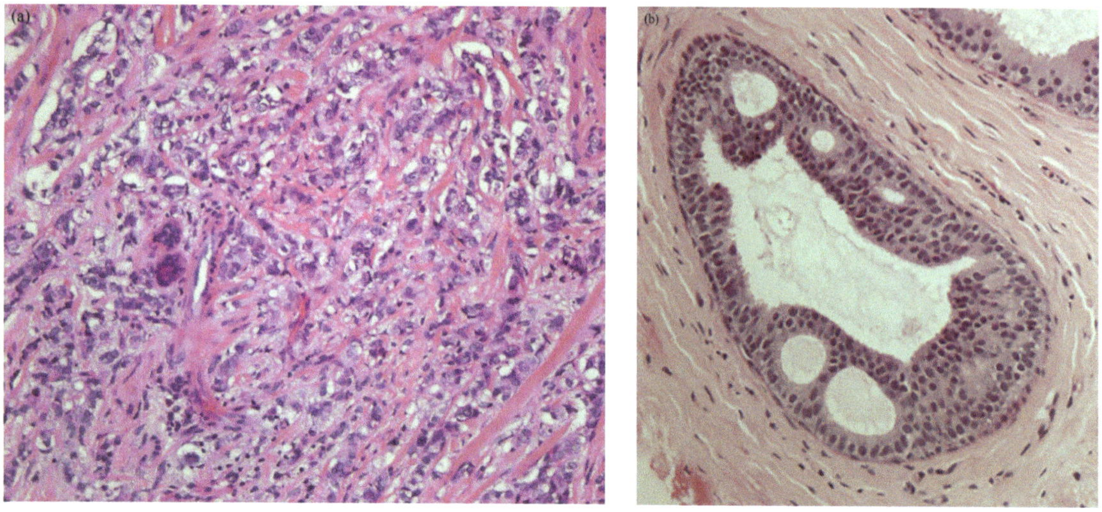

FIGURE 2.15
Core biopsy specimens showing histological appearances of (a) invasive cancer and (b) ductal carcinoma in situ.

preferred over manually guided methods to ensure optimal sampling and avoid the need for repeat biopsy. These techniques are especially amenable to sampling of palpable and impalpable lesions seen on ultrasound. Furthermore, smaller 18-gauge needles can assist biopsy of lesions within dense breast tissue and more confined areas such as the axilla. When performing an ultrasound-guided core biopsy, local anaesthetic (1% lignocaine or long-acting derivative) is injected around the intended biopsy site. A small incision measuring no more than 2–3 mm is made with an 11-blade scalpel to facilitate entry of the biopsy needle through the skin into the breast. This entry point should be pre-marked with a pen and made 1–2 cm away from the ultrasound transducer probe, thus allowing the operator to visualise the breast lesion. The ultrasound probe should be held with the non-dominant hand and the spring-loaded needle manipulated with the other hand (Figure 2.4a and b). It is helpful to enlist the assistance of a technician to stabilise the ultrasound probe thereby providing the operator with greater flexibility to manoeuvre the biopsy instrument. The needle should be directed to the edge of the area of concern and photo-documentation of the image completed. The patient should then be warned that the instrument is about to be fired to avoid audio-stress. Between two and four accurately placed needle passes will usually ensure an adequate sampling of the breast lesion. Results from the NHS breast screening programme confirm that core biopsy has both higher sensitivity and specificity compared with FNAC, with sensitivity 84.5% versus 81.5% and specificity 81.2% versus 58.4%, respectively.

Vacuum-assisted biopsy: Sometimes the standard techniques of core biopsy using needles ranging from 14-gauge to 18-gauge in size are inadequate to sample a lesion. Instead, a more invasive procedure employing an 11-gauge vacuum-assisted biopsy (VAB) device can achieve thorough sampling and yield larger volumes of tissue (the vacuum aids retrieval of these larger samples) (Figure 2.19). These vacuum-assisted techniques may be used at the outset or following an initial attempt at percutaneous biopsy using a standard gauge needle when they might avoid an otherwise open surgical diagnostic biopsy. These vacuum-assisted biopsy devices reduce the chance of histological underestimation associated with conventional core biopsy. Moreover, these vacuum-assisted techniques have recently evolved from being a purely diagnostic to a therapeutic procedure to completely remove a lesion using 7-gauge or 8-gauge needles—the so-called vacuum-assisted excision biopsy (VAE) (see the following).

Stereotactic-guided biopsy: These techniques are designed specifically to biopsy areas of micro-calcification detected on screening or incidentally during investigation of symptomatic disease (Figures 2.20 and 2.12). Areas of micro-calcification are often not visible on ultrasound and hence require stereotactic biopsy guided by mammography. Stereotactic devices calculate the position of a target lesion within the breast by localising coordinates in the horizontal, vertical, and depth axes from the surface of the breast. The mammograms are carefully reviewed on a dedicated workstation, and these coordinates used to determine the optimal directional approach

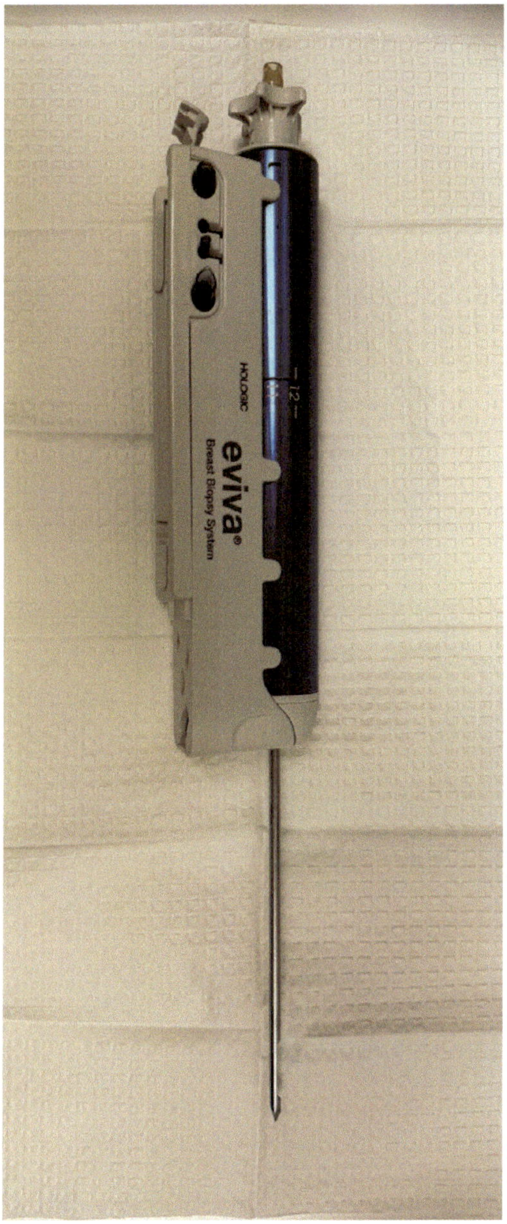

FIGURE 2.16
A range of needle sizes are employed for percutaneous biopsy; vacuum-assisted devices are usually 11-gauge (vacuum-assisted biopsy) or larger 7- or 8-gauge for vacuum-assisted excision.

to the lesion, taking account of the need to maintain the needle parallel to the chest wall in order to avoid a pneumothorax. Routine imaging at the start of the procedure permits calculation of the horizontal and vertical axes and two-angled images (15 degrees from the centre), then allow calculation of the depth of the lesion within the breast based on the principle of parallax. These coordinates will then guide the core-needle device to the targeted lesion on the breast. The patient is positioned prone on the procedure table, with the breast in the dependent position through an

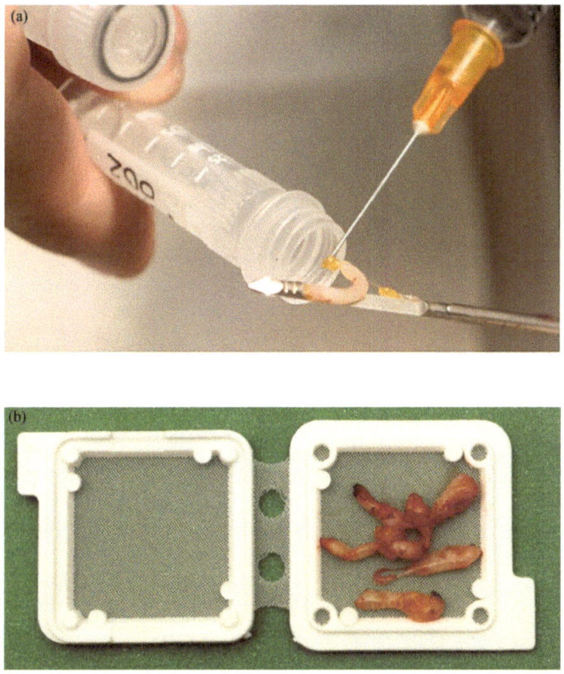

FIGURE 2.17
(a, b) Samples of tissue retrieved from ultrasound-guided standard 14-gauge needle core biopsy placed in a cassette prior to formal histopathological assessment.

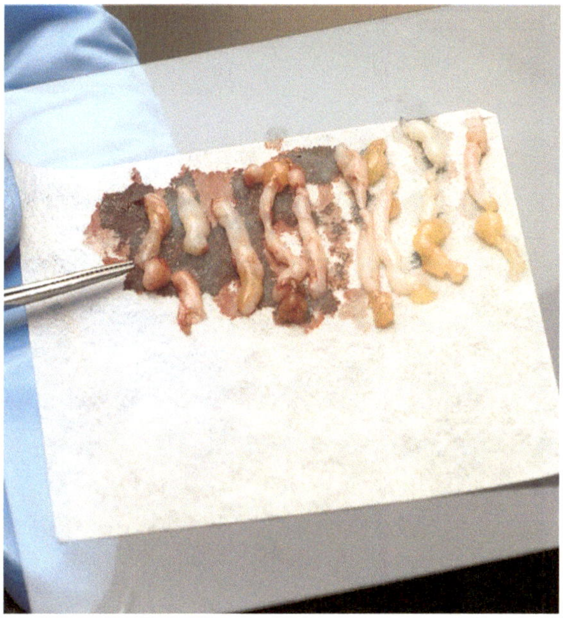

FIGURE 2.18
Samples from a large-gauge vacuum-assisted biopsy (VAB) (11-gauge needle). Multiple generous-sized cores of tissue leading to removal of a relatively large volume of tissue. VAB permits larger volumes of tissue to be retrieved and reduces the chance of under-diagnosis of invasive carcinoma and ductal carcinoma in situ (as non-invasive cancer and atypical ductal hyperplasia, respectively).

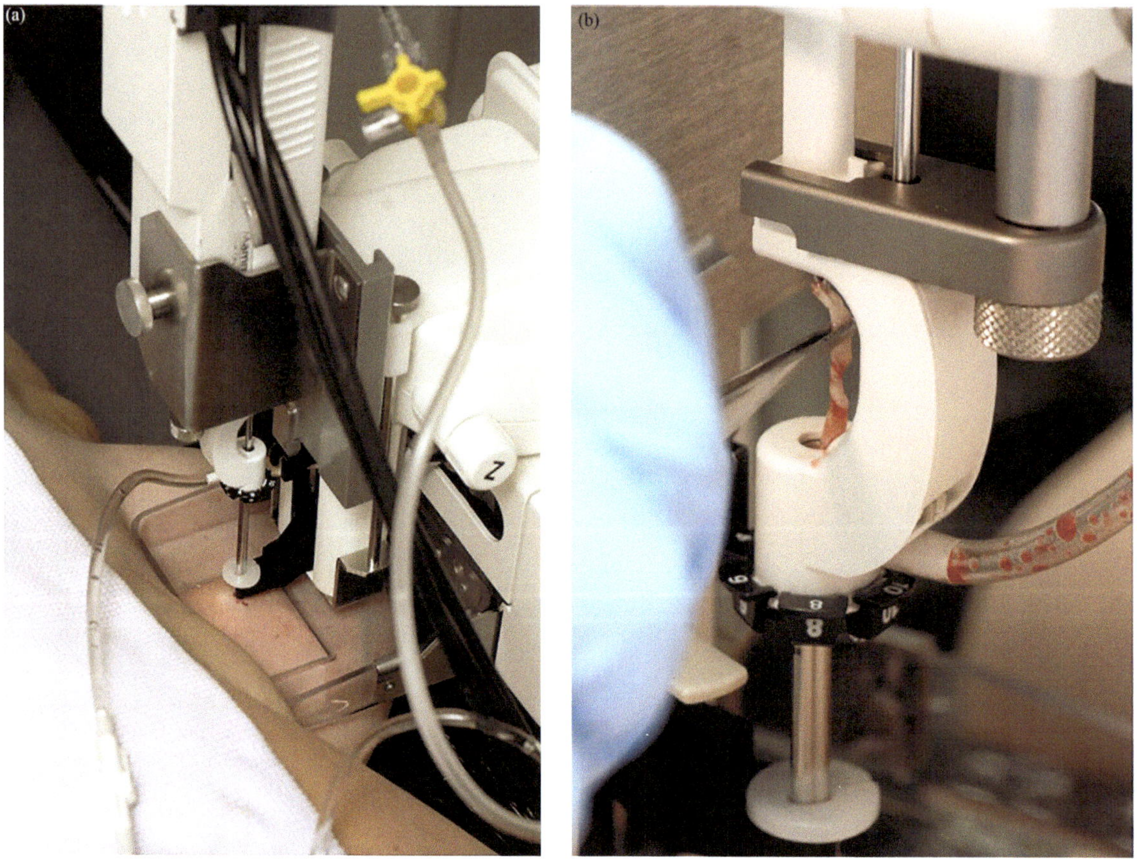

FIGURE 2.19
(a, b) Stereotactic machine with showing needle correctly positioned within breast based on localising coordinates in the horizontal, vertical and depth axes. Stereotactic biopsy using either standard gauge core or vacuum-assisted techniques permits accurate sampling of areas of microcalcification that are unlikely to be seen on ultrasound.

aperture on the stereotactic table. The needle is introduced through a small incision in the skin made with an 11-blade (after administration of local anaesthesia) and then manually advanced to the appropriate depth as calculated by the computer (that has been appropriately calibrated). Stereotactic images are taken to ensure correct position of the needle tip in relation to the breast lesion. The spring-loaded needle is then fired into the breast lesion and the location of the core biopsy checked with repeated stereotactic images. Multiple cores (up to six passes) should be obtained when sampling micro-calcifications and a specimen X-ray taken to confirm adequate sampling of the cluster. Use of large-gauge needles has increased the overall success rate of these stereotactic procedures for sampling calcifications (false negative rate of about 2%) and reduced the number of open (guided) diagnostic excision biopsies. When microcalcifications are readily visible on ultrasound, then ultrasound-guided biopsy will suffice and is an easier and less time-consuming biopsy to perform than stereotactic techniques.

Vacuum-assisted excision biopsy: Most lesions classified pathologically on core biopsy as B3 have prompted a diagnostic excision biopsy with or without localisation (wire, radioactive/magnetic seed, radiofrequency pellet or radar reflector). These B3 lesions are of uncertain malignant potential and include the following:

1. Atypical ductal hyperplasia with moderate degrees of atypia
2. Lobular neoplasia (atypical lobular hyperplasia; lobular carcinoma in situ (LCIS))
3. Papillary lesions
4. Columnar cell change with atypia
5. Phyllodes tumour

In addition to these histological diagnoses, surgical excision is also warranted when there is lack of concordance between the clinical, radiological, and core biopsy findings. LCIS is usually an incidental pathological finding in association with some other condition presenting symptomatically. There has been an

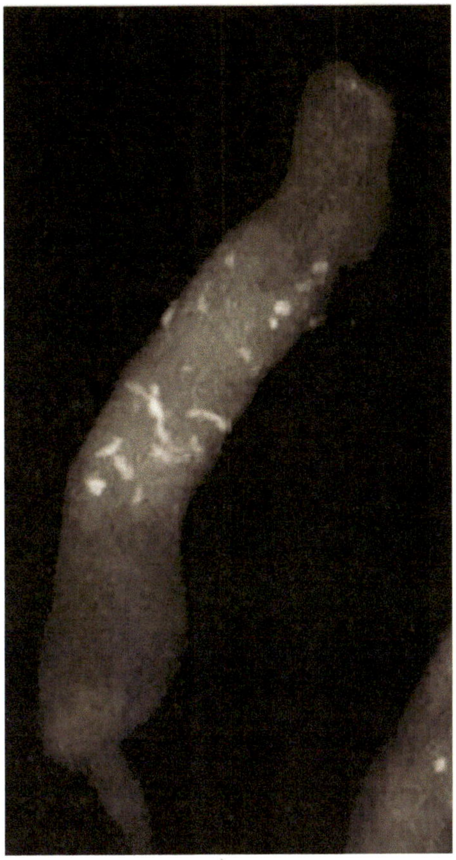

FIGURE 2.20
Specimen radiography of large cores of tissue from VAE showing microcalcification. Cores of tissue with calcification on specimen radiology confirm that adequate sampling has been undertaken after stereotactic biopsy of screen-detected/incidental microcalcification.

increasing trend in recent years for second-line VAB or vacuum-assisted excision of selected B3 lesions rather than a diagnostic surgical excision biopsy. Several of the above B3 lesions are potentially suitable for VAE that may spare patients the ordeal of an open surgical procedure under general anaesthesia. There is consensus that the following B3 lesions can be managed with VAE rather than diagnostic excision following either standard core biopsy or VAB:

1. Atypical ductal hyperplasia with moderate degrees of atypia
2. Lobular neoplasia (atypical lobular hyperplasia; lobular carcinoma in situ [LCIS])
3. Papillary lesions without atypia
4. Columnar cell change with atypia

Surgical excision biopsy with full histopathological evaluation should be performed for certain B3 lesions including cellular fibro-epithelial lesions, papillary lesions with atypia, and mucocele-like lesions that are all associated with a much higher upgrade rate to malignancy.

MRI-guided biopsy: The number of MRI abnormalities has increased significantly as a consequence of more widespread employment of MRI as part of the pre-operative workup of patients together with regular screening of higher-risk patients. These areas of enhanced uptake may be suspicious and represent multifocal, contralateral, or incidental disease and warrant further investigation. Some of these lesions will be visualised on a directed ('second look') ultrasound thereby permitting conventional image-guided biopsy. However, often this is not the case and MRI-guided biopsy is necessary for further tissue acquisition. A standard 14-gauge needle can be used but a larger bore 11-gauge needle is preferred and these MRI-guided techniques can be challenging and demand special training and equipment (high-strength field magnet, breast biopsy coil, and MRI-compatible titanium needles). An important aspect of MRI-guided biopsy is placement of the biopsy needle within the breast whilst the patient is outside the magnet and then MRI images taken to confirm the position of the needle. Biopsies are then taken with multiple passes to guarantee adequate sampling and a clip deployed to permit subsequent mammographic identification of the biopsy site (Figure 2.21).

2.5 Surgical Diagnostic Excision Biopsy

The greatest amount of tissue is obtained with open biopsy techniques (excision biopsy or wire-localised biopsy) and progressively decreasing amounts of tissue are yielded from large-bore needle biopsy (VAE, VAB) and standard core biopsy. The size of the skin incision corresponds to the amount of tissue required from the procedure which in turn depends upon whether this aims to completely excise a lesion or undertake diagnostic sampling. Thus, a very small incision is required for stereotactic VAB, but a slightly larger incision is necessary for standard core biopsy in which the needle must be manoeuvred within the tissue to obtain satisfactory samples. The largest incisions pertain to open biopsy procedures, but these incisions should be kept as small as possible for these diagnostic biopsies (as opposed to lumpectomy for cancer).

The process of acquiring tissue for histological examination under these circumstances demands a coordinated effort and cooperation between the surgeon and radiologist to ensure the appropriate area of breast tissue is excised corresponding to the radiological lesion. The crucial step is placement of the wire under image

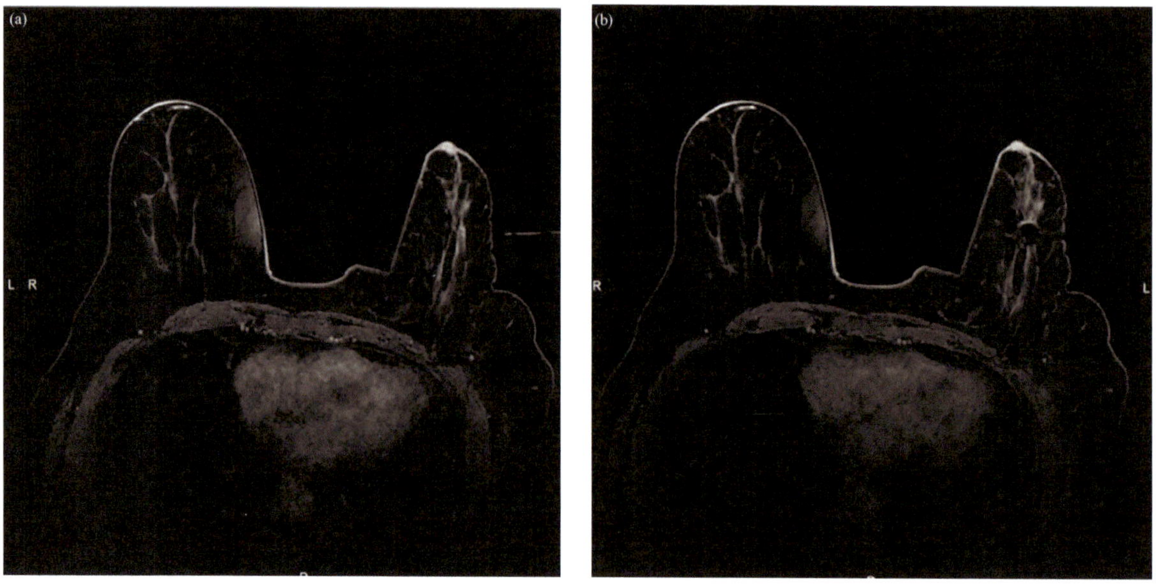

FIGURE 2.21
(a, b) MRI-guided biopsy requires special training and equipment. A clip is deployed following biopsy to permit subsequent localisation in the event of surgical diagnostic excision biopsy.

guidance within the radiology suite, although some surgeons with ultrasound competency perform their own localisations in the operating room. A variety of flexible hooked wires are available which are placed in the breast tissue via a rigid introducer needle under the guidance of bi-planar mammography or ultrasound. Mammograms with two views (antero-posterior and medio-lateral) should be obtained showing the position of the wire and its relationship to the lesion or deployed clip (from previous core biopsy) (Figure 2.22). The tip of the wire should lie within 2 cm of the lesion and the latter is ideally be transfixed by the wire. These localisation films should be carefully scrutinised and a three-dimensional image created that guides the surgical dissection. The surgeon may feel confident to proceed with excision biopsy when the wire transfixes the lesion, but the tip lies more than 2 cm from the lesion (although beware: this may lie within muscle and be difficult to retrieve). When the lesion has been localised with ultrasound only, it is helpful to place a clip within the lesion to confirm its removal on specimen radiography. Following wire localisation, the patient is either transported back to the ward or directly to the operating.

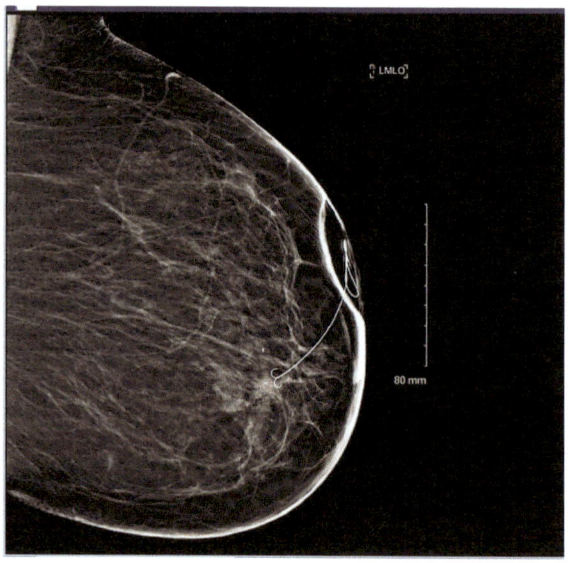

FIGURE 2.22
Needle localisation of impalpable, screen-detected lesion within the lower outer quadrant of the left breast. The tip of the wire lies close to the lesion and the post-biopsy clip in two-view mammography (within 2 cm).

2.6 Newer Technologies for Localisation of Impalpable Lesions

The most common method currently practiced in the United Kingdom for localisation of impalpable lesions is guide-wire localisation, and this remains the gold standard. However, there are associated technical problems relating to wire insertion and migration in addition to logistical issues and patient discomfort. The latter may result from geographical site differences for the procedures of localisation and surgery. Furthermore, wire insertion can incur much patient discomfort and impair overall patient experience. For these reasons, alternative techniques

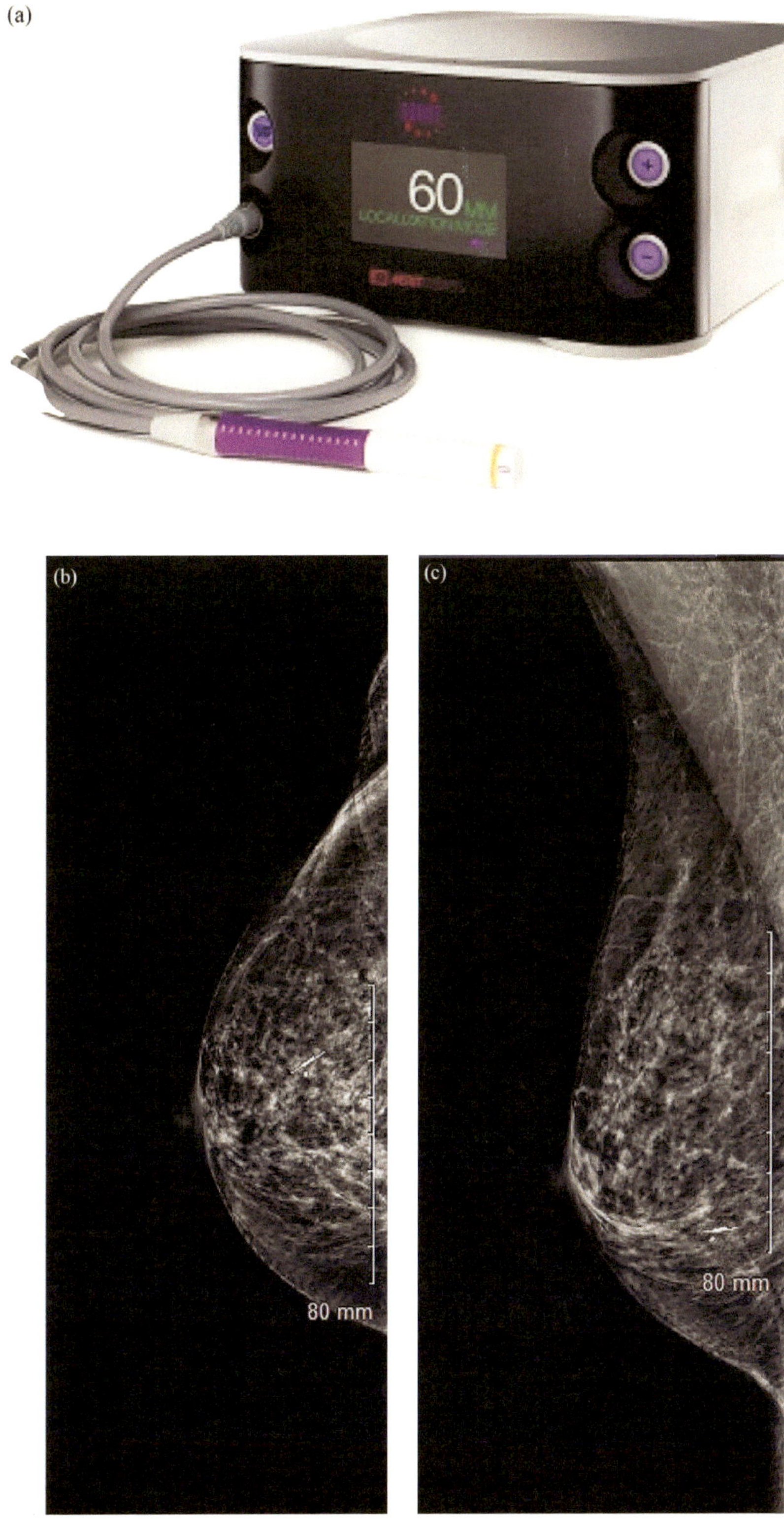

FIGURE 2.23
(a) SAVI-SCOUT uses non-radioactive technology to detect a reflector device within the breast using radar waves. A numerical signal is displayed on the monitor and indicates when the probe is close to the reflector; the reflector can be placed in the breast up to 30 days prior to surgery and is so small that patients cannot feel this. (b, c) The reflector is positioned so as to accurately localise a tumour and permit surgical removal in entirety. This avoids the need for wire localisation that can be associated with pain and discomfort as well as inconvenience in terms of theatre scheduling.

continue to be evaluated and more recently a range of novel technologies have emerged simultaneously that collectively present a choice of alternatives to wire-guided localisation (WGL) of breast lesions as well as biopsy-proven positive axillary lymph nodes. Novel techniques for localising impalpable lesions involve use of a range of devices that employ a seed/pellet/tag that can be inserted in the breast with ultrasound or stereotactic guidance well in advance of surgery (up to 30 days) and prior to commencement of neoadjuvant chemotherapy. Multiple devices can be placed for bracketing prior to resection of larger lesions. These newer devices that can be inserted into impalpable lesions to permit surgical identification include paramagnetic steel and iron oxide seeds (Magseed™), radar reflectors (SCOUT™), and radiofrequency tags (LOCalizer™) (Figure 2.23). Although these alternative methodologies are being widely adopted in several thousand cases around the world, clinical outcomes have not been formally evaluated to date. The majority of studies have evaluated one or another of these alternative devices in terms key performance indicators relative to WGL (in studies often sponsored by the relevant manufacturer of the device). Moreover, there are no large comparative studies examining the performance of these newer technologies against each other (as opposed to WGL).

Several studies are ongoing or planned that will collect valuable data on various different methods for localisation of impalpable breast lesions and clarify basic performance parameters relating to lesion identification and margin negativity rates. It is crucial that robust data is available to guide clinicians in use of the most appropriate device in terms of efficacy, patient comfort/convenience, and cost. There are pressures from the commercial sector to use cognate devices, and clinicians need to be confident that any particular method is non-inferior to WGL in terms of key performance indicators before making any decision on product choice—whether this be in a managed healthcare system or the private sector.

References

1) Wishart GC, Warwick J, Pitsinis V, et al. Measuring performance in clinical breast examination. Br J Surg. 2010. DOI: 10.1002/bjs.7108.
2) Britton P, Duffy SW, Sinnatamby R, et al. One-stop diagnostic clinics: How often are breast cancers missed? Br J Cancer. 2009;100:1873–1878.

3

Breast Cancer Staging and Imaging

Fiona Gilbert and Falak Masood

3.1 Introduction

A wide range of modalities are used in the diagnosis and staging of breast carcinoma. Conventional modalities include mammography and digital breast tomosynthesis (DBT), as well as ultrasound (US). New contrast-enhanced techniques are now available which provide useful functional as well as more accurate delineation of tumour extent, including dynamic-contrast-enhanced multiparametric magnetic resonance imaging (MRI) and contrast-enhanced mammography (CEM). Computerised tomography (CT) plays a vital role in staging cancers and assessing for distant site metastases. Increasingly nuclear medicine techniques such as positron emission tomography CT (PET-CT, using fluorodeoxyglucose-18 radiotracer; FDG-18) and bone scan (using technetium-99) have an invaluable role in staging breast cancers and for detection of distant metastases, as well as problem-solving for indeterminate areas seen on CT.

3.2 Digital Breast Tomosynthesis

Digital breast tomosynthesis (DBT) is an X-ray technique that permits viewing of breast tissue in narrow planes. The technique addresses one of the acknowledged limitations of digital mammography (DM) whereby superimposed fibroglandular tissue can obscure small cancers or mimic the radiological appearance of cancer. This technology has been widely adopted in many countries in both the symptomatic and screening setting. Comparative studies of screening and randomised controlled trials have demonstrated both an increase in cancer detection rates as well as reduced recall rates (1–5). Real-world data from a before and after analysis of 15 academic and private practice sites in the USA showed that the majority had reduced recall and improved cancer detection rates following adoption of DBT (6). However, the Norwegian To-Be RCT did not reveal any improvement in cancer detection rates amongst 26,000 women (7). The largest retrospective analysis involving more than one million women from five regions in the United States was published by Conant and colleagues (8). This showed that cancer detection rates were higher with DBT than 2D mammography (5.3/1000 vs 4.5/1000) and in particular there was a lower rate of false positive readings.

There have been concerns that some additional cancers found on DBT are intrinsically slower growing and may increase the rate of overdiagnosis (defined as detection of a cancer that would never have influenced a woman's lifespan had she not undergone screening). Although replacement of mammography by DBT results in detection of more cancers, this has not had any impact on mortality. To address whether or not these additional cancers found by DBT represent overdiagnosis, reduction in numbers of interval cancers can be assessed as an outcome measure. A time series analysis reveals that in the United States, 78,385 digital mammographies and 76,896 DBT examinations demonstrated an increase in cancer detection rates following the transition to DBT, but the number of interval cancers remained unchanged (1.1/1000) (9). The ReTomo Italian randomised controlled trial has confirmed an increase in cancer detection rates with the addition of DBT to 2D FFDM (101 in 13,356 and 61 in 13,521, respectively) but no significant reduction in interval cancers was observed (10). In a meta-analysis of five prospective DBT trials, including 129,969 DBT and 227,882 2D mammography examinations, cancer detection rates were 9.03/1000 and 5.95/1000, respectively. The pooled interval cancer rates of 1.56/1000 in the DBT arm and 1.75/1000 in the mammography arm were not significantly different (11). The UK PROSPECTS randomised controlled trial aims to recruit 100,000 women aged 50–70 years and will compare standard mammography with or without the addition of DBT (12). The US TMIST study

DOI: 10.1201/9781003394785-3

of 120,000 women aged 40–70 years is comparing the synthetic 2D and DBT with standard mammography. Both trials have interval cancer rates as the primary outcome measure. There is debate as to whether DBT has comparable added benefit in women with different breast densities. As DBT is able to reduce the overlapping effects of tissues, there is little potential benefit in fatty breasts with maximum benefit in those with BIRADS categories B and C. In women with dense breast tissue, DBT has been shown to be advantageous, with the TOMMY trial demonstrating improved sensitivity from the addition of DBT compared to full field digital mammography (FFDM) alone (93% vs 86%, $p = 0.03$) (13, 14). In this large study of assessment cases, DBT did not detect additional cancers in those patients with the densest breast tissue—BIRADS D category (14). However, sub-analysis of the recent TOSYMA trial involving more than 99,000 women showed DBT with synthesised mammography found 2.7/1000 more invasive cancers with dense breasts (BIRADS C and D) compared to 2D mammograms alone with the largest difference in those women with extremely dense breasts (BIRADS D) (15). This difference may be attributable to temporal improvement in the DBT acquisition technique and reconstruction algorithms.

The addition of DBT leads to a 200% increase in radiation dose. In efforts to reduce this to acceptable levels, many centres have stopped acquiring separate 2D FFDM and instead use synthetic images created from the DBT planes. Although earlier studies showed that calcification was not as well visualised on these synthetic images, subsequent reconstruction algorithms have shown improved resolution and use of synthetic images is now considered accepted practice and is associated with only a 20% increase in radiation dose compared to 2D mammography.

A number of studies have reported increased reading time due to the additional images available (2, 16, 17). This increase has ranged from 91 to 124 seconds, with most studies reporting a doubling of reading time compared to 2D mammography. Increased reading time has implications for an already over-stretched workforce involved in reading screening images. AI techniques can potentially improve cancer detection, decrease recall rates, and reduce reading time. Reader studies using AI algorithms have confirmed that reading times can be reduced and reader performance improved with an increase in cancer detection rates and similar or improved specificity (18). A systematic review and meta-analysis concluded that although there was strong evidence for comparable performance of AI to a radiologist in terms of reading 2D mammography, there remains insufficient published data in this area for DBT (19).

3.3 Breast Ultrasound Examination

Ultrasound is especially useful for younger women who tend to have denser breast tissue. However, this imaging modality is not a replacement for mammography. Ultrasound is less effective than mammography for detecting very small calcium deposits (microcalcifications) in the breast and, in consequence, is less sensitive in detecting ductal carcinoma in situ (DCIS) compared to mammography. Nonetheless, breast ultrasound can identify incidental benign breast conditions that might otherwise go unnoticed (20, 21).

Ultrasound can be a valuable problem-solving tool for symptomatic women, but it is relatively time-consuming and may result in false-positive findings. Because of this, breast ultrasound examination is a focused procedure and limited to the specific area or the part of the breast of concern to the clinician or patient.

Ultrasound is ideally suited for guiding interventional procedures, such as biopsies of solid breast masses, or aspiration of simple cysts and seromas.

The majority of breast cancers are identified either from routine screening mammography or following symptomatic presentation to breast clinics. When evaluating suspicious lesions, the conventional approach is with triple assessment, which involves three key components: clinical breast examination, imaging (mammography, ultrasound), and image-guided needle biopsy. Ultrasound plays a central role in the management of women with breast cancer and serve three primary purposes: determining the size and location of the tumour, guiding biopsy of cancerous tissue and evaluation of axillary lymph nodes (with or without needle biopsy) (22).

3.3.1 Indications and Contraindications to Breast Ultrasound Examination

In terms of breast ultrasound examination, there are no particular contraindications to a patient undergoing this procedure. However, the quality of the images can be impaired if a patient is unable to lie still/flat or reposition themselves on the examination table. Additionally, these types of examinations can be challenging for individuals with open wounds or damaged skin, and the presence of breast implants can obscure certain areas of the breast and limit accuracy. The duration of a complete examination typically ranges from five to twenty minutes. In cases of suspected breast cancer, a more detailed examination that encompasses the entire breast and the axilla on the ipsilateral side should be conducted.

The sensitivity of breast ultrasound is approximately 85% (23). Missed lesions tend to be invasive cancers that are either very small, located directly behind the nipple, or challenging to distinguish from normal tissue or fibrocystic changes. This is especially the case for lobular cancers, which constitute around 15% of invasive cancers. Furthermore, the calcifications of DCIS are often not visible on ultrasound (23). New ultrasound techniques, such as shear wave elastography, which measures the stiffness of breast lesions, may further improve the capability of ultrasound to differentiate benign from malignant breast masses (24, 25)

Ultrasound is frequently used to guide core biopsy of breast lesions whereby a sample of radiologically suspicious tissue is taken using a needle (usually 14 gauge for standard core biopsy). Even when lesions are palpable, the operator can see the needle passing into the lesion in real time, thus improving the accuracy of the procedure. Prior to biopsy, local anaesthetic is administered around the skin area near the lesion. In some cases, ultrasound is also used to insert wires to guide surgical resection or marker clip placement within the cancer before commencing neoadjuvant chemotherapy (NACT) that may result in a complete radiological response and necessitate resection of tissue around the marker clip (containing the tumour bed). Other applications include second look ultrasound after detection of additional lesions on MRI, evaluation of breast implants and response to upfront/primary systemic treatment (26).

3.3.2 Technique and Procedure of Breast Ultrasound Examination

Breast ultrasound is performed using an ultrasound scanner equipped with probes operating at a frequency of 10–13 MHz. The operator who conducts the examination provides clear instructions and an explanation of the entire procedure. Typically, a chaperone is present in the room to assist the operator, particularly during ultrasound-guided procedures.

During the procedure, the patient's upper torso is uncovered, and undergarments removed. A water-based gel is applied to the breast, and the probe is gently moved around the breast with minimal pressure. In cases where clinical abnormalities are detected in the axilla (underarm area), or as part of routine examination for women with a personal history of breast cancer, the axilla is also scanned. If enlarged lymph nodes are found in the axilla, adjacent lymph node areas, such as the neck and regions below the clavicle, may also be examined.

Advanced imaging techniques, such as Doppler and shear wave elastography, are performed without applying pressure. Utilisation of strain elastography involves only gentle probe movement and does not induce discomfort (26).

In the UK and most European countries, a structured reporting and classification system is in use. The most applied system is the Breast Imaging Reporting and Data System (BI-RADS) developed by the American College of Radiology. BI-RADS 1 means 'negative, no findings' (27).

3.3.3 Screening with Breast Ultrasound

Many studies have shown that whole breast ultrasound can be a useful supplemental screening tool in dense breasts, due to its accessibility, lack of intravenous (IV) contrast and ionising radiation, and better patient tolerance. Handheld ultrasound (HHUS) increases the cancer detection rate by 1.8–4.6 cancers per 1000 women screened, compared with mammography alone (28–32). However, the use of HHUS as a screening tool has some disadvantages, such as more prolonged scanning times, significant operator dependence and relatively higher recall rates (28, 33).

Automated breast ultrasound (ABUS) is a three-dimensional volume imaging technique, recently introduced as an alternative to handheld ultrasound (HHUS) for screening purposes and with similar diagnostic accuracy (33). ABUS should be performed by trained personnel (radiographers, technicians, or nurses) and provides optimal orientation and image documentation with better reproducibility. It is therefore more suitable for screening with an increase in the cancer detection rate of 1.9–7.7 cases per 1000 women compared to mammography alone (32). Furthermore, the coronal plane in ABUS can be helpful in local staging and guide treatment planning (Figure 3.1).

3.4 Magnetic Resonance Imaging (MRI)

Tumour neo-angiogenesis plays a key role in both local tumour growth and distant metastasis in breast cancer. Dynamic-contrast-enhanced MRI is a technique that uses an intravenous gadolinium-based contrast agent that decreases the local T1 time—leading to a high signal on T1-weighted images (34). Leaky vessels formed due to tumour neo-angiogenesis can then allow rapid extravasation of contrast agents, leading to local enhancement (35). Most MRI protocols used in clinical practice are multiparametric and include dynamic analysis of time-signal-intensity that allows valuable information on enhancement kinetics to be derived (36–38).

This functional information contributes to making contrast-enhanced breast MRI the most sensitive modality in the imaging of breast cancer (>90%; 39); it

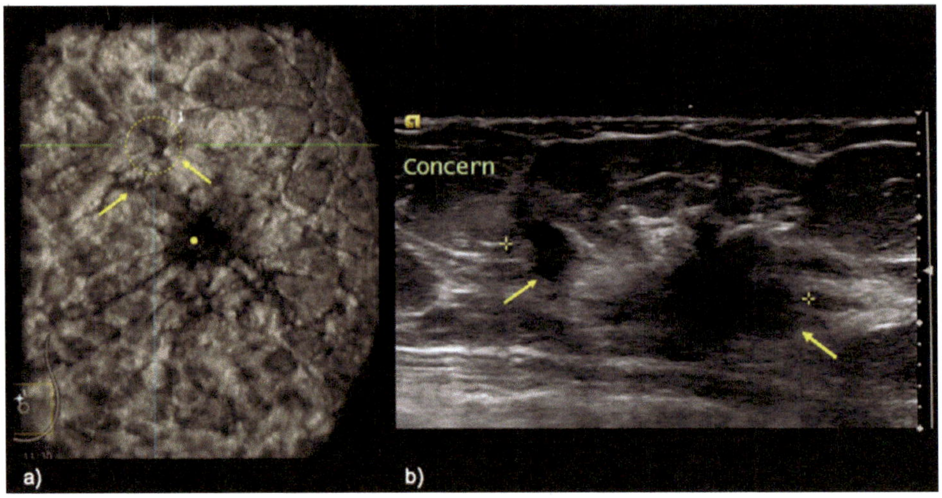

FIGURE 3.1
A multifocal grade II invasive carcinoma of no special type (NST) with intratumoural low-grade DCIS, presenting with (a) 'the retraction sign' (circle) and two foci of tumour, 18 mm and 6 mm (arrows), on ABUS coronal plane and (b) corresponding HHUS images.

is able to detect cancer not visible on mammography and ultrasound. Its role in diagnosis and management has therefore continued to expand.

Indications for MRI include staging of known cancer, the screening of very high-risk patients, response to chemotherapy in the neoadjuvant setting, including use as a problem-solving instrument (40, 41).

3.4.1 Applications

3.4.1.1 Pre-Operative Staging of Breast Cancer

Pre-operative local staging of a known breast cancer is a common indication for breast MRI (40, 41). MRI has a high sensitivity for cancer detection (close to 100%) and moderate specificity (up to 72%) (42, 43). In 15–30% of those patients with breast cancer breast MRI can lead to a change in treatment plans (44, 54). However, the detection of further disease in patients with a documented breast cancer has not translated into improved survival outcomes, and guidelines are notably highly variable in recommendations for when breast MRI is indicated in the pre-operative setting (45, 46).

Current indications for breast MRI imaging in the pre-operative setting include women with dense breasts (BIRADS C and D); women with diagnosis at a young age; women with hormone receptor-negative cancers and women with lobular cancers. (44, 47–50).

3.4.1.2 Staging Biopsy Proven Breast Cancers

Using breast MRI imaging, approximately 75% of cancers have a radiological size measurement within 1 cm from definitive pathologic size (51–53), and most studies demonstrate that size estimates based on MRI are more reliable than clinical examination, US, or mammography. MRI is less accurate for measuring the extent of larger cancers and areas of non-mass enhancement in comparison to mass lesions (51–53). MRI is particularly beneficial in staging invasive lobular carcinomas with good correlation between tumour size on MRI and on pathology (48–50).

3.4.1.3 Staging DCIS

MRI imaging can detect mammographically visible as well as occult foci of DCIS (55–58). In a prospective study of 593 patients with biopsy-proven invasive breast cancer who underwent breast MR (in addition to conventional) imaging, MRI imaging was found to have a sensitivity of 89% for diagnosis of DCIS pre-operatively and was significantly more accurate than conventional imaging with DCIS detected in 51.1% and 36.7% of cases, respectively. The superior sensitivity of MRI imaging over conventional modalities was more apparent with increasing relative size of DCIS components and increasing nuclear grade of the lesion (59). Pre-operative MRI in the DCIS setting can also find invasive components within DCIS, in particular where there is evidence of mass-like lesion, nipple-areolar complex involvement or a hetereogeneous enhancement pattern (60).

3.4.1.4 Detection of Mammographic Occult Lesions in Pre-Operative Setting

Detection of mammographic occult lesions in the affected breast is a common finding. Meta-analysis of

50 studies demonstrated that 67% of additional findings at pre-operative MRI are malignant and in 20% of cases the additional disease detected changes the treatment plan (61). Findings that potentially change the surgical treatment plan should be confirmed histologically with core biopsy prior to primary treatment. MRI is associated with a high frequency of incidental findings, and therefore, a multi-parametric protocol is useful in characterising lesions that are definitely benign and do not require any (unnecessary) biopsy. In the case of indeterminate lesions, MRI directed 'second look' US examination allows the option of ultrasound-guided biopsy in more than half (57.5%) of lesions (62). Lesions that are suspicious and occult on ultrasound and mammogram should be sampled with MRI-guided biopsy.

3.4.1.5 Using MRI to Plan Surgery and Re-Excision

Increased accuracy of staging with MRI has not translated into improved surgical outcomes of patients. As outlined earlier, women undergoing MRI have a higher likelihood of a change in treatment plan with meta-analyses demonstrating an odds ratio of 1.39 for higher likelihood of undergoing mastectomy (54).

A nationwide British prospective randomised controlled trial looking at the comparative effectiveness of MRI in breast cancer (COMICE trial) compared outcomes between patients where surgeons were and were not able to use better staging information available from pre-operative MRI. This trial found nearly identical re-excision rates of 19% in both arms (63) and additional lesions often prompted mastectomy as these were presumed to be malignant (MRI biopsy was not commonly available at the time the trial was conducted). In contrast, a Swedish trial has shown that MRI findings can reduce re-excision rates from 15% to 5% in women undergoing breast conservation surgery (Gonzalez et al. 2014).

Nonetheless, for lobular cancers, there is clear evidence that information from MRI helps reduce re-excision rates without increasing rates of mastectomy (64–67).

3.4.1.6 Detection of Contralateral Breast Cancer

Breast MRI can demonstrate occult contralateral disease in between 5.5 and 9.3% of women with known unilateral breast cancer with 28–37% of these findings (i.e. 2–4%) representing malignancy (Plana et al. 2012). These cancers detected in the contralateral breast are small (mostly under 1 cm) and are exclusively non-invasive disease (DCIS) in one-third of cases. Density of breast tissue and other risk factors are not associated with increased likelihood of detecting a contralateral cancer (68).

3.4.2 Supplemental Screening

Those with a lifetime risk for developing breast cancer of greater than 20% are classified as high-risk (69). This includes carriers of genetic mutations, such as BRCA1, BRCA2, PALB2, TP53, PTEN, CHEK2, CDH1, ATM, and STK11, as well as those who have undergone chest irradiation before the age of 30 years (often in the context of lymphoma treatment). Annual screening MRI (and mammography if over 40) is recommended in this subset of women (70). Most literature on use of MRI for screening focussed on high-risk population, in particular BRCA1/2 carriers in whom MRI has been shown to have high sensitivity (75.2–100%) and specificity (82–98.4%) (71).

Limited evidence has been available hitherto to recommend for or against screening with MRI in intermediate risk women (those with a lifetime risk of breast cancer between 15 and 20%, personal history of breast cancer, dense breasts, or history of high-risk lesions). However, evidence is emerging that supports a role for MRI, especially in women previously treated with breast-conserving surgery for cancer and under 50 years of age at the time of breast cancer diagnosis (70, 72, 73). MRI screening is not recommended for women with an average lifetime risk of breast cancer (below 15%) (69).

3.4.3 Evaluation of Response to Neoadjuvant Chemotherapy

Evaluating residual tumour size in the neoadjuvant chemotherapy (NAC) setting is important from both the oncology perspective (ensuring response to a specific regimen) and from the surgical perspective (ensuring negative margins are achieved when breast-conserving surgery is planned and accurately delineating tumour extent). MRI has been shown to be more accurate than both conventional mammography and ultrasound and can distinguish more effectively post-treatment fibrosis and post-biopsy change from residual tumour more effectively in the context of response to NAC. In turn, this information can improve surgical planning (74, 75).

3.4.4 Assessment of Symptomatic Patients as a Problem-Solving Tool

MRI has developed as a useful problem-solving tool in clinical practice due to its high sensitivity (99%) combined with a high negative predictive value (100%) and ability to distinguish benign and malignant disease

(76, 77). The indications for use of MRI include the following situations:

- Conventional imaging (with ultrasound and mammography) is inconclusive or normal.
- Suspicion of an occult cancer (unexplained clinically suspicious examination findings).
- Suspicious nipple discharge.
- Suspicious lesions (BIRADS 4 and above) which are not amenable to biopsy.
- Discordant radiologic-pathologic findings.
- Cancer of unknown primary origin (particularly in the scenario of axillary carcinoma of unknown primary origin in the breast). In general, a negative breast MRI excludes malignancy (77).

The role of MRI in characterising calcifications is more controversial, and MRI has lower sensitivity for diagnosing DCIS. Therefore, MRI is unable to exclude non-invasive cancer with sufficient confidence and the decision to perform biopsy in these cases is be based on mammographic features and index of suspicion (78).

3.5 Contrast-Enhanced Mammography

Contrast-enhanced mammography (CEM) was introduced commercially in 2011 and is an emerging technique that utilises contrast to visualise the vascularity of breast lesions. CEM is superior to conventional mammography for the identification of breast cancer, particularly in women who have dense breasts. CEM has the advantage over mammography of investigating physiological and morphological abnormalities in a manner that is similar to breast MRI (79). CEM can achieve comparable sensitivity to breast MRI at lower costs and wider accessibility[2].

3.5.1 Technique

After administration of an iodinated contrast agent over a two-minute period, a single breast compression is performed during a dual-energy exposure on the standard mediolateral oblique and craniocaudal projections. This permits images with low energy (LE) and high energy (HE) to be generated. The LE image would function similarly to the full-field digital mammography (FFDM) image (80). The HE image, produced at a higher tube voltage, is not appropriate for diagnostic applications and used to create a recombined image. The latter is obtained using a subtraction technique to highlight the regions of the breast that have taken in contrast media (80).

3.5.2 Clinical Indications and Applications

3.5.2.1 Assessing Findings on Screening FFDM

CEM is increasingly used to evaluate abnormalities seen on screening mammography and to assess the probability of malignancy (81). A systematic review and meta-regression of 60 CEM studies showed that CEM interpretation yielded a sensitivity of 95% and a specificity of 81%. A subgroup analysis of nine studies for patients with dense breasts showed a pooled sensitivity of 95% and a pooled specificity of 78% (82).

3.5.2.2 Supplemental Screening

CEM is a potential alternative to breast MRI in women who are at increased risk of developing breast cancer and women with dense breasts. A prospective pilot study compared MRI to CEM in 307 women with an intermediate or high risk of breast cancer. Out of three cancers detected during the initial screening, MRI identified three and CEM identified two of them, while none were identified on FFDM. The specificity of CEM was compared to MRI at 94.7% and 94.1%, respectively (80, 81, 83). In another retrospective study of 611 women with intermediate breast cancer risk, dense breasts (C or D) were reported in 93.1% of them, and CEM has shown an incremental cancer detection rate of 13.1 out of 1000 (80, 81, 84). While the preliminary studies are promising, the evidence is still limited, and clinical trials are ongoing to evaluate the role of CEM in screening (85).

3.5.2.3 Assessment of Symptomatic Patients

In a reader study of 100 CEM examinations performed in patients with palpable breast abnormalities (73% of them had breast cancer), CEM was significantly superior to mammography in sensitivity (95% vs 84%) and specificity (81% vs 63%), respectively (80, 81, 86). Another study showed no significant differences in the performance between CEM and ultrasound in 115 symptomatic women (89% of them had palpable masses) (80, 87).

3.5.2.4 Pre-Operative Staging of Breast Cancer

CEM could be useful to evaluate tumour size and the extent of disease for local staging of breast cancer prior to surgery. Studies have shown good correlation between the CEM index tumour size and histopathology size (88). Although CEM might be inferior to breast MRI at detecting additional unilateral and contralateral tumour foci, it has demonstrated a higher specificity and positive predictive values (PPV) (89–91).

3.5.2.5 Evaluation of Response to Neoadjuvant Chemotherapy

Many small CEM studies showed promise in the evaluation of response to NACT. A meta-analysis of six studies involving a total of 328 patients showed equivalent diagnostic accuracy for CEM and MRI in the prediction of pathologic complete response with an AUC of 0.85 (95% CI 0.82–0.88) (92, 93). A prospective study of 110 patients investigated CEM as an alternative to breast MRI in the assessment of residual disease after NACT and showed a PPV of 81% and an NPV of 50% for CEM. Moreover, there was no statistically significant difference in performance parameters between CEM and MRI (93).

3.6 Staging Investigations

Accurate disease staging is important in breast cancer patients for fully informed decision-making, in terms of treatment planning and for establishing prognosis (94). Staging investigations are employed for some newly diagnosed breast cancers, at the time of locoregional recurrence and to monitor response of metastatic disease to palliative therapies.

Identification of distant metastatic disease in newly diagnosed breast cancer patients profoundly alters patient management in terms of the type of surgery and chemotherapy offered. The incidence of widespread metastases in this group of patients is low (approximately 4%) and selecting appropriate patients for full staging investigations is challenging (98, 99). Optimisation of staging criteria is fundamental not only to diagnose metastatic disease but also to minimise false-positive results, patient anxiety, workload of staff, and treatment delays. Current guidelines are unclear and lack consistency in terms of timing and type of staging investigations and practice varies greatly between units (94).

Common sites of distant metastatic disease include bone, lung, and liver. CT thorax, abdomen, and pelvis is the initial staging investigation of choice due to its specificity and convenience (95, 96). CT can accurately diagnose bone metastases and can safely replace bone scintigraphy if the femoral necks are included in the field of view (96, 97).

Most authorities agree that routine staging is not recommended for asymptomatic early breast cancer patients, owing to the low prevalence of distant metastatic disease in the absence of symptoms such as back pain or cough (up to 2%) (98–100). The risk of distant metastasis increases with larger tumour size, higher histological grade, and extensive lymph node involvement, with a 15–20% risk of distant metastasis in patients with stage III and above (96, 100). For this reason, CT staging should be offered to patients with symptoms of possible metastatic disease, to asymptomatic patients with T3–T4 disease (>5 cm), and to those with more than 4 abnormal lymph nodes at imaging or after surgery.

The incidence of locoregional recurrence after initial breast cancer treatment is 3–10% and this is associated with increased risk of distant metastasis (101). Synchronous metastases occur in up to 15–30% of patients with a locoregional recurrence and up to 35% of patients with isolated lymph node recurrence (102). Adequate pre-operative staging is imperative for tailoring optimal treatment plans, as the presence and extent of metastatic disease determines the curative or palliative intent of treatment (102). CT thorax-abdomen and pelvis is the first choice for staging these patients. (Figures 3.2 and 3.3).

CT is the primary test to evaluate visceral metastasis and first line for brain metastasis. This is also the imaging of choice for monitoring treatment response in patients with established metastatic disease. In

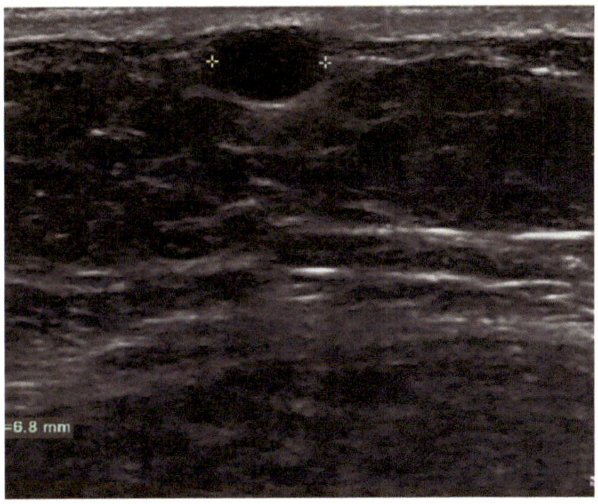

FIGURE 3.2
A 58-year-old patient had been treated 3 years before for grade 3 invasive carcinoma NST, ER/PR positive, HER2 negative (previous right WLE, SLNB Adjuvant RT, on tamoxifen). The patient presents symptomatic for new lump in the right breast. Recent (1 month before) bilateral mammography was normal. Ultrasound shows a 7 mm hypoechoic mass (asterisks). Ultrasound-guided biopsy shows invasive carcinoma NST, provisional grade 2. ER 8, PR 5, HER-2 negative. A CT staging was performed—Figure 3.3.

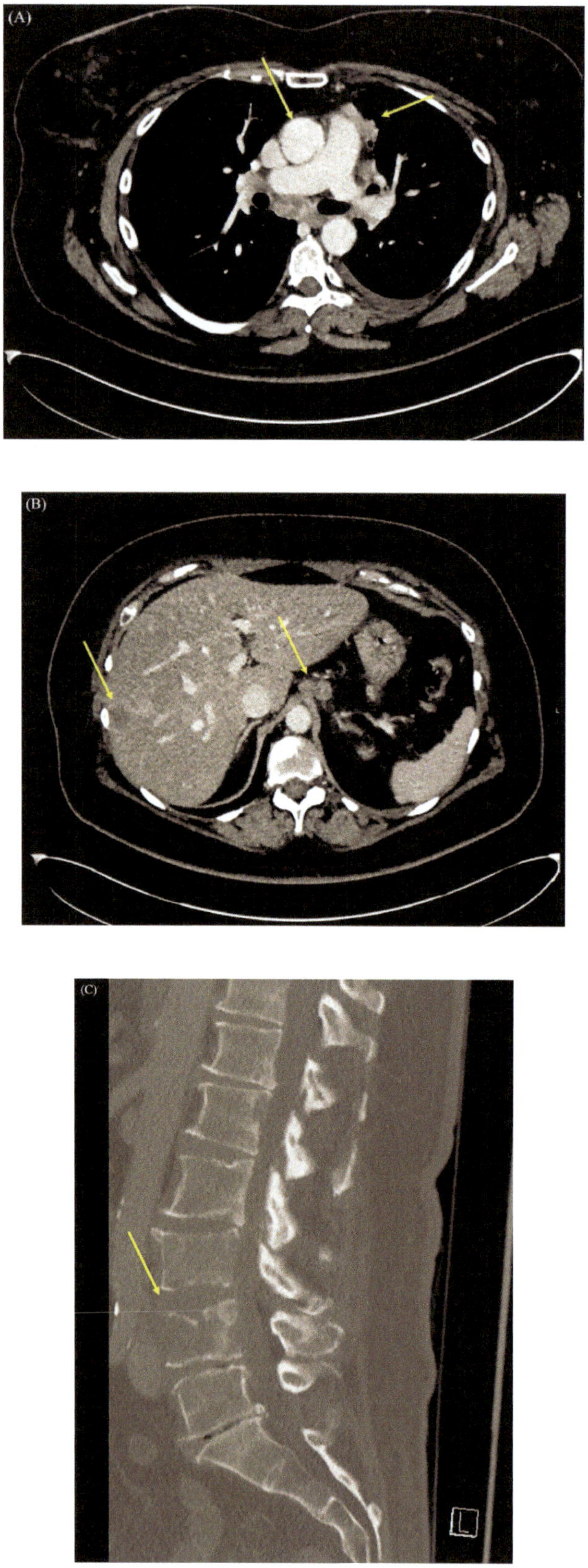

FIGURE 3.3
(Same patient as Figure 3.2) CT staging reveals multiple metastases within (A) lung and mediastinum, (B) liver and abdominal nodes, and (C) bone.

some cases, other advanced imaging techniques are recommended.

CT is highly sensitive for detection of bone lesions, when these involve the cortical bone, but less accurate when tumour is confined to the marrow space are difficult to detect on CT. For this reason, CT is considered to have high specificity but low sensitivity for bone metastases. When there is clinical suspicion of bone disease or the need to evaluate inconclusive bone lesions, further types of imaging are indicated.

Bone scan has high sensitivity but lower levels of specificity for diagnosis of bone metastasis. Accumulation of radionuclide relates to increased local blood flow and osteoblastic activity; for this reason, osteolytic lesions can yield false negative results (100). MRI has high sensitivity and specificity for bone lesions and is used for problem-solving in doubtful cases (100); it can differentiate between healthy and pathological bone marrow as a non-invasive effective test, with higher sensitivity than bone scan for osseous metastases (100).

MRI has higher sensitivity than CT for detection of brain metastasis due to higher soft tissue resolution and improved detection of parenchymal and leptomeningeal disease (100). Brain MRI is indicated in the presence of clinical symptoms suggestive of cerebral disease and negative CT results. Inconclusive liver findings on CT scan might be resolved with a dedicated liver MRI that employs a hepatobiliary contrast agent.

Whole-body MRI (WB-MRI) is assuming an increasingly important role in breast cancer staging as it performs better in treatment response evaluation compared to CT, has comparable performance to FDG-PET/CT, and has a useful diagnostic role in non-FDG avid tumours (103).

Hybrid techniques that combine morphological and functional information are the most sensitive and specific diagnostic tests for metastases. There is increasing evidence that FDG-PET/CT detects distant metastases with higher sensitivity than conventional imaging, although in cases of lobular cancer and low-grade tumours, it can be less sensitive (100). For this reason, current guidelines suggest that patients with inflammatory breast cancer are staged with FDG-PET/CT due to superior performance in detection of locoregional and distant metastasis (104). PET/CT can also be used for problem-solving when CT findings are inconclusive.

FDG-PET/CT has high levels of sensitivity and specificity for diagnosis of bone metastases that exceeds that for combined CT and bone scan. Nonetheless, low-grade and lobular cancers can lead to false negative results. FDG-PET/MRI is a promising technique with similar diagnostic performance to WB-MRI and

PET/CT (100). It combines the high soft tissue resolution of MRI with its multi-parametric ability.

Breast cancer is an heterogenous disease and imaging that provides not only morphological but also functional data is likely to be especially valuable in clinical practice in the coming years (105). Recently, new radio-tracers have been introduced for hybrid imaging, but these are currently used only in a research setting. In the future, targeted PET radiotracers (which for instance detect HER2 expression or ER receptor expression) may improve breast cancer characterisation and treatment for a better personalised approach (105).

In conclusion accurate disease staging is key in decision-making for correct patient management. Multiple imaging techniques are available with different diagnostic accuracy and availability. Optimisation of staging criteria in terms of timing and correct diagnostic technique is a challenging but necessary task that not only ensures appropriate management but also potentially minimises patient anxiety, workload, and treatment delays. Shared decision-making within the multidisciplinary team is crucial for high-quality and effective patient care.

References

1) Michell MJ. Breast screening review—a radiologist's perspective. Br J Radiol. 2012;85(1015):845–7.
2) Wallis MG, Moa E, Zanca F, et al. Two-view and single-view tomosynthesis versus full-field digital mammography: High-resolution X-ray imaging observer study. Radiology. 2012; 262(3):788–96.
3) Svahn TM, Chakraborty DP, Ikeda D, et al. Breast tomosynthesis and digital mammography: A comparison of diagnostic accuracy. Br J Radiol. 2012;85(1019):e1074–82.
4) Gilbert FJ, Tucker L, Young KC. Digital breast tomosynthesis (DBT): A review of the evidence for use as a screening tool. Clin Radiol. 2016;71(2):141–50.
5) Monticciolo DL, Newell MS, Moy L, et al. Breast cancer screening in women at higher-than-average risk: Recommendations from the ACR. J Am Coll Radiol. 2018;15(3 Pt A):408–14.
6) Friedewald SM, Young VA, Gupta D. Lesion localization using the scroll bar on tomosynthesis: Why doesn't it always work? Clin Imaging. 2018;47:57–64.
7) Hofvind S, Hovda T, Holen ÅS, et al. Digital breast tomosynthesis and synthetic 2D mammography versus digital mammography: Evaluation in a population-based screening program. Radiology. 2018;287(3):787–94.
8) Conant EF, Talley MM, Parghi CR, et al. Mammographic screening in routine practice: Multisite study of digital breast tomosynthesis and digital mammography screenings. Radiology. 2023;307(3):e221571.
9) Bahl M, Gaffney S, McCarthy AM, et al. Breast cancer characteristics associated with 2D digital mammography versus digital breast tomosynthesis for screening-detected and interval cancers. Radiology. 2018;287(1):49–57.
10) Pattacini P, Nitrosi A, Giorgi Rossi P, et al. A randomized trial comparing breast cancer incidence and interval cancers after tomosynthesis plus mammography versus mammography alone. Radiology. 2022;303(2):256–66.
11) Houssami N, Zackrisson S, Blazek K, et al. Meta-analysis of prospective studies evaluating breast cancer detection and interval cancer rates for digital breast tomosynthesis versus mammography population screening. Eur J Cancer. 2021;148:14–23.
12) Conant EF, Barlow WE, Herschorn SD, et al; Population-based Research Optimizing Screening Through Personalized Regimen (PROSPR) Consortium. Association of digital breast tomosynthesis vs digital mammography with cancer detection and recall rates by age and breast density. JAMA Oncol. 2019;5(5):635–42.
13) Gilbert FJ, Tucker L, Gillan MG, et al. Accuracy of digital breast tomosynthesis for depicting breast cancer subgroups in a UK retrospective reading study (TOMMY trial). Radiology. 2015;277(3):697–706.
14) Gilbert FJ, Tucker L, Gillan MG, et al. The TOMMY trial: A comparison of TOMosynthesis with digital mammography in the UK NHS Breast Screening Programme—a multicentre retrospective reading study comparing the diagnostic performance of digital breast tomosynthesis and digital mammography with digital mammography alone. Health Technol Assess. 2015;19(4):i–xxv, 1–136.
15) Weigel S, Heindel W, Hense HW, et al. Breast density and breast cancer screening with digital breast tomosynthesis: A TOSYMA trial subanalysis. Radiology. 2023;306(2):e221006.
16) Skaane P, Bandos AI, Gullien R, et al. Comparison of digital mammography alone and digital mammography plus tomosynthesis in a population-based screening program. Radiology. 2013;267(1):47–56.
17) Zuley ML, Bandos AI, Ganott MA, et al. Digital breast tomosynthesis versus supplemental diagnostic mammographic views for evaluation of noncalcified breast lesions. Radiology. 2013;266(1):89–95.
18) Conant EF, Barlow WE, Herschorn SD et al. Association of digital breast tomosynthesis vs digital mammography with cancer detection and recall rates by age and breast density. JAMA Oncol. 2019;5(5):635–42.
19) Yoon JH, Strand F, Baltzer PAT, et al. Standalone AI for breast cancer detection at screening digital mammography and digital breast tomosynthesis: A systematic review and meta-analysis. Radiology. 2023;307(5):e222639.
20) Bae MS, Moon WK, Chang JM, et al. Breast cancer detected with screening US: Reasons for non-detection at mammography. Radiology. 2014;270:369–77.
21) Hooley RJ, Scoutt LM, Philpotts LE. Breast ultrasonography: State of the art. Radiology. 2013;268(3):642–59.
22) Evans A. Screening and beyond. In: Breast Ultrasound. ESR & EUSOBI, 2016:80–85. Available at: https://www.eusobi.org/breast-imaging-publications-and-guidelines/
23) Britton P, Warwick J, Wallis MG, et al. Measuring the accuracy of diagnostic imaging in symptomatic breast patients: Team and individual performance Br J Radiol. 2012;85:415–22.
24) Evans A, Trimboli RM, Athanasiou A, et al. Breast ultrasound: Recommendations for information to women and referring physicians by the European Society of Breast Imaging. Insights Imaging. 2018;9(4):449–61.
25) Berg W, Cosgrove D, Doré C, et al. Shear-wave elastography improves the specificity of breast US: The BE1 multinational study of 939 masses. Radiology. 2012;262:435–49.
26) Evans A, Whelehan P, Thomson K, et al. Differentiating benign from malignant solid breast masses: Value of shear wave elastography according to lesion stiffness combined with gray scale ultrasound according to BI-RADS classification. Br J Cancer. 2012;10;107:224–9.
27) Mendelson EB, Bhm-Velez M, Berg WA, et al. ACR BI-RADS ultrasound. In: ACRBI-RADS Atlas, Breast Imaging Reporting and Data System. American College of Radiology, 2013.
28) Gilbert FJ, Hickman SE, Baxter GC, et al. Opportunities in cancer imaging: Risk-adapted breast imaging in screening. Clin Radiol. 2021;76:763–73.
29) Berg WA, Blume JD, Cormack JB, et al. Combined screening with ultrasound and mammography vs mammography alone in women at elevated risk of breast cancer. J Am Med Assoc. 2008;299:2151–63.

30) Corsetti V, Houssami N, Ferrari A, et al. Breast screening with ultrasound in women with mammography-negative dense breasts: Evidence on incremental cancer detection and false positives, and associated cost. Eur J Cancer. 2008;44:539–44.
31) Ohuchi N, Suzuki A, Sobue T, et al. Sensitivity and specificity of mammography and adjunctive ultrasonography to screen for breast cancer in the Japan Strategic Anti-cancer Randomized Trial (J-START): A randomised controlled trial. Lancet. 2016;387:341–8.
32) Berg WA, Vourtsis A. Screening breast ultrasound using handheld or automated technique in women with dense breasts. J Breast Imaging. 2019;1:283–96.
33) Allajbeu I, Hickman SE, Payne N, et al. Automated breast ultrasound: Technical aspects, impact on breast screening, and future perspectives. Curr Breast Cancer Rep. 2021;13:141–50.
34) Knopp MV, Weiss E, Sinn HP, et al. Pathophysiologic basis of contrast enhancement in breast tumors. J Magn Reson Imaging. 1999;10(3):260–6.
35) Carmeliet P, Jain RK. Angiogenesis in cancer and other diseases. Nature. 2000;407(6801):249–57.
36) Marino MA, Helbich T, Baltzer P, et al. Multiparametric MRI of the breast: A review. J Magn Reson Imaging. 2018;47(2):301–15.
37) Kaiser WA, Zeitler E. MR imaging of the breast: Fast imaging sequences with and without Gd-DTPA. Preliminary observations. Radiology. 1989;170(3 Pt 1):681–6.
38) Rahbar H, Partridge SC. Multiparametric MR imaging of breast cancer. Magn Reson Imaging Clin N Am. 2016;24(1):223–38.
39) Menezes GL, Knuttel FM, Stehouwer BL, et al. Magnetic resonance imaging in breast cancer: A literature review and future perspectives. World J Clin Oncol. 2014;5(2):61–70.
40) Mann RM, Kuhl CK, Kinkel K, et al. Breast MRI: Guidelines from the European Society of Breast Imaging. Eur Radiol. 2008;18(7):1307–18.
41) Sardanelli F, Boetes C, Borisch B, et al. Magnetic resonance imaging of the breast: Recommendations from the EUSOMA working group. Eur J Cancer. 2010;46(8):1296–316.
42) Bluemke DA, Gatsonis CA, Chen MH, et al. Magnetic resonance imaging of the breast prior to biopsy. JAMA. 2004;292(22):2735–42.
43) Heywang-Köbrunner SH, Bick U, Bradley WG Jr, et al. International investigation of breast MRI: Results of a multicentre study (11 sites) concerning diagnostic parameters for contrast-enhanced MRI based on 519 histopathologically correlated lesions. Eur Radiol. 2001;11(4):531–46.
44) Houssami N, Abraham LA, Kerlikowske K, et al. Risk factors for second screen-detected or interval breast cancers in women with a personal history of breast cancer participating in mammography screening. Cancer Epidemiol Biomarkers Prev. 2013;22(5):946–61.
45) National Institute for Health and Care Excellence. Early and locally advanced breast cancer: Diagnosis and management. NICE guideline [NG101], 2018. Available at: https://www.nice.org.uk/guidance/ng101.
46) Federatie Medische Specialisten. Borstkanker—MRI bij PA-bevestigde borstkanker, 2018. Available at: https://richtlijnendatabase.nl/richtlijn/borstkanker/diagnostiek/preoperatieve_stadiering/mr.html.
47) Lee JM, Abraham L, Lam DL, et al. Cumulative risk distribution for interval invasive second breast cancers after negative surveillance mammography. J Clin Oncol. 2018;36(20):2070–77.
48) Parvaiz MA, Yang P, Razia E, et al. Breast MRI in invasive lobular carcinoma: A useful investigation in surgical planning? Breast J. 2016;22(2):143–50.
49) Selvi V, Nori J, Meattini I, et al. Role of magnetic resonance imaging in the preoperative staging and work-up of patients affected by invasive lobular carcinoma or invasive ductolobular carcinoma. Biomed Res Int. 2018;2018:1569060.
50) Mann RM, Veltman J, Barentsz JO, et al. The value of MRI compared to mammography in the assessment of tumour extent in invasive lobular carcinoma of the breast. Eur J Surg Oncol. 2008;34(2):135–42.
51) Yoo EY, Nam SY, Choi HY, et al. Agreement between MRI and pathologic analyses for determination of tumor size and correlation with immunohistochemical factors of invasive breast carcinoma. Acta Radiol. 2018;59(1):50–57.
52) Haraldsdóttir KH, Jónsson Þ, Halldórsdóttir AB, et al. Tumor size of invasive breast cancer on magnetic resonance imaging and conventional imaging (mammogram/ultrasound): Comparison with pathological size and clinical implications. Scand J Surg. 2017;106(1):68–73.
53) Rominger M, Berg D, Frauenfelder T, et al. Which factors influence MRI-pathology concordance of tumour size measurements in breast cancer? Eur Radiol. 2016;26(5):1457–65.
54) Houssami N, Turner RM, Morrow M. Meta-analysis of preoperative magnetic resonance imaging (MRI) and surgical treatment for breast cancer. Breast Cancer Res Treat. 2017; 165(2):273–83.
55) Orel SG, Mendonca MH, Reynolds C, et al. MR imaging of ductal carcinoma in situ. Radiology. 1997;202(2):413–20.
56) Knuttel FM, Menezes GL, van Diest PJ, et al. Meta-analysis of the concordance of histological grade of breast cancer between core needle biopsy and surgical excision specimen. Br J Surg. 2016;103(6):644–55.
57) Lee HJ, Park JH, Nguyen AT, et al. Prediction of the histologic upgrade of ductal carcinoma *in situ* using a combined radiomics and machine learning approach based on breast dynamic contrast-enhanced magnetic resonance imaging. Front Oncol. 2022;12:1032809.
58) Kuhl CK, Schrading S, Bieling HB, et al. MRI for diagnosis of pure ductal carcinoma in situ: A prospective observational study. Lancet. 2007;370(9586):485–92.
59) Kuhl CK, Strobel K, Bieling H, et al. Impact of preoperative breast MR imaging and MR-guided surgery on diagnosis and surgical outcome of women with invasive breast cancer with and without DCIS component. Radiology. 2017;284(3): 645–55.
60) Lee CW, Wu HK, Lai HW, et al. Preoperative clinicopathologic factors and breast magnetic resonance imaging features can predict ductal carcinoma in situ with invasive components. Eur J Radiol. 2016;85(4):780–9.
61) Plana MN, Carreira C, Muriel A, et al. Magnetic resonance imaging in the preoperative assessment of patients with primary breast cancer: Systematic review of diagnostic accuracy and meta-analysis. Eur Radiol. 2012;22(1):26–38.
62) Spick C, Baltzer PA. Diagnostic utility of second-look US for breast lesions identified at MR imaging: Systematic review and meta-analysis. Radiology. 2014;273(2):401–9.
63) Turnbull L, Brown S, Harvey I, et al. Comparative effectiveness of MRI in breast cancer (COMICE) trial: A randomised controlled trial. Lancet. 2010;375(9714):563–71.
64) Gonzalez V, Sandelin K, Karlsson A, et al. Preoperative MRI of the breast (POMB) influences primary treatment in breast cancer: A prospective, randomized, multicenter study. World J Surg. 2014;38(7):1685–93.
65) Lobbes MB, Vriens IJ, van Bommel AC, et al. Breast MRI increases the number of mastectomies for ductal cancers, but decreases them for lobular cancers. Breast Cancer Res Treat. 2017;162(2):353–64.
66) Sinclair K, Sakellariou S, Dawson N, et al. Does preoperative breast MRI significantly impact on initial surgical procedure and re-operation rates in patients with screen-detected invasive lobular carcinoma? Clin Radiol. 2016;71(6):543–50.
67) Mann RM, Loo CE, Wobbes T, et al. The impact of preoperative breast MRI on the re-excision rate in invasive lobular carcinoma of the breast. Breast Cancer Res Treat. 2010;119(2):415–22.
68) Lehman CD, Gatsonis C, Kuhl CK, et al. MRI evaluation of the contralateral breast in women with recently diagnosed breast cancer. N Engl J Med. 2007;356(13):1295–303.
69) Saslow D, Boetes C, Burke W, et al. American Cancer Society guidelines for breast screening with MRI as an adjunct to mammography. CA Cancer J Clin. 2007;57(2):75–89.
70) Monticciolo DL, Newell MS, Moy L, et al. Breast cancer screening in women at higher-than-average risk: Recommendations from the ACR. J Am Coll Radiol. 2018;15(3 Pt A):408–14.
71) Kriege M, Brekelmans CT, Boetes C, et al; Magnetic Resonance Imaging Screening Study Group. Efficacy of MRI and mammography for breast-cancer screening in women with a familial or genetic predisposition. N Engl J Med. 2004;351(5):427–37.

72) Gweon HM, Cho N, Han W, et al. Breast MR imaging screening in women with a history of breast conservation therapy. Radiology. 2014;272(2):366–73.
73) Lehman CD, Lee JM, DeMartini WB, et al. Screening MRI in women with a personal history of breast cancer. J Natl Cancer Inst. 2016;108(3):djv349.
74) Marinovich ML, Houssami N, Macaskill P, et al. Meta-analysis of magnetic resonance imaging in detecting residual breast cancer after neoadjuvant therapy. J Natl Cancer Inst. 2013;105(5):321–33.
75) Scheel JR, Kim E, Partridge SC, et al. MRI, clinical examination, and mammography for preoperative assessment of residual disease and pathologic complete response after neoadjuvant chemotherapy for breast cancer: ACRIN 6657 trial. Am J Roentgenol. 2018;210(6):1376–85.
76) Reig B, Kim E, Chhor CM, et al. Problem-solving breast MRI. Radiographics. 2023;43(10):e230026.
77) Bennani-Baiti B, Bennani-Baiti N, Baltzer PA. Diagnostic performance of breast magnetic resonance imaging in non-calcified equivocal breast findings: Results from a systematic review and meta-analysis. PLoS One. 2016;11(8):e0160346.
78) Schnall M, Orel S. Breast MR imaging in the diagnostic setting. Magn Reson Imaging Clin N Am. 2006;14(3):329–37, vi.
79) James J, Tennant S. Contrast-enhanced spectral mammography (CESM). Clin Radiol 2018;73(8):715–23.
80) Jochelson MS, Lobbes MBI. Contrast-enhanced mammography: State of the art. Radiology. 2021;299(1):36–48.
81) Ghaderi KF, Phillips J, Perry H, et al. Contrast-enhanced mammography: Current applications and future directions. Radiographics. 2019;39(7):1907–20.
82) Cozzi A, Magni V, Zanardo M, et al. Contrast-enhanced mammography: A systematic review and meta-analysis of diagnostic performance. Radiology. 2022;302(3):568–81.
83) Jochelson MS, Pinker K, Dershaw DD, et al. Comparison of screening CEDM and MRI for women at increased risk for breast cancer: A pilot study. Eur J Radiol. 2017;97:37–43.
84) Sorin V, Yagil Y, Yosepovich A, et al. Contrast-enhanced spectral mammography in women with intermediate breast cancer risk and dense breasts. Am J Roentgenol. 2018;211(5):W267–74.
85) ClinicalTrials.gov. Breast screening—Risk adaptive imaging for density (BRAID), 2019 [cited 2020 Jun 15]. Available at: https://clinicaltrials.gov/ct2/show/NCT04097366
86) Tennant SL, James JJ, Cornford EJ, et al. Contrast-enhanced spectral mammography improves diagnostic accuracy in the symptomatic setting. Clin Radiol. 2016;71(11):1148–55.
87) Lu Z, Hao C, Pan Y, et al. Contrast-enhanced spectral mammography versus ultrasonography: Diagnostic performance in symptomatic patients with dense breasts. Korean J Radiol. 2020;21(4):442–49.
88) Fallenberg EM, Dromain C, Diekmann F, et al. Contrast-enhanced spectral mammography versus MRI: Initial results in the detection of breast cancer and assessment of tumour size. Eur Radiol. 2014;24:256–64.
89) Taylor DB, Burrows S, Saunders CM, et al. Contrast-enhanced mammography (CEM) versus MRI for breast cancer staging: Detection of additional malignant lesions not seen on conventional imaging. Eur Radiol Exp. 2023;7(1):8.
90) Jochelson MS, Dershaw DD, Sung JS, et al. Bilateral contrast-enhanced dual-energy digital mammography: Feasibility and comparison with conventional digital mammography and MR imaging in women with known breast carcinoma. Radiology. 2013;266(3):743–51.
91) Lee-Felker SA, Tekchandani L, Thomas M, et al. Newly diagnosed breast cancer: Comparison of contrast-enhanced spectral mammography and breast MR imaging in the evaluation of extent of disease. Radiology. 2017;285(2):389–400.
92) Kaiyin M, Lingling T, Leilei T, et al. Head-to-head comparison of contrast-enhanced mammography and contrast-enhanced MRI for assessing pathological complete response to neoadjuvant therapy in patients with breast cancer: A meta-analysis. Breast Cancer Res Treat. 2023;1–9.
93) Hogan MP, Horvat JV, Ross DS, et al. Contrast-enhanced mammography in the assessment of residual disease after neoadjuvant treatment. Breast Cancer Res Treat. 2023;198(2):349–59.
94) Chand N, Cutress RI, Oeppen RS, et al. Staging investigations in breast cancer: Collective opinion of UK breast surgeons. Int J Breast Cancer. 2013;2013:506172.
95) Tennant S, Evans A, Macmillan D, et al. CT staging of locoregional breast cancer recurrence. A worthwhile practice? Clin Radiol. 2009;64(9):885–90.
96) James JJ, McMahon MA, Tennant SL, et al. CT staging for breast cancer patients with poor prognostic tumours. Breast. 2012;21(6):735–8.
97) Groves AM, Beadsmoore CJ, Cheow HK, et al. Can 16-detector multislice CT exclude skeletal lesions during tumour staging? Implications for the cancer patient. Eur Radiol. 2006;16(5):1066–73.
98) Schneider C, Fehr MK, Steiner RA, et al. Frequency and distribution pattern of distant metastases in breast cancer patients at the time of primary presentation. Arch Gynecol Obstet. 2003;269(1):9–12.
99) Roszkowski N, Lam SS, Copson E, et al. Expanded criteria for pretreatment staging CT in breast cancer. BJS Open. 2021;5(2):zraa006.
100) Pesapane F, Downey K, Rotili A, et al. Imaging diagnosis of metastatic breast cancer. Insights Imaging. 2020;11(1):79.
101) Murata T, Yoshida M, Shiino S, et al. A prediction model for distant metastasis after isolated locoregional recurrence of breast cancer. Breast Cancer Res Treat. 2023;199(1):57–66.
102) Poodt IGM, Schipper RJ, de Greef BTA, et al; Sentinel Node and Recurrent Breast Cancer (SNARB) Research Group. Screening for distant metastases in patients with ipsilateral breast tumor recurrence: The impact of different imaging modalities on distant recurrence-free interval. Breast Cancer Res Treat. 2019;175(2):419–28.
103) Kosmin M, Padhani AR, Gogbashian A, et al. Comparison of whole-body MRI, CT, and bone scintigraphy for response evaluation of cancer therapeutics in metastatic breast cancer to bone. Radiology. 2020;297(3):622–29.
104) van Uden DJP, Prins MW, Siesling S, de Wilt JHW, Blanken-Peeters CFJM, Aarntzen EHJG. [18F]FDG PET/CT in the staging of inflammatory breast cancer: A systematic review. Crit Rev Oncol Hematol. 2020;151:102943. doi: 10.1016/j.critrevonc.2020.102943. Epub 2020 May 7. PMID: 32416347.
105) Romeo V, Helbich TH, Pinker K. Breast PET/MRI hybrid imaging and targeted tracers. J Magn Reson Imaging. 2023;57(2):370–86.

4

Principles of Breast Cancer Screening

Jonathan J. James and Nisha Sharma

4.1 Introduction

Breast cancer is the commonest malignancy in the UK with around 55,000 women diagnosed per year. Population screening aims to reduce mortality by detecting the disease at an earlier stage, leading to improvements in patient survival. A series of randomised control trials beginning in the mid-1960s suggested that regular screening using mammography could lead to a reduction in breast cancer mortality. In 1986, the UK National Health Service (NHS) commissioned a review of the available evidence under the leadership of Professor Sir Patrick Forrest. The Forrest Report led the UK to set up the world's first population-based breast screening programme, with mammographic screening provided free at the point of delivery for the eligible population beginning in 1988.

Although the incidence of breast cancer has been rising, mortality rates have been falling since the early 1990s. Screening alone cannot explain all the reduction in breast cancer mortality, with improvements in the range of available treatments and the delivery of breast services making substantial contributions too. Over the last 30 years, breast cancer screening has evolved and become common place across the developed world, but there remains an ongoing debate over the mortality benefit, potential harms, and cost-effectiveness of these programmes.

4.2 The Evidence for Population Screening

Randomised controlled trials (RCTs) provide the most reliable evidence for the effectiveness of breast cancer screening by comparing the breast cancer mortality in women who were screened to a control group who are not invited. The most cited trials are the New York Health Insurance plan (HIP), Malmo I and II, Swedish Two Counties, Canada I and II, Stockholm, Goteborg (Gothenburg), Edinburgh, and the UK Age Trial. All these RCTs took place over 30 years ago, with most dating from the 1970s and '80s, with the earliest (HIP) starting in 1963. Clearly there has been considerable change in mammographic techniques and treatment of breast cancer over that time. Consequently, the precise mortality reduction attributable to screening is controversial, particularly as there was contamination of the control groups over time with some trials offering screening to the unscreened population between 4 and 10 years after randomisation. However, meta-analysis has consistently shown a 20% reduction in mortality in women invited for screening [1, 2].

There is definitive evidence from the RCTs for a mortality reduction in women aged between 50 and 70 years, and hence, this is the group offered screening in most European population-based programmes. Only the Swedish Two Counties Trial recruited women over the age of 70 years and the numbers of women screened in this age group are low. Consequently, the RCTs provide little evidence for the routine screening of women over the age of 70 years. Nonetheless, screening women over 70 years of age would seem an attractive option with increasing breast cancer incidence in an ageing population and the improved sensitivity and specificity of screening mammography. However, in older women, the chance of finding and treating a breast cancer that would not have become apparent in the women's lifetime or led to a reduction in life expectancy is greater. This is termed overdiagnosis and is a major harm of screening.

Eight of the RCTs invited women aged between 40 and 49 years for screening. Meta-analysis of these studies has shown a mortality reduction of 15–18% for women who were between the age of 40–49 years at the time of randomisation [3]. Screening younger women presents additional problems. Firstly, breast cancer is only half as common in women in their '40s compared to those in their '50s, and the potential gain from screening is lower. However, breast cancer remains an important cause of death in younger women and therefore more life years can be gained by reducing

DOI: 10.1201/9781003394785-4

breast cancer mortality in this age group. Secondly, breast tissue is denser in younger women, and so the sensitivity of screening mammogram is lower. Thirdly, tumours in younger women progress more rapidly, and hence, for screening to be effective, the interval between screening mammograms may need to be reduced. This interval is determined by the lead time; defined as the time between mammographic detection by screening and symptomatic presentation. In the Swedish Two Counties trial, the lead time for women 40–49 years of age was 1.7 years compared to a lead time of 2.6–3.8 years for women aged 50 to 74 years [4]. For screening to be effective, the screening interval should be less than the lead time. In the 40–49 age group, the dual effect of a lower breast cancer incidence and the need for annual screening has raised concerns about cost-effectiveness.

4.3 The Benefits and Harms of Breast Cancer Screening

The benefit of breast cancer screening arises from finding small, high-grade invasive breast cancers that are lymph node negative. In contrast, some low-grade cancers, particularly tubular carcinomas are so slow growing that finding these cancers by screening is unlikely to save lives. Around 20% of cancers detected by screening in the UK are non-invasive (namely, ductal carcinoma in situ [DCIS]), typically manifesting on mammography as areas of microcalcification (Figure 4.1). The rise in incidence of DCIS mirrors the introduction of mammographic screening. Only around 40% of women with a diagnosis of DCIS will go on to develop invasive disease if left untreated [5]. The detection of high-grade DCIS is likely to be worthwhile as it is known to be a precursor of high-grade invasive disease. In the UK screening programme, it has been shown that for every three screen-detected cases of DCIS, there was one fewer invasive interval cancer in the next 3 years [6]. The merit of detecting low-grade DCIS is more controversial with only 16% progressing to invasive over 10 years compared to a 60% 10-year progression rate for high-grade DCIS [7]. Even when low-grade DCIS does progress, the carcinoma is often of low histological grade. Consequently, the finding of some cancers is likely to lead to overdiagnosis, defined as either invasive or non-invasive disease which would not have become apparent clinically in a women's lifetime unless detected by screening. The effectiveness of screening relates to the balance between mortality reduction and the level of overdiagnosis.

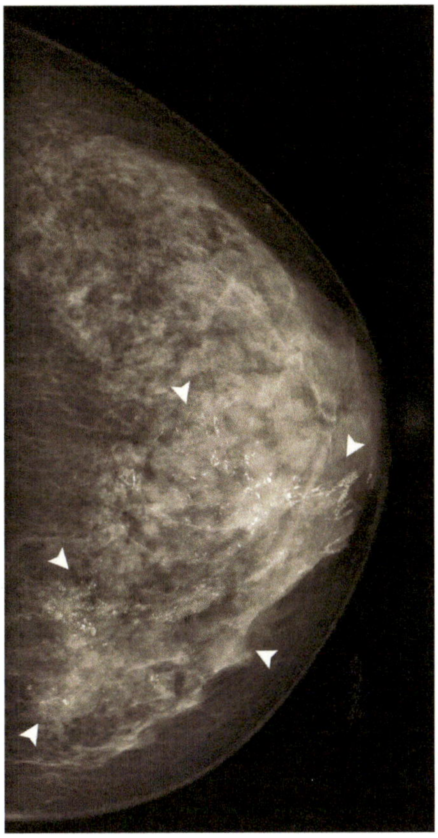

FIGURE 4.1
Ductal carcinoma in situ (DCIS). This cranio-caudal (CC) mammogram demonstrates an extensive area of pleomorphic microcalcifications in the medial aspect of the left breast (arrowheads). Biopsy demonstrated extensive high-grade DCIS and the patient underwent mastectomy.

The debate around the benefits and harms of screening has become increasingly polarised, and as a consequence, the UK government set up an independent panel under the chairmanship of Sir Michael Marmot to review the literature, seek expert testimony, and provide an objective and independent assessment of the benefits and harms of screening [1, 2]. Known as the Marmot Report (2012), it concluded that breast screening in the UK did confer significant benefit and should continue, with women invited to participate over a 20-year period benefitting from a 20% mortality reduction. On the negative side, 11% of the cancers diagnosed in the lifetime of the population of women invited for screening constituted overdiagnosis. For an individual woman who participated in the screening programme and had a cancer diagnosed, the probability of overdiagnosis is 19%. What this means for the UK screening programme is for every 10,000 women screened over a 20-year period between the ages of 50 and 70 years, 681 cancers will be detected of which 129 will represent overdiagnosis, with 43 deaths from breast cancer prevented [1, 2].

The harm to patients from overdiagnosis relates to over-treatment. Once diagnosed, cancers must be treated and this exposes women to the emotional and physical side effects of surgery, radiotherapy, and long-term hormone treatments. In recent years there has been considerable interest in identifying those lesions that require treatment and which ones can be left alone, be actively monitored, or undergo minimally invasive therapies. A good example of this is providing surveillance rather than surgery to women diagnosed with lower-grade DCIS. Several trials are being undertaken worldwide. In the UK, the Low-Risk DCIS trial (LORIS) randomised women with a diagnosis of low- and intermediate-grade DCIS to either active monitoring or surgery [8]. With a primary end point of ipsilateral invasive breast cancer free survival, the trial aims to establish whether women can safely avoid surgery and without any detrimental effect to their physical and psychological well-being.

Many small, biologically favourable cancers diagnosed through screening have an excellent prognosis and are at risk of overdiagnosis and over-treatment. Vacuum-assisted biopsy (VAB) techniques are frequently used to sample breast lesions under ultrasound, X-ray, or MRI guidance. A large-bore needle is used enabling larger volumes of breast tissue to be removed for pathological assessment, reducing sampling errors and the under-staging of disease within the breast. The same devices used for VAB are now frequently used to excise breast lesions of uncertain malignant potential (B3 lesions) as an alternative to diagnostic surgical excision—an approach known as vacuum-assisted excision (VAE). VAE could potentially be used to excise small breast cancers. In the UK, the SMALL trial is underway and is a randomised trial of VAE versus surgery for the treatment of small, biologically favourable screen detected breast cancers [9]. A biologically favourable breast cancer would be a grade 1 tumour measuring less than 15 mm in size that is strongly hormone receptor positive, HER2 negative and without evidence of lymph node involvement on pre-operative axillary ultrasound.

4.4 The Screening Process and Assessment

In the UK, women between the ages of 50 and 70 years are invited to attend for a screening mammogram every three years. Recent performance metrics for the programme are shown in Table 4.1. Women over the age of 70 years can self-refer for screening every three years but do not receive a routine invite. Screening is with two view (medio-lateral oblique and cranio-caudal projections), full field digital mammography performed of each breast (Figure 4.2). Mammograms are performed by female radiographers in one of the 80 static screening centres in England or on a mobile van designed to take screening to remote locations and improve uptake (Figure 4.3). Double reading of screening mammograms is standard practice in the UK and most European countries and is acknowledged to improve cancer detection rates by 6–15% as well as keep recall rates low [10–12]. Discrepancies between reader opinions are dealt either through arbitration by an independent third reader or consensus depending on local screening centre protocols.

TABLE 4.1

UK National Health Service Breast Screening Programme: Performance in England 2018–2020

	2018/2019	2019/2020
Number of women invited	2,943,251	2,909,626
Acceptance rate (% of invited)	70.8%	69.1%
Total number of women screened (invited and self-referrals)	2,234,523	2,123,603
Number of women recalled for assessment	84,559	76,440
Women recalled for assessment (%)	3.8%	3.6%
Number of cancers detected	19,558	17,771
Cancer detected per 1000 women screened	8.8	8.4
Number of in situ cancers detected	4,128	3,742
Number of invasive cancers less than 15 mm	7,888	7,092

Source: NHS BSP Annual Review 2018/2019, NHS BSP Annual Review 2019/2020, NHS BSP Publications, Sheffield, UK, under Open Government Licence.

The traditional role of the radiographer in breast cancer screening is to produce consistently high-quality mammograms to maximise breast tissue coverage and so optimise cancer detection. Over the last 20 years, a reorganisation of the radiographer workforce has been undertaken to address increasing demands of the UK breast screening programme to screen more women and tackle radiology workforce shortages. This has led to innovative ways of working and the development of advanced radiographer practitioners and consultant radiographers. These physician extender roles undertake some of the work traditionally done by a radiologist and might include reading screening mammograms, breast ultrasound, image-guided biopsy, and clinical assessment. In the UK, advanced practice training can only be undertaken by fully registered, graduate radiographers who already have experience performing the traditional role of the breast radiographer. Training is overseen by a university and undertaken as an accredited module

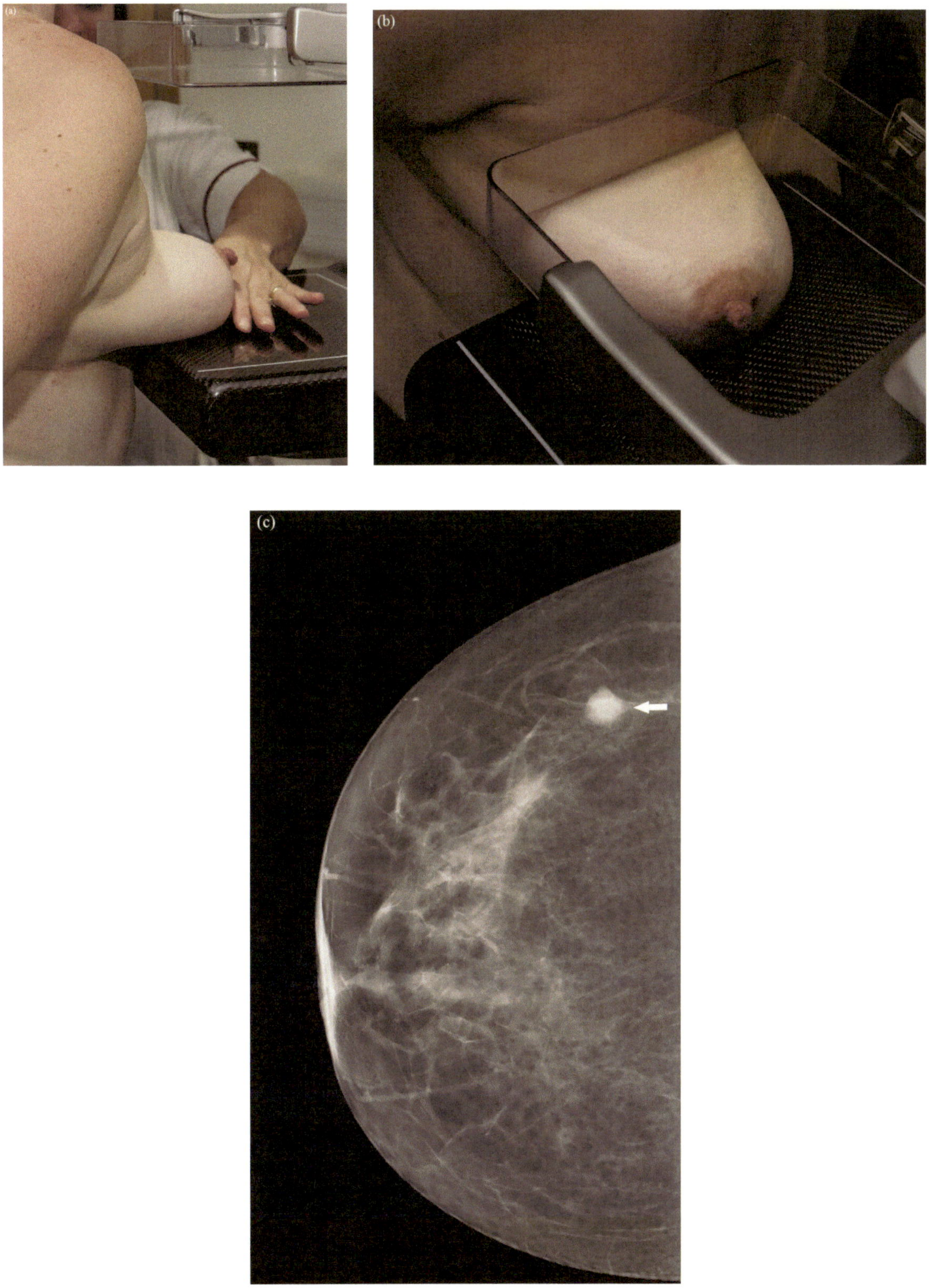

FIGURE 4.2
Screening mammography. Positioning for the cranio-caudal (CC) view is achieved by pulling the breast up and forward from the chest wall, with compression applied from above (a). A well-positioned CC view should have the nipple in profile and demonstrate all the breast tissue medially and most of the lateral aspect of the breast except for the axillary tail (b). (c) is the resulting right CC mammogram demonstrating a dense, well-defined mass (arrow) in the lateral aspect of the breast that was a grade 3 ductal carcinoma on biopsy.

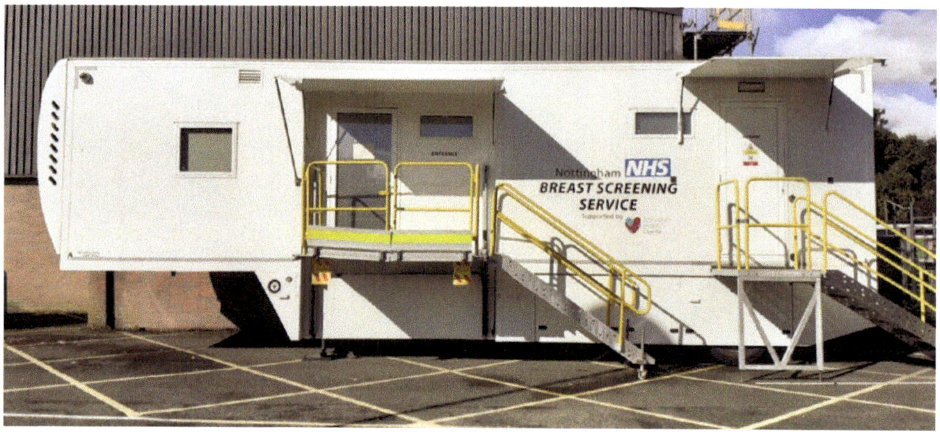

FIGURE 4.3
Mobile screening van. Many women in the UK have their screening mammograms performed on mobile vans.

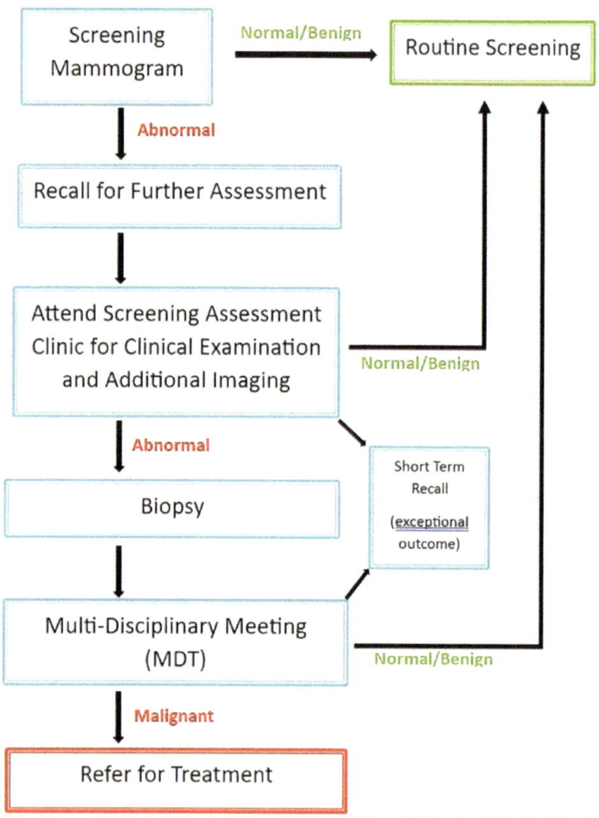

FIGURE 4.4
The screening assessment process.

at Masters level lasting a minimum of 12 months. In England, 78% breast screening units employ at least one advanced radiographer practitioner, with the average employing between three and four [13]. All readers have their performance monitored and there is no difference in cancer detection rates or recall rates between radiologists and radiographer readers [14].

The UK breast screening programme requires all readers to interpret a minimum of 5000 mammograms per year. There is evidence to suggest that higher-volume readers have an increased sensitivity for detecting breast cancer than lower-volume readers [15]. Years of reading experience is also an important performance indicator, with more experienced readers having lower recall rates and consequently an increased positive predictive value for recall cases. For the same number of years of reading experience there is no difference between the performance of radiologists and non-radiologist readers in the UK screening programme [14].

Many European countries have a broadly similar approach to mammographic screening, inviting a similar age group as the UK with double reading also the standard of care. Most European programmes operate a two-year screening interval for women over the age of 50, which is based on the lead-time calculations from randomised control trials. In this respect, the UK is something of an outlier with a three-year screening interval. Reducing this interval in the UK may be beneficial as higher interval cancer rates are observed in the third year after screening.

In the UK, around 4% of women will be recalled for further investigation after a screening mammogram, these typically include extra mammography images such as spot compression views or digital breast tomosynthesis, ultrasound, and clinical examination. The screening assessment process is shown in Figure 4.4. The purpose of screening assessment is to distinguish real lesions from superimposition of normal breast tissue, characterise a lesion, and facilitate image-guided biopsy where necessary under ultrasound or X-ray guidance (Figure 4.5). Percutaneous biopsy is typically performed with a 14-gauge core-needle under ultrasound guidance for mass lesions or larger bore vacuum-assisted biopsy (VAB) under X-ray guidance for microcalcifications. In the UK, 1 out of every 4 women recalled to a screening assessment clinic will

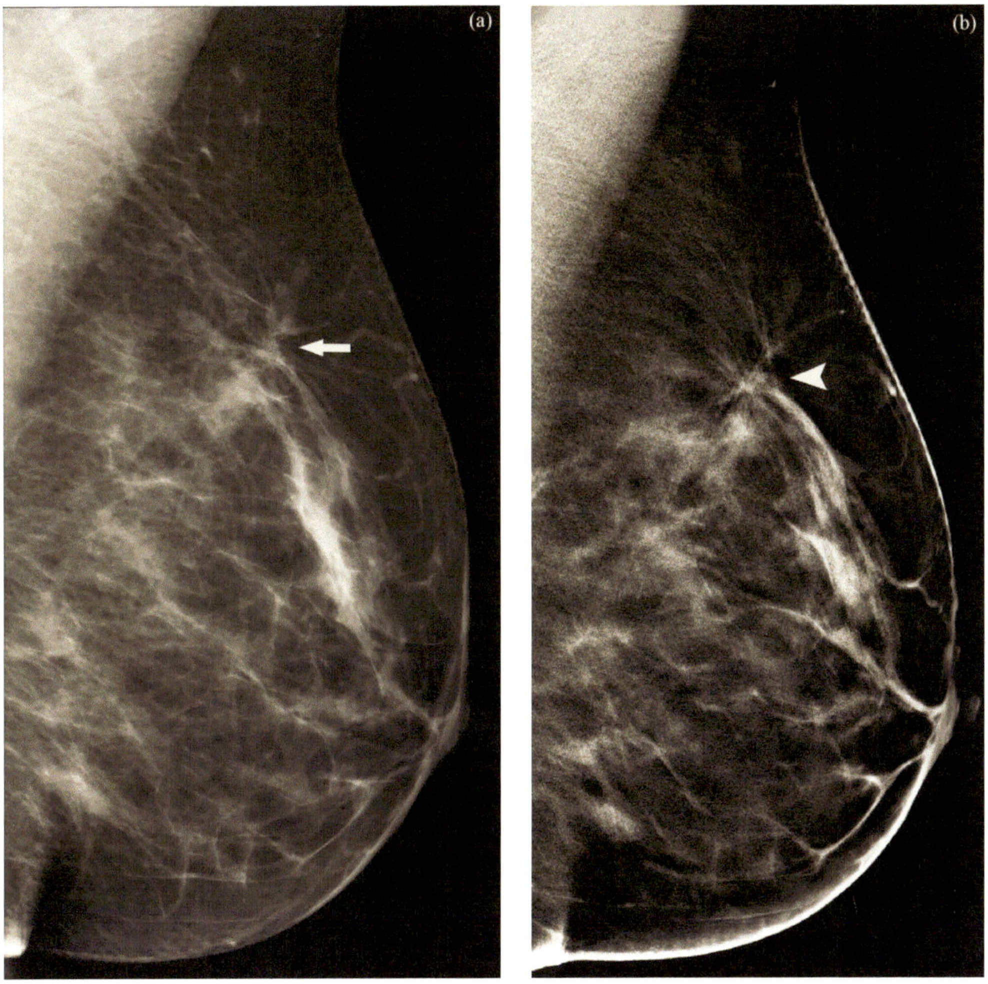

FIGURE 4.5
Screening assessment. (a) shows a left medio-lateral oblique screening mammogram from a 55-year-old who attended screening. Following double reading, a possible abnormality (arrow) was identified and so the woman was recalled for further assessment. (b) is a single slice from the digital breast tomosynthesis examination performed at the screening assessment clinic confirming the presence of a spiculate mass (arrowhead), which was a histological grade 2 ductal carcinoma on ultrasound-guided core biopsy.

have a cancer diagnosis and will be referred for treatment. Also, 3 out of 4 will not have cancer and will receive a routine invite for the next screening round three years later. There is a short-term recall option for women when the assessment process has failed to make a definitive diagnosis with women offered a one-year follow-up appointment. Short-term recall is only used in exceptional circumstances as it is associated with significant patient anxiety and is the outcome for less than 1 in 1000 women.

4.5 Alternative Screening Modalities

Since the programme began, mammography has been the modality of choice for breast cancer screening. It is relatively cheap, quick to perform and interpret, acceptable to women and sensitive for invasive and in situ disease. Over the years mammography has undergone something of a revolution. Initially the mammographic image was recorded on film, but at the beginning of the 21st century, digital technology became available. Screening programmes worldwide quickly began to benefit from the more efficient image acquisition, storage and display that digital could offer. As well as these logistical advantages, the Digital Mammographic Imaging Screening Trial (DMIST) demonstrated that the digital image offered improved diagnostic accuracy over film-based mammography for some groups, such as women under the age of 50 years, those with dense breast tissue, and pre- or peri-menopausal women [16].

Despite digital leading to improvements in image quality, mammography still has some limitations as a screening tool. It has low sensitivity for women with dense breasts due to tumour masking and reduced specificity when breast lesions are simulated by the summation of normal glandular breast tissue. The development of digital technology has enabled the development of digital breast tomosynthesis (DBT). This advanced mammographic technique generates pseudo-3D imaging by constructing thin slices through the breast from multiple low-dose digital projections, potentially increasing the sensitivity and specificity of screening mammography. Studies have demonstrated the potential of DBT to improve cancer detection rates and lower recall rates particularly in high recall environments [17]. Consequently, breast cancer screening with DBT has been widely adopted in North America with 84% of screening centres having DBT systems. Nonetheless, there is little evidence to date that increases in cancer detection associated with DBT translates into reduction in the interval cancer rate, which is an important measure of the effectiveness of any screening modality. The conspicuity of spiculate lesions and architectural distortions is particularly good with DBT (Figure 4.5). These radiological features are often associated with low-grade, good prognostic tumours. There is concern that additional breast cancers detected with DBT may represent overdiagnosis, and for this reason, adoption of DBT as a routine screening modality in European population-based screening programmes is more limited. Research into the cost-effectiveness of DBT as a screening tool is ongoing including the Tomosynthesis Mammographic Imaging Screening Trial (TMIST) in North America and the PROSPECTS study in the UK.

It was hoped that DBT screening might be most effective in women with denser breasts who are not currently well served by conventional 2D mammography. DBT screening does offer improvements in sensitivity and specificity across a range of breast densities, except for the 10% of women with an exceptionally dense background parenchymal pattern for whom there is little evidence of improved cancer detection rates [18]. DBT typically requires a small amount of fat around the lesion for cancers to be visualised. The use of a contrast agent is probably required to increase cancer detection in those women with an extremely dense background pattern. This permits visualisation of abnormal vasculature associated with malignancy and hence increases sensitivity. The two techniques currently available are contrast-enhanced breast MRI and contrast-enhanced mammography (CEM).

4.6 AI and Breast Screening

There is good evidence for the use of mammography as a breast cancer screening tool, but false negative and false positive interpretations can be problematic. These occur when readers either miss abnormalities or misinterpret the image leading to a reduction in both the sensitivity and specificity of screening. Over the past few years, attempts have been made to enlist computer assistance to improve readers diagnostic accuracy.

In 1998, computer-aided detection (CAD) gained regulatory approval as a method to improve the sensitivity of mammographic interpretation. CAD systems used mathematical models developed by computer software engineers to determine whether an imaging feature associated with cancer, such as a mass, distortion, asymmetry, or microcalcifications, were present on a mammogram, with marks or prompts placed on the image by the CAD system to prevent observational oversights by the reader. CAD systems were widely used by radiologists to aid interpretation of mammograms, especially in countries such as the USA, where single reading of screening mammography was the norm. By contrast, these CAD systems were neither popular nor widely used in European countries where screening programmes have relied on double reading of screening mammograms to improve cancer detection rates and ensure recall rates remain low. However, human double reading is expensive and can be difficult to achieve with increasing demand for screening and workforce shortages. In 2008, the role of CAD was investigated in the UK screening programme. The Computer-Aided Detection Evaluation Trial II (CADET II) found that a single reader using a CAD system was able to achieve the same cancer detection rate as double reading. However, this was achieved at the expense of an increase in false positive interpretations, leading to a 16% increase in recall rate [19]. Consequently, CAD was not considered a cost-effective alternative to human double reading. Furthermore, by 2015, concerns had been raised internationally that, despite $400 million dollars a year being spent on use of CAD in the USA, there was no evidence that this had led to an improvement in the diagnostic accuracy of screening mammography [20].

In recent years, old-fashioned CAD has been superseded by artificial intelligence (AI) algorithms based on machine learning technology whereby a computer works out how to identify the presence of breast cancer on a mammogram using artificial neural networks. These algorithms have shown great promise with a diagnostic accuracy for interpretation of mammograms, exceeding that of CAD and achieving or even surpassing human performance in retrospective studies [21]. Nonetheless, it remains unclear at the present time how AI will be used in breast cancer screening. Firstly, it could be used in a similar way to old-fashioned CAD as a clinical decision support tool, with marks placed on the image by the algorithm to indicate potential areas of concern. One of the problems with traditional CAD systems was the high number of false marks on the image that distract the reader. The new generation of AI systems are associated with a significant reduction in false prompts (around 70%) with no loss of sensitivity [22]. Secondly, AI could act as a triaging tool for screening mammograms. Retrospective studies have consistently demonstrated the ability of these systems to correctly identify a subset of women with normal mammograms. This has the potential to reduce workload by removing some cases from human reading altogether or allocating low-risk cases to be read by a single reader. Thirdly, AI could be used as an independent reader and replace a human reader in the double reading workflow. Each of these potential roles are currently under investigation, but evidence from prospective studies on real-life screening populations is needed before these products are ready for real-world deployment.

Apart from image interpretation, other potential roles for AI include the assessment of mammographic image quality at the time of acquisition, measuring a woman's lifetime breast cancer risk and even improving appointment scheduling. It seems likely that AI will impact many aspects of breast-screening programmes in the future.

4.7 Quality Assurance

Quality assurance (QA) is an important part of any screening programme. In the UK, performance data for each breast screening unit has been published since the programme began in 1988. Minimum standards and targets are defined and measured for all components of the programme, including administration of the scheme, reader performance, biopsy, pathological assessment, and surgical management.

In recent years there has been considerable interest in development of more individualised performance assessment in all aspects of medicine. Traditionally performance metrics for the readers of screening mammograms have been produced nationally and at screening centre level, but this can mask poor individual performance. Measuring performance has the potential to improve service quality by providing supportive training to readers, informing the public and spotting potential problems early. However, collecting and interpreting real-life performance data is problematic due to its retrospective nature. For instance, an accurate measure of individual reader sensitivity, defined as the proportion of patients with breast cancer reported as positive on a screening mammogram, will not be known for several years until interval cancer data becomes available. Likewise, specificity is the proportion of disease-free patients the reader reports as negative, but this will not become apparent until after the next screening round at the earliest. An individual reader will only detect a relatively small number of cancers with resultant statistical instability around small case numbers. Consequently, it may take many years for poor performance to become apparent through the clinical audit of real-life performance data. Test-set-based external quality assurance (EQA) schemes are used by some programmes to provide a more reproducible measure of reader performance. In the UK, the EQA scheme is known as PERFORMS (Personal Performance in Mammographic Screening) and has been running for over 30 years with all readers completing interpretation of a cancer enriched test-set of 60 screening mammography cases at least once a year. Individual reader performance can then be compared with their peers nationally. It is known that scores in the PERFORMS scheme correlate with real-life performance metrics, predicting and identifying poor reader performance [23].

4.8 Interval Cancers

Interval cancers are an inevitable part of any screening programme. These are cancers that arise symptomatically after a normal screening result and before the next screening round takes place. Longer screening round lengths are inevitably associated with higher the numbers of interval cancers. An excess of interval cancers is seen in women with dense parenchymal background patterns [4]. Interval cancers show no difference in histological grade and lymph nodes stage compared to symptomatic cancers in the non-screened population. Moreover, they have a similar prognosis with reported survival rates of 79.1% for women with an interval cancer and 76.8% for women in non-screened cancer groups which are worse than figures for breast cancers detected through screening [24].

National Health Service Breast Screening Programme (NHSBSP) has a three yearly screening interval and interval cancer rates are approximately

3 per 1000 women screened. For instance, in the screening programme in England, typically 2.2 million women are screened every year in England with detection of around 18,000 cancers; 6000 women will present with an interval cancer. Identifying and reviewing interval cancers is part of the QA process and is an important programme performance metric. It is also a valuable education tool for readers, increases detection of more subtle cancers, and ultimately improves the service offered to women. The UK screening programme formally classifies all interval cancers into one of three groups—*satisfactory, satisfactory with learning points*, and *unsatisfactory* [25]. Around 80% of interval cancers are in the satisfactory group and are true negatives, developing since the last screen with no detectable signs of cancer on the screening mammogram. In 13% of cases, the cancer was visible on a screening mammogram with hindsight but was not recalled because the signs of cancer were relatively subtle. This latter group is classified as satisfactory with learning points and provides the greatest educational opportunities for readers. Of the interval cancers, 7% are in the unsatisfactory classification. These are false negatives and were visible on the last screening mammograms and would have been considered detectable by most readers but were missed. This later group, represent a tiny minority of interval cases. They are now notifiable safety incidents under UK Duty of Candour Legislation, and a formal apology made to the women concerned [26].

4.9 Screening High-Risk Groups

Many countries use MRI as a supplemental screening tool for women with the highest risk of developing breast cancer. In the UK, women with a lifetime risk of more than 40% or 8 times the risk of women in the general population are defined as very high-risk and offered screening MRI. This would include those with genetic mutations (e.g. BRCA1, BRCA2, PALB2, or TP53) or women who received mantel chest irradiation at a young age to treat lymphoma. There is high quality (level 1) evidence for the effectiveness of MRI screening in these patient groups. The cancer detection rate among known BRCA1 and BRCA2 carriers is 26.2 per 1000 women screened compared to 5.4 per 1000 in those women who are high-risk but not mutation carriers [27].

In recent years, there has been considerable interest in the use of MRI in women with intermediate risk factors, particularly those with dense breast tissue. Breast density has been traditionally classified into one of four groups using the Breast Imaging Reporting Data System (BIRADS) density categories: A is used for almost entirely fatty breasts accounting for 10% of women, B for scattered areas of fibroglandular density (40% of women), C for heterogeneously dense (40% of women), and D for extremely dense breast tissue (10% of women). Women who are extremely dense (BIRADS D) have approximately double the breast cancer risk of women with entirely fatty breasts (BIRADS A). It will be mandated across all American states from September 2024 that women with heterogeneously dense or extremely dense breast tissue on screening mammography are duly informed in order that supplementary screening with other imaging modalities can be discussed. In addition to an increased breast cancer risk, women with dense breasts are more prone to a false negative mammographic interpretation as a consequence of tumours being obscured by dense glandular breast tissue. The Dutch Dense Tissue and Early Breast Neoplasm Screening (DENSE) trial showed supplemental screening with dynamic-contrast-enhanced breast MRI had a cancer detection rate of 16.5 per 1000 for women with dense breasts [28]. Interval cancer rates are an important predictor of the effectiveness of a screening modality. The DENSE trial has importantly demonstrated a fall in interval cancer rates from 5.0 per 1000 in the mammography only group to 2.5 per 1000 in the MRI invitation cohort. On the downside, MRI has the disadvantage of being associated with false positive findings. In the DENSE trial, the recall rate was 9.5% with a false positive rate of 8%. A better understanding of the effectiveness and relative benefit of supplemental screening in the context of intermediate risk groups is required. For instance, does the tumour biology of the extra cancers detected reflect faster growing lesions and justify the greater number of false positive results, the risk of overdiagnosis, and increased expenditure? To reduce costs, abbreviated MRI protocols with shorter acquisition and interpretation times are currently under investigation.

Other imaging modalities have been suggested in order to provide a more personalised approach to breast cancer screening rather than a 'one size fits all' mammography policy that is offered in many countries. Whole breast ultrasound (handheld or automated) has been suggested as a supplemental screening tool for women with dense breasts. Screening ultrasound does find additional cancers in this group of women after a negative mammogram. This rate of detection is 4.4 per 1000 examinations but is offset by the disadvantage of an increase in the number of false positives with ultrasound recall rates of up to 14% [29]. Contrast-enhanced mammography (CEM) is also a potential tool for screening women at increased risk. CEM combines iodinated contrast agents and mammography to image

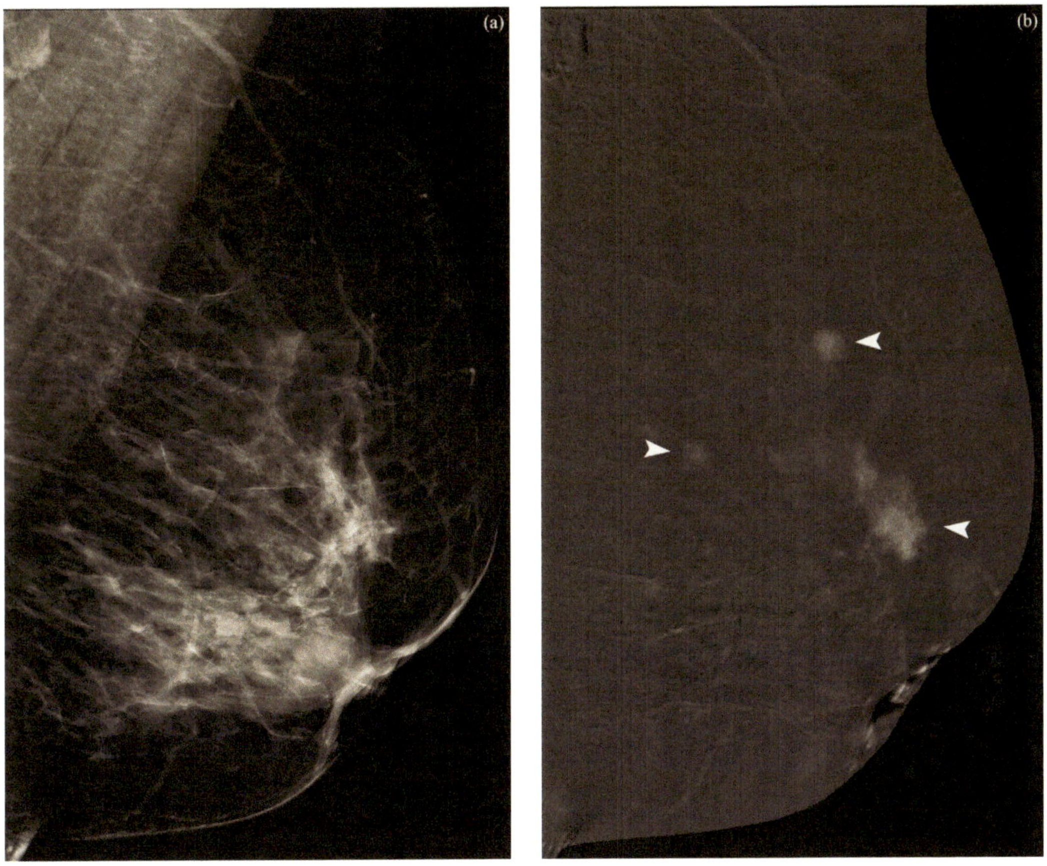

FIGURE 4.6
Contrast-enhanced mammography (CEM). CEM consists of two sets of images: a low-energy image looking like a standard mammogram (a) and a recombined image (b) showing areas of enhancement representing abnormal vasculature associated with malignancy. No abnormality is demonstrated on the low-energy image (a), but multifocal carcinoma (arrowheads) is demonstrated on the recombined image (b).

the abnormal vasculature associated with malignancy in a similar way to breast MRI (Figure 4.6). In a recent meta-analysis, the diagnostic performance of CEM and MRI for staging breast cancer were found to be equivalent with sensitivities of 96% and 97%, respectively, and both modalities having a specificity of 77% [30]. CEM is a potentially cheaper and more readily available alternative to MRI and is preferred by patients. Clinical trials, such as the Breast Screening Risk Adaptive Imaging for Density (BRAID) trial in the UK, are currently underway to assess the effectiveness of CEM as a screening tool in the populations of women who are not well served by standard screening mammography.

References

1. Independent UK Panel on Breast Cancer Screening. The benefits and harms of breast cancer screening: An independent review. Lancet. 2012;380:1778–86.
2. Marmot MG, Altman DG, Cameron DA, et al. The benefits and harms of breast cancer screening: An independent review. Br J Cancer. 2013;108:2205–40.
3. Tabar L, Fagerberg G, Chen HH, et al. Efficacy of breast cancer screening by age. New results from the Swedish Two-County Trial. Cancer. 1995;75(10):2507–17.
4. Ray KM, Joe BN, Freimanis RI, et al. Screening mammography in women 40–49 years old: Current evidence. Am J Roentgenol. 2018;210(2):264–70.
5. Cowella CF, Weigelta B, Sakr RA, et al. Progression from ductal carcinoma in situ to invasive breast cancer: Revisited. Molec Oncol. 2013;6:859–69.
6. Duffy SW, Dibden A, Michalopoulos D, et al. Screen detection of ductal carcinoma in situ and subsequent incidence of invasive interval breast cancers: A retrospective population-based study. Lancet Oncol. 2016;17:109–14.
7. Co M, Cheng KCK, Yeung YH, et al. Clinical outcomes of conservative treatment for low-risk ductal carcinoma in situ: A systematic review and pooled analysis. Clin Oncol. 2023;35:255–61.
8. Francis A, Thomas J, Fallowfield L, et al. Addressing overtreatment of screen detected DCIS; the LORIS trial. Eur J Cancer. 2015;51:2296–303.
9. Morgan J, Potter S, Sharma N, et al. The SMALL trial: A big change for small breast cancers. Clin Oncol. 2019;31:659–63.
10. Harvey SC, Geller B, Oppenheimer RG, et al. Increase in cancer detection and recall rates with independent double interpretation of screening mammography. AJR. 2003;180(5):1461–67.

11. Ciatto S, Ambrogetti D, Bonardi R, et al. Second reading of screening mammograms increases cancer detection and recall rates. Results in the Florence screening programme. J Med Screen. 2005;12(2):103–6.
12. Blanks RG, Wallis MG, Moss SM. A comparison of cancer detection rates achieved by breast cancer screening programmes by number of readers, for one and two view mammography: Results from the UK National Health Service breast screening programme. J Med Screen. 1998;5(4):195–201.
13. Royal College of Radiologists, The breast imaging and diagnostic workforce in the United Kingdom: Results of a survey of breast screening programme units and radiology departments. [internet] 2016. Available at: https://www.rcr.ac.uk/system/files/publication/field_publication_files/bfcr162_bsbr_survey.pdf.
14. Chen Y, James JJ, Michalopoulou E, et al. Performance of radiologists and radiographers in double reading mammograms: The UK National Health Service Breast Screening Program. Radiology. 2023;306:102–9.
15. Hoff SR, Myklebust T, Lee CI, et al. Influence of mammographic volume on radiologists' performance: Results from BreastScreen Norway. Radiology. 2019;292:289–96.
16. Pisano ED, Gatsonis C, Hendrick E, et al. Diagnostic performance of digital versus film mammography for breast-cancer screening. N Engl J Med. 2005;353:1773–83.
17. Marinovich ML, Hunter KE, Macaskill P, et al. Breast cancer screening using tomosynthesis or mammography: A meta-analysis of cancer detection and recall. J Nat Cancer Inst. 2018;110:942–49.
18. Østerås BH, Martinsen ACT, Gullien R, et al. Digital mammography versus breast tomosynthesis: Impact of breast density on diagnostic performance in population-based screening. Radiology. 2019;293:60–68.
19. Gilbert FJ, Astley SM, Gillan MGC, et al. Single reading with computer-aided detection for screening mammography. N Engl J Med. 2008;359:1675–84.
20. Lehman CD, Wellman RD, Buist DSM, et al. Diagnostic accuracy of digital screening mammography with and without computer-aided detection. JAMA Intern Med. 2015;175(11):1828–37.
21. Hickman SE, Woitek R, Le EPV, et al. Machine learning for workflow applications in screening mammography: Systematic review and meta-analysis. Radiology. 2022;302:88–104.
22. Mayo RC, Kent D, Sen LC, et al. Reduction of false-positive markings on mammograms: A retrospective comparison study using an artificial intelligence-based CAD. J Digit Imaging. 2019;32(4):618–24.
23. Chen Y, James JJ, Cornford EJ, et al. The relationship between mammography readers' real-life performance and performance in a test set–based assessment scheme in a National Breast Screening Program. Radiol Imaging Cancer. 2020;2(5):e200016.
24. Mette Kalager M, Tamimi RM, Bretthauer M, et al. Prognosis in women with interval breast cancer: Population based observational cohort study. BMJ. 2012;345:e7536.
25. Public Health England. Breast screening: Reporting, classification and monitoring of interval cancers and cancers following previous assessment. [Internet] updated 2011. Available at: https://www.gov.uk/government/publications/breast-screening-interval-cancers/breast-screening-reporting-classification-and-monitoring-of-interval-cancers-and-cancers-following-previous-assessment.
26. Care Quality Commission. Regulation 20: Duty of Candour. [Internet] 2022. Available at: https://www.cqc.org.uk/guidance-providers/regulations-enforcement/regulation-20-duty-candour
27. Kriege M, Brekelmans CT, Boetes C, Besnard PE, Zonderland HM, Obdeijn IM, Manoliu RA, Kok T, Peterse H, Tilanus-Linthorst MM, Muller SH. Efficacy of MRI and mammography for breast-cancer screening in women with a familial or genetic predisposition. N Engl J Med. 2004 Jul 29;351(5):427–37.
28. Bakker MF, De Lange SV, Pijnappel RM, et al. Supplemental MRI screening for women with extremely dense breast tissue. N Engl J Med. 2019;381:2091–102.
29. Melnikow J, Fenton JJ, Whitlock EP, et al. Supplemental screening for breast cancer in women with dense breasts: A systematic review for the U.S. Preventive Services Task Force. Ann Intern Med. 2016;164:268–78. doi: 10.7326/M15-1789
30. Neeter LMFH, Robbe MMQ, van Nijnatten TJA, et al. Comparing the diagnostic performance of contrast enhanced mammography and breast MRI: A systematic review and meta-analysis. J Cancer. 2023;14:174–82.

5

Lesions of Uncertain Malignant Potential

B3 Lesions

Nuala Healy and Fleur Kilburn-Toppin

5.1 Introduction

Breast needle core biopsies are classified into one of five categories, ranging from B1 (normal breast tissue) through to B5 (malignant). Whilst a definitive benign or malignant diagnosis is possible for most breast lesions, a proportion of these will fall into the borderline category of B3. These are lesions that are benign on histology but are either heterogeneous in nature (meaning the area sampled may not be representative of the whole lesion) or they have an increased risk of association with malignancy (1).

The terminology of B3 lesions has changed over time. Currently lesions classified as B3 include (i) atypical intraductal epithelial hyperplasia (AIDEP)/atypical ductal hyperplasia (ADH); (ii) non-pleomorphic/classical lobular (in situ) neoplasia (LN), which includes atypical lobular hyperplasia (ALH) and lobular carcinoma in situ (LCIS); (iii) flat epithelial atypia (FEA;) (iv) radial scar with or without epithelial atypia; (v) cellular fibroepithelial lesion where a phyllodes tumour cannot be excluded; (vi) mucocele-like lesions; and (vii) other rarer abnormalities (2). Radiologically, B3 lesions can have a wide variety of appearances including clustered microcalcification, masses or distortion (Table 5.1). Imaging features can overlap with those of benign lesions as well as malignancy, for example, the mammographic distortion seen with a radial scar (3). They can often be mammographically occult and found coincidentally in biopsies of screen detected lesions (4). On ultrasound examination, they may appear as a mass or ill-defined hypoechoic area and they can present clinically with symptoms such as a palpable mass or nipple discharge, such as in the case of papillomas (5).

In the United Kingdom (UK), it is estimated that approximately 7% of lesions are categorised as B3, with rates varying between different countries (6). The proportion of lesions classified as B3 varies between 3.3 and 12.6% in the UK alone, and this is considered due to both variation in histological classification by pathologists and to differences in recall and biopsy rates by radiologists (7). B3 lesions are often diagnosed through mammographic breast screening, with an increased frequency in recent years largely attributed to the enhanced sensitivity of digital mammography. The latter can detect small microcalcifications that are sometimes associated with B3 lesions (8). Another factor that may contribute to an increase in diagnosis of B3 lesions are changes in methods of sampling, with increasing use of vacuum-assisted biopsy (VAB). These percutaneous biopsy techniques are employed particularly for mammographically detected microcalcifications, as well as other radiological abnormalities such as areas of distortion. VAB involves use of a larger needle (12 gauge to 7 gauge) than a conventional core biopsy needle with assistance of a vacuum to retrieve specimens. As a diagnostic procedure, VAB can yield larger volumes of tissue than core biopsy, allowing the pathologists to make a definitive diagnosis with less chance of missing ductal carcinoma in situ (DCIS) or invasive cancer (9). In some cases a lesion may be entirely removed with VAB if very small, but this is not an intended aim of VAB.

One of the concerns regarding B3 lesions is their 'uncertain malignant potential', and upgrade to malignancy at the site of the lesion. The overall upgrade rate of B3 lesions to either in situ or invasive cancer overall is approximately 20–30% (5) but is highly dependent on lesion type and presence or absence of atypia (6). The upgrade rate for malignancy can vary from less than 2% for fibroepithelial lesions and up to 40% for epithelial atypia/AIDEP (10). Most upgrades are to in situ rather than invasive cancer and involve cancers that are often low-grade and hormone-receptor-positive with a consequently better prognosis. Nonetheless, upgrade to higher grades of both invasive and non-invasive malignancy does occur (11). Furthermore, the rate of progression to eventual malignancy can take place over a prolonged period of time. As well as

DOI: 10.1201/9781003394785-5

TABLE 5.1

Imaging Features of B3 Lesions, with Typical Appearances on Mammography, US, and MRI

B3 Lesion	Mammographic Appearances	US Appearances	MRI Appearances
Atypical ductal hyperplasia (ADH)	Focal mass, microcalcifications (granular, and cluster or ductal in distribution), asymmetric density.	Mass or ill-defined hypoechoic area.	Non-specific. If visible can demonstrate mass or non-mass enhancement.
Columnar cell lesions (CCC)	Mass or clustered, amorphous microcalcifications.	Often normal but can present as a hypoechoic mass.	Usually normal.
Complex Sclerosing lesion (CSL)	Spiculate mass with radiolucent centre or architectural distortion, often visible only on a single view. May have associated microcalcifications.	Up to a third are normal on US. Otherwise variable appearance ranging from hypoechoic, irregular mass, or focal area of shadowing.	May be normal or demonstrate a lesion with or without enhancement.
Lobular neoplasia (LN)	Often occult and incidentally found. Microcalcifications are often associated with adjacent benign tissues.	Hypoechoic lesion or non-specific altered echogenicity.	If identified on MRI, associated with non-mass enhancement.
Papillary lesions	Often normal, but can showed dilated ducts or retroareolar mass. Microcalcifications present in 25%.	Hypoechoic nodule, often in duct, or complex cystic lesion. Vascularity in stalk.	Well-defined enhancing mass or irregular lesion often associated with dilated ducts.

risk of upgrade to malignancy, some B3 lesions such as LCIS and ADH are associated with an increased risk of cancer developing in either breast and demand careful imaging surveillance (5, 12).

Historically, surgical diagnostic biopsy was performed for all B3 lesions to obtain adequate amounts of tissue and ensure no coexisting malignancy. However, a number of studies have demonstrated that radiologically guided vacuum-assisted excision (VAE) using a 7- or 8-gauge needle is a satisfactory method for more extensive sampling of lesions and obtaining a greater volume of tissue for histological evaluation (13). VAE has the benefit of not requiring an operation and is well tolerated by patients. It can reduce rates of histological underestimation of malignancy at surgery and permit women to avoid an additional diagnostic surgical biopsy prior to any therapeutic procedure. Furthermore, VAE may be used to entirely remove a lesion as definitive therapeutic excision, especially if this is small (less than 15 mm). Although VAE may not be suitable for all lesions, for example, when close to the nipple or too large for representative sampling, approximately 80% of women can be spared open surgical biopsy (11).

In order to be of equivalent diagnostic accuracy to a surgical excision, it is recommended that approximately 4 g of tissue is removed at vacuum excision (equating to a total of 12 biopsies with a 7-gauge needle) (14). Both UK and European guidelines recommend the use of VAE for B3 lesions without atypia due to the low upgrade rate of malignancy in this group (5, 12). VAE with atypia is a more challenging group, as the type of atypia will affect the upgrade rate. UK guidelines recommend all B3 lesions should be managed with VAE except for papillomas with atypia, fibroepithelial lesions and spindle cell lesions (5). European guidelines differ slightly in terms of management of ductal lesions with atypia for which surgical excision rather than VAE is recommended (12, 15).

B3 lesions require careful discussion at a multidisciplinary meeting (MDT); surgical excision is no longer the only available option, and management of these lesions has become more complex. Radiological pathological concordance is paramount and, when in doubt, will affect the usual management plan. From a radiological perspective, deployment of marker clips at the time of biopsy allows accurate identification of the sampled area and ensures concordance with radiological findings. In those cases with more extensive radiological abnormalities, a decision must be made on whether to sample the most radiological suspicious lesion or multiple areas (16). Diagnosis can be challenging from the pathologist's perspective, with significant inter-observer variation, but with improved levels of concordance amongst specialised breast pathologists. When reviewing cases at the MDT, consideration of whether there are similar changes in the initial diagnostic biopsy and subsequent excision specimen is essential, and whether the original biopsy site is present to ensure the correct area has been sampled. Table 5.2 illustrates the management strategies

TABLE 5.2

Upgrade Rates and Comparison of Management Recommendations from Three Key Published Guidelines Regarding B3 Lesions (5, 10, 15)

B3 Lesion	Upgrade Rate to Malignancy	Management According to UK Guidelines	Management According to the Second International Consensus Guidelines	European Management Guidelines
Atypical ductal hyperplasia (ADH)	5–50%	VAE	Surgical excision	Surgical excision. VAE could be considered if <15 mm.
Columnar cell lesions (CCC)	0–5%	VAE	VAE	If no ADH imaging surveillance. If ADH is present, VAE or surgical excision.
Complex sclerosing lesion (CSL)	0–40% 10% (without atypia) 36% (with atypia)	VAE	If visible on imaging, VAE.	If no atypia—VAE. If atypia—surgical excision, but VAE could be considered.
Lobular neoplasia (LN)	0–40% (12% for ALH and 22% for LCIS)	VAE	If visible on imaging, VAE, but if discordance, surgical excision.	VAE but surgical excision if discordance.
Papillary lesions	10% (without atypia) 27–36% (with atypia)	If no atypia—VAE. If atypia—surgical excision.	If visible on imaging, VAE, but if too large, surgical excision.	If no atypia—VAE. If atypia—surgical excision.

for B3 lesions as proposed by three separate sets of guidelines.

In general, lesions associated with epithelial atypia have an increased risk of developing cancer in either breast, and therefore, annual mammographic surveillance is recommended for 5 years (5, 15). Women with LCIS or ADH may derive protection from development of invasive cancer by use of selective oestrogen receptor modulators (SERMs), such as tamoxifen (17). A notable problem with therapies for chemoprevention is lack of compliance and poor uptake (18). The latest EUSOMA guidance recommends that women with atypical hyperplasia or LCIS should be offered primary prevention but that there is currently insufficient evidence for recommending chemoprevention for other B3 lesions (15). Lifestyle factors, such as obesity, smoking, alcohol consumption, and physical activity, are associated with an increased risk of breast cancer, and there is likely some benefit in lifestyle modification for women with a B3 diagnosis (19). Indeed, the most recent EUSOMA guidance recommends discussion of lifestyle interventions for women deemed to be at increased risk of breast cancer based on possession of a B3 lesion (15).

Despite existence of online risk prediction tools for women with B3 lesions, such as the Tyrer Cuzick model (20), the performance of these models for women with indeterminate lesions is debatable. With the advent of machine learning and artificial intelligence (AI), nomograms have been developed to attempt to more accurately determine if surgery can be safely avoided in women with B3 lesions. These incorporate radiological images, histopathology, and breast cancer risk factors (21). Whilst mammography remains the principal modality for both diagnosis and follow-up of B3 lesions, contrast-enhanced MRI has shown promise in a number of studies in terms of excluding the presence of coexisting malignancy due to a very high negative predictive value (22). Similar results have been reported for contrast-enhanced mammography.

One of the greatest challenges pertaining to B3 lesions is communication with patients. There is inevitably an element of uncertainty at the initial B3 diagnosis and a complex range of management options exists due to the heterogeneous nature of this group of lesions together with variable patient factors. The concept of risk can be difficult to explain, and in particular, there is an immediate risk of upgrade as well as a potential long-term risk of breast cancer. Shared decision-making in these instances is key, as well as providing adequate time for explanation of these complex scenarios. It has been recommended by EUSOMA that breast centres should develop tailored written information to help patients understand the impact of B3 lesions and how this affects their future breast cancer risk (15).

5.2 Atypical Ductal Hyperplasia (ADH)/Atypical Intraductal Epithelial Proliferation (AIDP)

Atypical ductal hyperplasia (ADH) is also known as atypical intraductal epithelial proliferation (AIDP). This is a borderline breast lesion on pathology, with histological changes identical to low-grade DCIS at a cellular level and differentiation between ADH and DCIS is based exclusively on size. Thus, ADH involves only a single duct or the lesion diameter is less than 2 mm. Any lesion more extensive than this is classified as DCIS.

ADH is one of the most frequently diagnosed B3 lesions of the breast. On mammographic imaging ADH can be associated with microcalcifications, a focal mass or asymmetric density (10, 23). The microcalcifications are typically granular in nature and can either form a cluster or exhibit a ductal distribution (Figures 5.1 and 5.2). On ultrasound, ADH is often visualised as a mass or an ill-defined hypoechoic area. ADH, if visible on MRI, typically has nonspecific features, with either mass or non-mass enhancement (14).

On pathological analysis ADH is defined as a small focus of a low-grade, epithelial intraductal proliferation, not exceeding a maximum diameter of 2 mm (2, 10). The 2019 WHO classification of breast tumours recommends referring to this lesion as atypical ductal hyperplasia (ADH). However, an alternative term, atypical intraductal epithelial proliferation (AIDEP) is often used, possibly better reflecting the uncertain nature of the lesion (2, 24, 25). As mentioned, size is the main discriminator from DCIS, and this can be difficult to determine on pre-operative CNB or VAB (2, 14). Therefore, additional sampling of the lesion is required, either with VAE or diagnostic excision.

ADH demonstrates clonal proliferation in almost all cases, with overexpression of the oestrogen receptor (ER) and loss of basal cytokeratins (2, 25). Both clonal proliferation and immunohistochemistry can prove useful in differentiating ADH from usual type ductal hyperplasia (UDH), the main differential diagnosis.

The rate of ADH upgrade to DCIS or invasive cancer is between 5% and 50% but is highly variable and difficult to predict (14, 25–27). Upgrade is higher in cases with discordant imaging and pathology findings, those with mass lesions on imaging and those where the original diagnosis was based on standard core-needle biopsy. A meta-analysis of 93 articles aimed to determine whether imaging or patient factors could confidently predict absence of any upgrade to malignancy and thus avoidance of surgery (28). This study involved more than 6000 cases of ADH, with the majority (5,911/6458) managed with surgical excision alone and the remaining 547 cases managed with imaging follow-up. The authors concluded that excision should be recommended for all patients with ADH found at

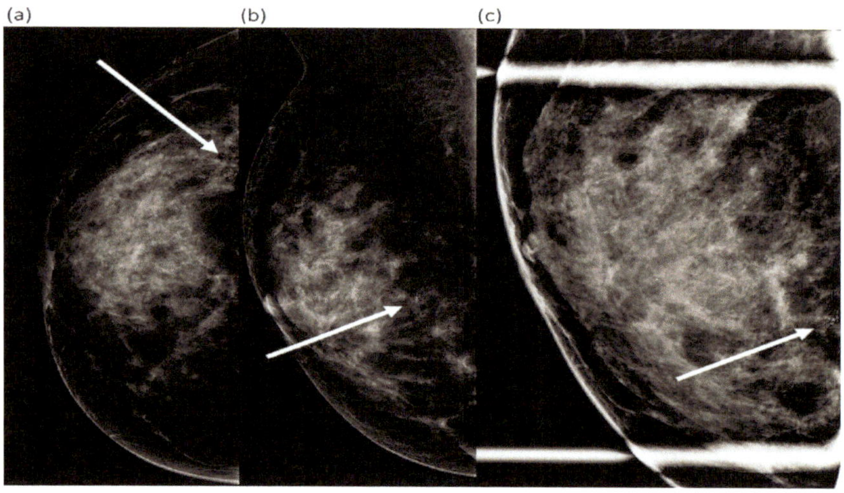

FIGURE 5.1
A 45-year-old undergoing annual mammography for high-risk family history was noted to have 10 × 7 mm cluster of new, granular microcalcifications at the posterior extent of the right breast on mammogram. This is demonstrated on CC view (a), MLO view (b), and better appreciated on magnification view (c). Stereotactic biopsy was not possible due to posterior location. US biopsy of an area of altered echogenicity demonstrated area of ADH and VAE of this area showed high-grade DCIS. Right mastectomy revealed 50 mm high-grade DCIS.

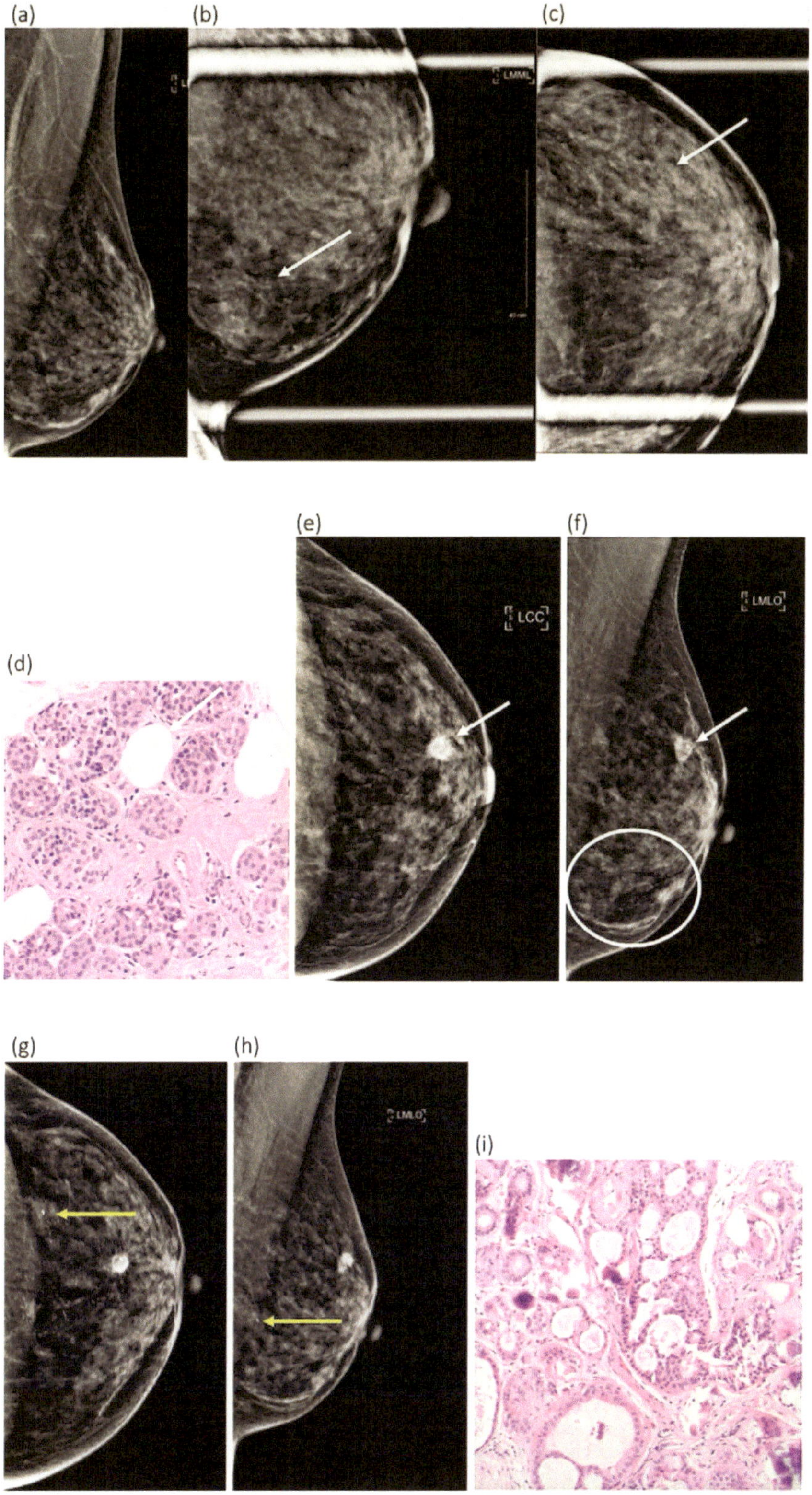

FIGURE 5.2
A 57-year-old woman recalled from screening for developing microcalcification in the left inferolateral breast seen on lateral view (a), and magnification views (b, c) extending over approximately 5 cm. Vacuum-assisted biopsy was performed, which demonstrated LCIS (d). However, post-clip mammograms (e, f) demonstrated the clip actually lies distant to the area of concern (circle) in the superior breast (arrow), highlighting the importance of clip placement and subsequent mammography. A further VAB was performed of another area of microcalcification, with post-clip mammograms now confirming correct targeting (g, h). Pathology demonstrated a small focus of ADH with associated microcalcification (i).

needle biopsy, but noted that the studies included in this meta-analysis were quite heterogeneous.

The main area of controversy is whether these lesions can be managed with a less invasive VAE rather than diagnostic surgery. As previously discussed, an important issue to consider is the size of the lesion. According to the UK National Health Service Breast Screening Programme (NHS BSP) Working Group guidelines, VAE is the recommended method for detailed secondary assessment of most ADH cases irrespective of whether initially diagnosed on CNB or primary diagnostic VAB (5). By contrast, the Second International Consensus Conference on lesions of uncertain malignant potential in the breast recommends that all ADH lesions should be surgically excised to ensure adequate sampling of the area (10). Current European guidelines recommend either surgical excision or VAE for lesions measuring less than 15 mm but certainly surgical excision for those lesions exceeding15 mm in size (15).

5.3 Columnar Cell Lesions

Columnar cell lesions represent a spectrum of epithelial changes in the breast characterised by enlarged terminal duct lobular units lined by columnar epithelium. This group of lesions includes columnar cell change (CCC), columnar cell hyperplasia (CCH), and flat epithelial atypia (FEA). Whereas CCC and CCH are considered benign lesions, FEA may be associated with higher-grade lesions, such as ADH, lobular neoplasia (LN), DCIS, or invasive carcinoma. FEA is also considered to be a precursor to low-grade DCIS and invasive carcinoma.

Columnar cell lesions typically present on mammography as clustered, amorphous, or fine pleomorphic microcalcifications (29, 30). In some cases, these may present as a mass on mammography or ultrasound. Figure 5.3 is a representative case of FEA.

According to the current WHO classification, columnar cell lesions include CCC and CCH without atypia; when atypia is present, the lesion is called flat epithelial atypia (FEA) (2). Columnar cell lesions are clonal alterations of the terminal duct lobular unit (TDLU) characterised by enlarged, variably dilated acini lined by columnar epithelial cells. FEA is characterised by low-grade cytological atypia with one to several layers of mildly atypical cuboid to columnar cells in a flat architecture. Nuclei are round and uniform with inconspicuous nucleoli, similar to the nuclei that characterise low-grade DCIS (2).

FEA shares molecular changes of the so-called low-grade molecular pathways with other lesions, such as ADH, low-grade DCIS, or classical LN, and also including tubular carcinoma, invasive cribriform carcinoma, classical invasive lobular carcinoma (ILC), and low-grade invasive ductal carcinoma (2, 31). FEA is often associated with these lesions.

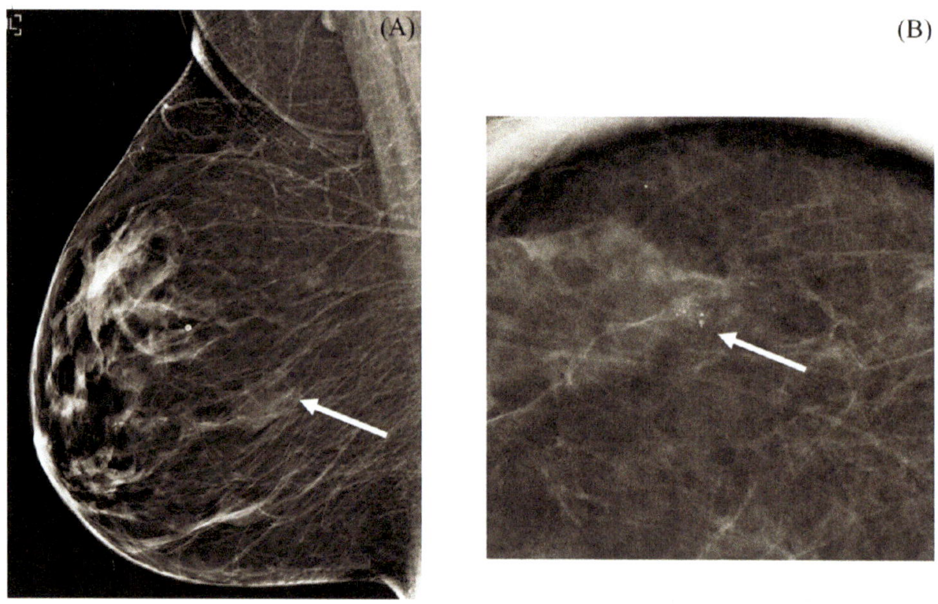

FIGURE 5.3
(A) 56-year-old recalled from screening for new 6 mm cluster of calcifications in the posterior central right breast. (B) Magnification views confirm 6 mm cluster of granular calcifications. Stereotactic biopsy of the microcalcifications showed FEA and subsequent VAE did not show evidence or atypia or malignancy.

For pure FEA the risk of local recurrence and progression to carcinoma is low. When FEA is associated with other lesions like ADH, DCIS, and LN, the risk associated with the higher-risk lesion should be adopted when counselling patients about treatment options.

A meta-analysis of 42 studies involving a total of 2482 cases of pure FEA without other high-risk lesions, calculated a pooled upgrade rate of 5% for pure FEA on CNB after surgical excision or 2-year imaging follow-up (32). Several other and mostly earlier meta-analyses reported slightly different upgrade rates following surgical excision ranging from 1% to 16% (10, 33, 34).

Radiological follow-up is the preferred management option espoused by several independent research groups for pure FEA diagnosed on VAB and this is supported by published guidelines (10). If there is a mass, residual microcalcifications, or discordance between imaging and pathology, then further sampling should be considered (10, 35–37). If the lesion is not deemed pathologically to be pure FEA and there are additional high-risk lesions present such as ADH or LN, further tissue sampling is warranted as these are predictors of histological upgrade to malignancy. German guidelines recommend that surgery can be omitted if there is near complete removal of the mammographic abnormality or if the lesion is considered to be small (<2 TDLU) in the VAB sample (38). The NHS BSP recommends VAE as a suitable alternative to surgical excision with the latter reserved for cases of radio-pathological discordance or if there is upgrade to DCIS or invasive cancer on VAE (5). European guidelines recommend that pure FEA can be safely managed with surveillance alone, unless there is associated ADH in which case a VAE or surgical excision is recommended (15).

5.4 Radial Scar (RS) or Complex Sclerosing Lesion (CSL)

A radial scar is also known as a complex sclerosing lesion (CSL). These lesions are typically seen on tomosynthesis or a mammogram as a spiculate lesion with a radiolucent centre or an area of architectural distortion, often only visible on a single mammographic view. The spicules associated with the lesion can be quite long and are iso-dense to the adjacent parenchyma. The parenchymal deformity seen on mammography may also be associated with indeterminate microcalcifications.

Ultrasound appearances can be variable and challenging to interpret. These can range from a hypoechoic, irregular mass or non-specific shadowing, with up to one third of CSL lesions showing no sonographic abnormality (39–41).

MRI features can be non-specific, ranging from no obvious abnormality on MRI or the presence of a lesion without enhancement to a discrete mass lesion with suspicious enhancement (41, 42). As MRI has a high negative predictive value, this imaging modality can exclude any underlying invasive malignancy associated with CSL, although cannot reliably differentiate between CSL with and without atypia (43–45). Examples of CSL are shown in Figures 5.4 and 5.5.

According to the WHO classification, radial scar and a CSL essentially represent the same entity (2). They both have a stellate configuration with a central fibro-elastotic core and lack a reactive fibroblastic stroma. There are peripherally entrapped glandular structures and cysts that are often radially orientated. A radial scar is typically less than 10 mm in size, while a CSL tends to be larger. A number of lesions may coexist alongside CSL, including apocrine metaplasia, usual type ductal hyperplasia, sclerosing adenosis, and microcalcifications.

Reported upgrade rates of CSL to DCIS or invasive disease range widely in the literature, from zero to almost 40% (46–49). The gauge of the needle used and number of passes can impact the upgrade rate on histology (48, 50). Studies have shown that CSL upgrades rates are higher when there is associated atypia. Data from the NHSBSP suggests upgrade to malignancy occurs in 36% of cases with atypia versus 10% without atypia (5). Similar findings were observed in a study by Groen and colleagues where a RS without and with atypia had upgrade rates of 9% and 33%, respectively (51).

As with all B3 lesions there must be good correlation between radiology and final histology, with MDT input for each case. German guidelines recommend no surgical excision if the lesion is less 5 mm in size and has been almost completely excised with VAB (38). The Second International Consensus Conference on lesions of uncertain malignant potential in the breast recommend therapeutic vacuum-assisted biopsy followed by imaging surveillance (10). UK guidelines recommend thorough sampling of the area with VAE (>4 g of tissue), when CSL is detected on initial biopsy (core or VAB) (5). If there is no atypia on VAE or the original specimen, then the patient should undergo routine mammographic screening. Following MDT discussion, if atypia is identified on either biopsy or VAE, without histological upgrade, annual mammography for 5 years should be offered, following MDT discussion (5). European guidelines advocate VAE as optimum management for a CSL without atypia, but

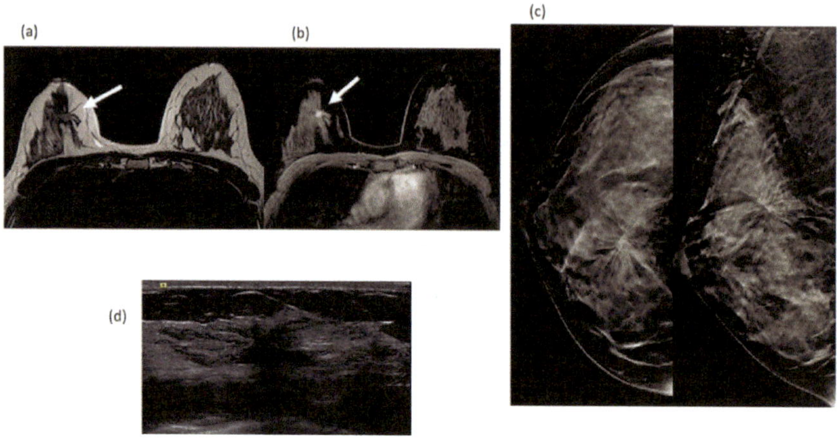

FIGURE 5.4
A 28-year-old BRCA patient undergoing first screening MRI which demonstrates (a) a spiculate mass in the right upper inner quadrant on T2 weighted imaging, with (b) central enhancement on T1 post-contrast imaging. (c) Tomosynthesis demonstrated a spiculate lesion on both CC and MLO views. (d) US biopsy shows a hypoechoic area of shadowing and parenchymal distortion. The histology of US-guided biopsy demonstrated a CSL with no atypia. Subsequent VAE showed similar findings with no evidence upgrade. Bilateral risk reducing mastectomy performed within a year did not demonstrate any evidence of malignancy.

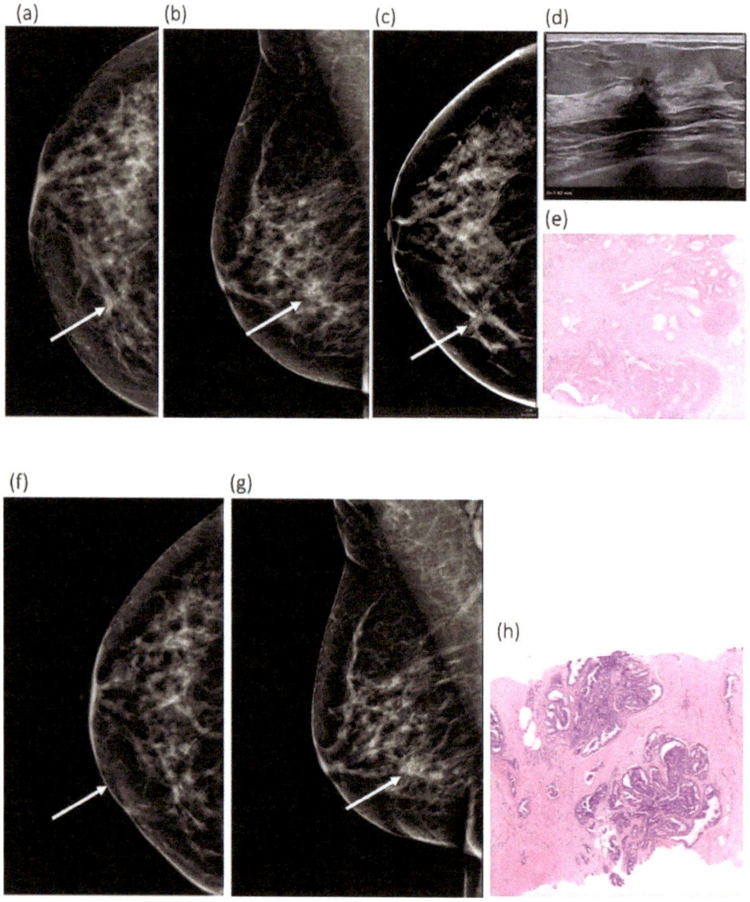

FIGURE 5.5
A 54-year-old recalled from screening for a new area of distortion and associated microcalcification seen on the right CC and MLO view (a, b). Tomosynthesis views better demonstrate the associated distortion (c). US confirmed a small 7 mm hypoechoic area in the right medial breast (d). Core biopsy of the lesion demonstrated a radial scar/complex sclerosing lesion with focal atypical intraductal proliferation (e). Clip placement at the time of biopsy helped to confirm the subtle area of distortion had been correctly targeted (f, g). Subsequent VAE demonstrated upgrade to low-grade DCIS (h).

in the presence of atypia, surgical excision is recommended but VAE could be considered (15).

5.5 Lobular Neoplasia (LN)

Classical lobular neoplasia (LN) comprises a spectrum of lesions and is classified by the WHO as classical LCIS or atypical lobular hyperplasia (ALH). Pleomorphic LCIS (PLCIS) and florid LCIS are regarded as comparable to DCIS, and therefore designated B5a, rather than B3. Morphological changes are similar for ALH and LCIS but more than 50% of the acini in a terminal ducto-lobular unit must be expanded by epithelial cells for diagnosis of LCIS, with less extensive involvement of acini designated ALH (5, 10).

Both ALH and LCIS are considered risk factors for development of invasive malignancy. Patients with ALH have a 4–5 times greater relative risk of malignancy than the general population, but this risk is 8–10 times greater for LCIS (52). Although LN was originally considered to be just a marker of risk for developing carcinoma, epidemiological and morphological evidence suggest that it is also a non-obligate precursor of malignancy. Moreover, despite the risk of developing malignancy being increased for both breasts, this is three times greater in the ipsilateral breast containing the original LN, with invasive lobular carcinoma occurring more frequently that ductal carcinoma (53).

Many LN lesions have no characteristic imaging features, and LN is often mammographically occult. Microcalcification may be present, but tends to be identified in adjacent benign breast tissue that is separate from the lobular neoplastic architecture, thus rendering LN an incidental finding on biopsy (4) Upgrade rates are notably higher (13–18%) for LN associated with mass lesions and calcifications (8, 54). On ultrasound examination, LN may present as a hypoechoic lesion or non-specific altered echogenicity. When these B3 lesions are detected on MRI or CEM, the characteristic finding is non-mass enhancement. An example of LCIS is provided in Figure 5.6.

On histological examination, the lobular cells tend to be discohesive, often with eccentric nuclei and intracytoplasmic vacuoles. The distinction between ALH and LCIS is quantitative as described above. Pleomorphic LCIS is diagnosed when the lesion comprises high-grade nuclei (B5a). Pleomorphic LCIS and florid LCIS can be associated with luminal calcification and comedo-necrosis and therefore identified mammographically. Although classical LCIS tends to be strongly and uniformly positive for ER and negative for HER2, cases of pleomorphic LCIS can be ER negative and HER2 positive. This feature can help distinguish between these two types of LCIS in challenging cases (55–57). A defining feature of LN is inactivation of the E-cadherin gene leading to diminished or absent E-cadherin expression on immunohistochemistry (58). In some cases, expression of this cell adhesion molecule can be heterogeneous, and in such cases, a lobular phenotype can be confirmed by negative β-catenin or cytoplasmic P120 staining (59, 60).

The upgrade rate of LN to malignancy varies considerably in the literature, with average rates of 27% for LN (range 0–40%), 12% for ALH, and 22% for LCIS (7, 61, 62). A recent meta-analysis involving 16 studies calculated pooled risks for upgrade to any malignancy following the diagnosis of LN, ALH, or LCIS of 3.1%, 2.5% and 5.8%, respectively (63). Several recent studies suggest that when a diagnosis of pure LN is made based on CNB, and no other lesions are present, such as ADH, papilloma, or radial scar, the upgrade rate is less than 5% (64). A prospective multi-institutional trial (TBCRC 20) aimed to determine the rate of upgrade to cancer after excision for pure LCIS diagnosed on CNB. Women diagnosed with LCIS who received no surgery (as reported to the SEER registry) had a subsequent 10-year incidence of cancer development of 13.9%, and breast cancer specific survival was not impacted by the choice of surgical procedure (65).

Once a diagnosis of LCIS is established with CNB, the need for further excision is a matter of debate. The surgical management of patients with LCIS has changed dramatically over the past few decades. Thus, in the 1960s–'70s most patients with classical LCIS underwent mastectomy, and in many cases this was bilateral. Management has changed over time and mastectomy is now performed in only 10–20% of cases and most women with classical LCIS undergo local surgical excision in the contemporary era (66–68). Guidelines recommend that cases of classical LN should be managed with VAE and imaging follow-up if there is radiological and pathological concordance (5, 10, 15). If lesions are designated B5a on histology then surgical excision with clear margins is mandatory.

5.6 Papillary Lesions

There is a spectrum of papillary lesions of the breast ranging from benign entities and those with atypia, including benign papilloma and papilloma with ADH, to malignant lesions such as papillary carcinoma in situ and invasive papillary carcinoma. Papillary lesions can present with either bloody nipple discharge or be detected incidentally on imaging.

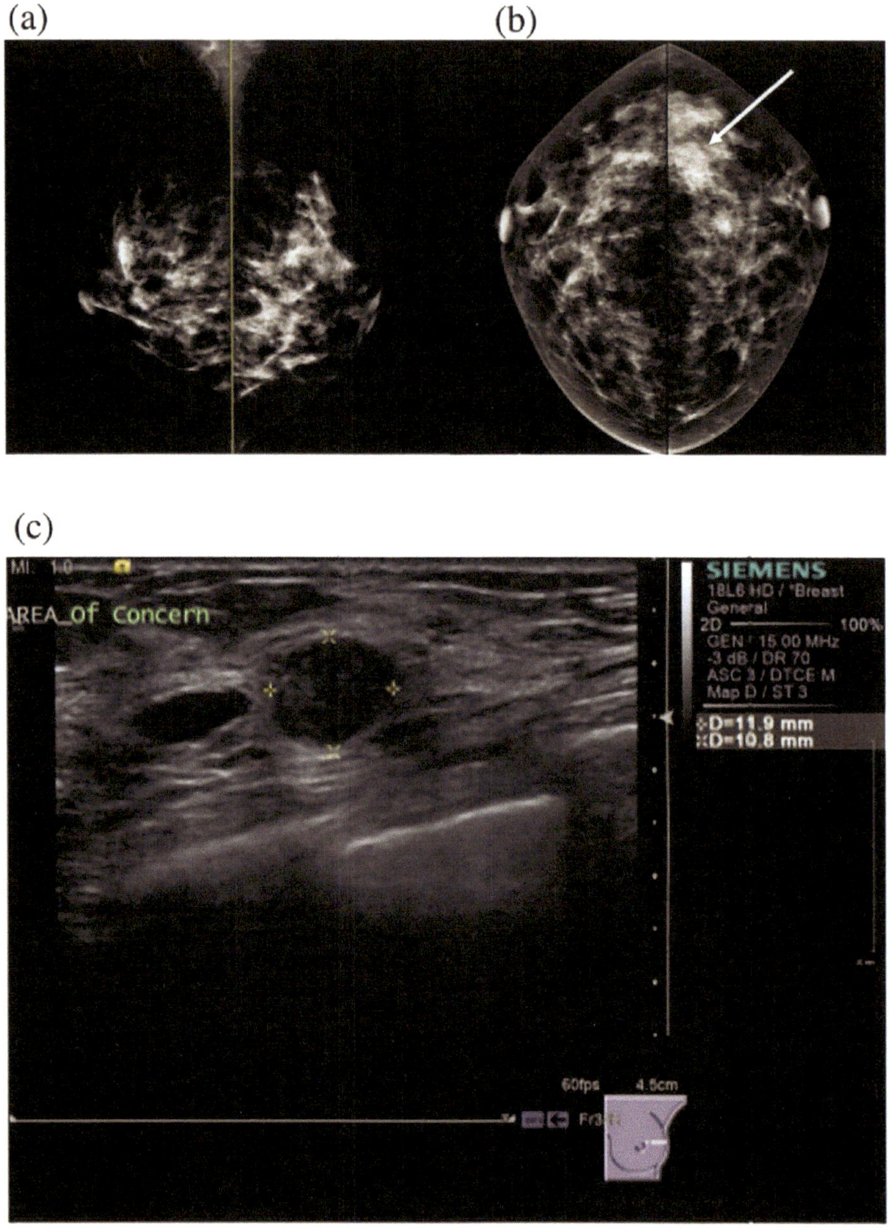

FIGURE 5.6
A 42-year-old presenting symptomatically with a palpable lump in the left lateral breast. (a, b) Mammograms demonstrated a possible density, seen only on the CC view (b). (c) US of the area of concern demonstrated a 12 mm solid mass. Core biopsy demonstrated features of LCIS colonising a fibroepithelial lesion (B3). Surgical excision was performed, with final pathology of a fibroadenoma with classical LCIS, and LCIS also in background breast parenchyma. Five-year follow-up mammography was recommended.

Mammography is often normal but may reveal dilated ducts or a well-defined retroareolar mass. In 25% of cases there are clustered calcifications on mammography which can be pleomorphic in nature (69). Papillary lesions may appear as a complex cystic lesion on ultrasound or as a well-defined hypoechoic nodule, often within a dilated duct. Colour Doppler may demonstrate vascularity within the stalk (70). These lesions may appear as well-defined, enhancing masses on MRI or irregular lesions associated with dilated ducts. It is impossible to distinguish from imaging alone those lesions which are benign from those that have atypia or malignancy. Examples of papillary lesions are provided in Figures 5.7 and 5.8.

An intraductal papilloma is a benign lesion of papillary architecture. It comprises a fibrovascular core that is covered by normal luminal epithelial cells with associated myoepithelium. Intraductal papillomas can be

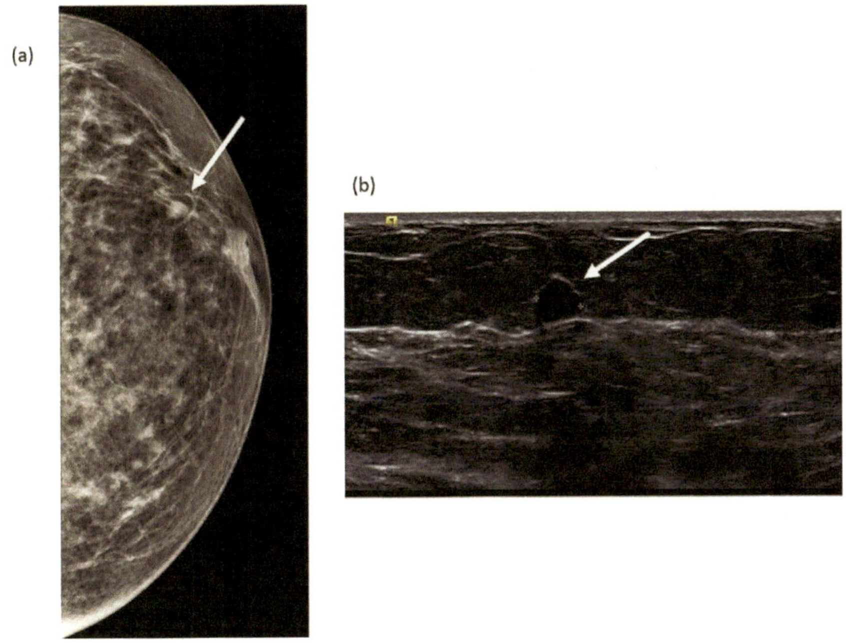

FIGURE 5.7
(a) 67-year-old recalled from screening for 6 mm new density just lateral to the left nipple. (b) Ultrasound shows relatively well-defined 6 mm hypoechoic mass. Ultrasound-guided biopsy demonstrated a papillary lesion without atypia. Subsequent VA E did not show any evidence of malignancy.

associated with hyperplasia, apocrine metaplasia, squamous metaplasia, infarction, or fibrosis with distortion (71). If a papilloma is associated with 3 mm or more of associated non-high-grade atypia, this is considered to be DCIS (72). Therefore, assessment of lesions with atypia is essential to differentiate between a papilloma with atypia and DCIS within a papilloma. Multiple peripheral papillomas are more likely to be associated with atypia and/or DCIS compared with solitary intraductal papillomas (73). The combination of basal cytokeratins (CK5, CK14), myoepithelial (SMM), and ER immunohistochemistry can help distinguish benign papillomas from those with atypia and/or papillary DCIS.

Atypia is the strongest predictor of upgrade of intraductal papilloma to in situ or invasive carcinoma. Upgrade to malignancy is observed in less than 10% of papillomas without atypia but this increases to 27–36% for lesions with atypia (74–76). A meta-analysis identified a number of predictive factors for upgrade to malignancy, including bloody nipple discharge or palpable mass at presentation, mass or microcalcifications on mammography, peripheral location within the breast, BI-RADS 4B or higher, radio-pathological discordance, and lesion size exceeding 1 cm (77). According to this meta-analysis, upgrade rates associated with these predictive factors ranged from 7.3 to 31.1%.

If CNB identifies an intraductal papilloma without atypia and the radiological and pathological findings are concordant, VAE is an acceptable management strategy (15). The majority of retrospective studies have confirmed improvement of diagnostic accuracy with VAE, and women can be safely offered imaging surveillance after percutaneous needle excision (78, 79). If a CNB or a VAB identifies a papilloma with atypia (i.e. ADH), then surgical excision is necessary to permit evaluation of the intact lesion and determine the extent of continuous atypia (using a 3 mm cutoff value for diagnosis of DCIS (5, 15, 76, 80). Large papillary lesions without atypia or lesions where VAB is not technically feasible should be surgically excised (10). Multiple papillomas have a threefold increased risk of invasive cancer and a sevenfold risk if ADH or LN is present and therefore long-term imaging surveillance is recommended (10).

5.7 Miscellaneous

There are a number of less commonly encountered entities that are classified as B3 lesions and incorporated under the umbrella term of 'miscellaneous lesions'. These encompass a broad spectrum of lesions including atypical apocrine adenosis, mucocele-like lesions and several stromal spindle and myofibroblastic proliferations. As outcome data is limited on these lesions, they should be managed on an individual basis following multidisciplinary team discussion.

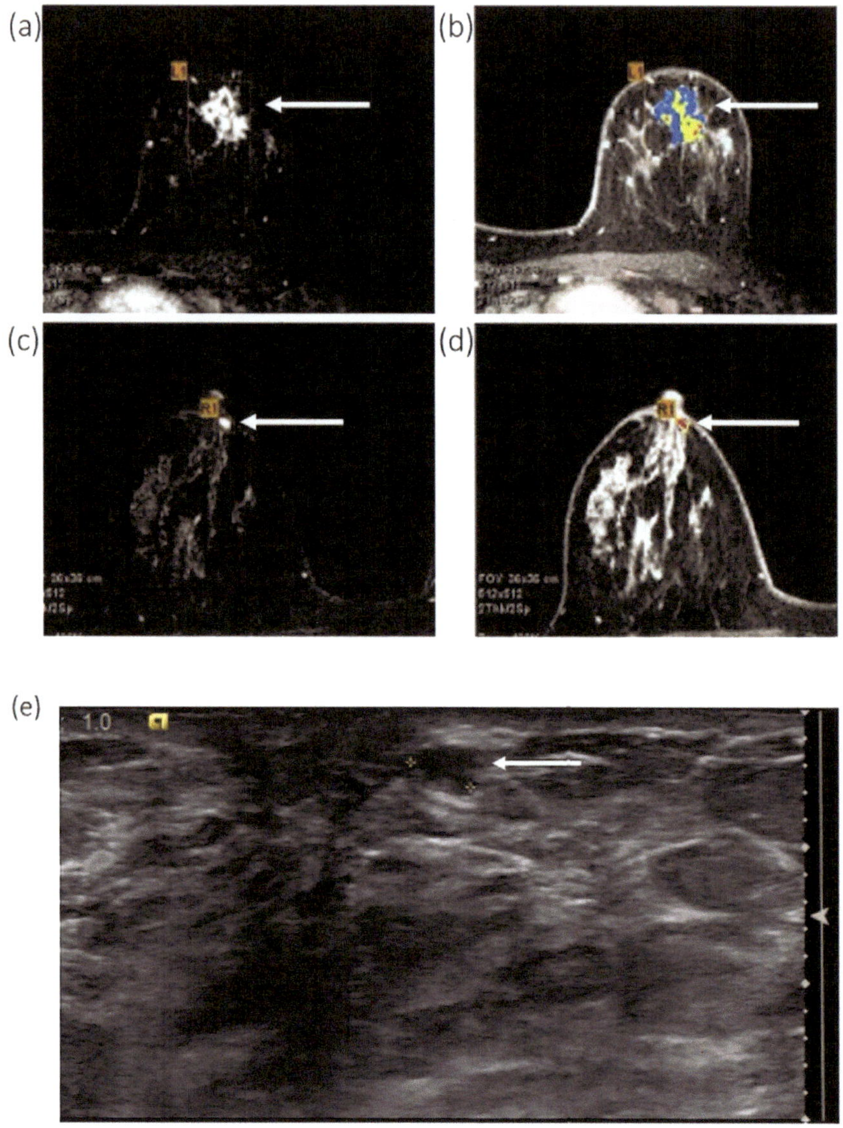

FIGURE 5.8
A 60-year-old patient with a biopsy proven grade 2 invasive carcinoma of the left breast as seen on MRI (a, b), performed to assess suitability for conservation. MRI also demonstrated a further small 5 mm mass near the nipple demonstrating type 3 curve (arrows in c, d). Second look US was performed which demonstrated a small oval mass near the nipple (arrow on e), core biopsy confirmed a papillary lesion with columnar cell change and usual type hyperplasia but no atypia (B3). The patient was able to undergo conservation for her left breast malignancy.

5.7.1 Atypical Apocrine Adenosis

Atypical apocrine adenosis is a glandular proliferation that can display similarity to low-grade apocrine DCIS. Differentiation between the two entities is usually challenging and can only be reliably determined following evaluation of the surgical specimen (10). Immunohistochemistry is not particularly helpful, as ER and basal cytokeratins are negative in most cases, and androgen receptors are positive both in adenosis and in low-to-intermediate-grade DCIS. However, when there is strong HER2 expression (score 3+) this is strong evidence for high-grade DCIS (10).

5.7.2 Mucocele-Like Lesions

Mucocele-like lesions are defined as free mucus pools within the stroma of the breast tissue. These pools are devoid of any epithelial structures and often occur close to ruptured ducts (2). Mucinous adenocarcinoma, the main differential diagnosis, needs to be excluded on histology (2). Cytokeratins can prove useful and when there is no evidence of epithelial cells in the free mucus pools, the upgrade rate to malignancy is low (<2%) (2, 38). If a mucinous carcinoma has been excluded with immunohistochemistry and there is concordance between imaging and pathology findings, these cases can be managed with surgical excision or therapeutic VAE (5).

5.7.3 Fibroepithelial Lesions

Fibroepithelial lesions are breast lesions composed of both epithelial and stromal components, and comprise the common fibroadenoma and the less frequently encountered phyllodes tumour (<1% of all breast neoplasms). Phyllodes tumours are fibroepithelial neoplasms that typically present at a later stage than fibroadenomas, usually in the fourth to fifth decades. Imaging features of phyllodes tumours are often similar to a fibroadenoma on conventional imaging, with a well-circumscribed oval mass on mammography or ultrasound. Larger lesions may have ill-defined margins and cystic areas on ultrasound. Phyllodes tumour should be considered if there is rapid growth of a benign lesion. Although malignancy is infrequent, no imaging features exist to differentiate benign from malignant lesions. Unless they are completely excised, these lesions tend to recur irrespective of whether benign, borderline, or malignant (5, 7, 81). Therefore, all phyllodes tumours, as well as rare fibroepithelial lesions that are classified as B3 on pathology, require complete surgical excision (82).

5.8 Imaging Surveillance Following B3 Diagnosis

Following a B3 diagnosis with subsequent VAE or surgical excision and MDT discussion, most centres perform mammographic surveillance for 5 years. However, this is a complex issue with many other factors to consider, such as patient age, breast density, family history of malignancy, size of B3 lesion, presence of other high-risk lesions, etc. The UK NHSBSP guidelines recommend follow-up with annual mammography for all lesions except papillary lesions without atypia, radial scar without atypia or mucocele-like lesion without atypia (11). The American College of Radiology guidelines recommend considering surveillance with breast MRI in cases of ADH, ALH, and LCIS (83). Although there are limited guidelines and studies on surveillance in cases of B3 lesions, some authors recommend surveillance with MRI for cases of ADH and LN (14, 84).

5.9 Primary Prevention and B3 Lesions

Primary prevention is the use of some form of pharmacological treatment to decrease the risk of invasive breast cancer in women without a personal history of breast cancer. There are a limited number of primary prevention studies that include B3 lesions, with the majority focussed on family lineage as a risk factor. Most primary prevention strategies target ER-positive cancers and achieve their effects through one of two mechanisms—either reduction of oestrogen levels and hormonal stimulation of breast tissue (oophorectomy, aromatase inhibitors) or competitive blockage of hormone binding to the ER (selective ER modulators [SERMs]—tamoxifen and raloxifene). The majority of B3 lesions, including ADH, are hormone receptor positive and, therefore, potentially amenable to primary preventative approaches (85, 86).

Several studies of both pre- and post-menopausal women have included limited numbers of women with LCIS and atypias and shown a reduction in breast cancer risk amongst subgroups of patients with high-risk lesions (14, 75–90). It should be noted that the numbers of women with B3 lesions were very small in all these studies with evidence that primary prevention strategies lead to a reduction in the proportion of 'good prognosis' tumours but with minimal impact on overall survival. Although current guidelines (91, 92) recommend that women at increased breast cancer risk should be offered primary prevention therapy, this is in the context of elevated risk based on family history of the disease for which there is a stronger evidence base than for cases of atypias that are poorly represented numerically in these studies.

References

1. Lee AHS, Anderson N, Carder P, et al. Guidelines for non-operative diagnostic procedures and reporting in breast cancer screening. Royal College of Pathology, 2016.
2. WHO Classification of Tumours, WHO. Breast tumours. 5th edn. International Agency for Research of Cancer, 2019.
3. Cohen MA, Newell MS. Radial scars of the breast encountered at core biopsy: Review of histologic, imaging, and management considerations. AJR. 2017;209(5):1168–77.
4. Maxwell AJ, Clements K, Dodwell DJ, et al. The radiological features, diagnosis and management of screen-detected lobular neoplasia of the breast: Findings from the Sloane Project. Breast. 2016;27:109–15.
5. Pinder SE, Shaaban A, Deb R, et al. NHS breast screening multidisciplinary working group guidelines for the diagnosis and management of breast lesions of uncertain malignant potential on core biopsy (B3 lesions). Clin Radiol. 2018;73(8):682–92.
6. Bianchi S, Caini S, Renne G, et al. Positive predictive value for malignancy on surgical excision of breast lesions of uncertain malignant potential (B3) diagnosed by stereotactic vacuum-assisted needle core biopsy (VANCB): A large multi-institutional study in Italy. Breast. 2011;20(3):264–70.
7. El-Sayed ME, Rakha EA, Reed J, et al. Predictive value of needle core biopsy diagnoses of lesions of uncertain malignant potential (B3) in abnormalities detected by mammographic screening. Histopathology. 2008;53(6):650–7.

8. Rakha EA, Lee AH, Jenkins JA, et al. Characterization and outcome of breast needle core biopsy diagnoses of lesions of uncertain malignant potential (B3) in abnormalities detected by mammographic screening. Int J Cancer. 2011;129(6):1417–24.
9. Cullinane C, Byrne J, Kelly L, et al. The positive predictive value of vacuum assisted biopsy (VAB) in predicting final histological diagnosis for breast lesions of uncertain malignancy (B3 lesions): A systematic review & meta-analysis. Eur J Surg Oncol. 2022;48(7):1464–74.
10. Rageth CJ, O'Flynn EAM, Pinker K, et al. Second International Consensus Conference on lesions of uncertain malignant potential in the breast (B3 lesions). Breast Cancer Res Treat. 2019;174(2):279–96. Erratum in: Breast Cancer Res Treat. 2019;176(2):481–2.
11. Sharma N, Cornford E, Cheung S, et al. The impact of vacuum-assisted excision in the management of indeterminate B3 lesions in the NHS Breast Screening Programme in England. Clin Radiol. 2021;76(6):470.
12. Elfgen C, Leo C, Kubik-Huch RA, et al. Third international consensus conference on lesions of uncertain malignant potential in the breast (B3 lesions). Virchows Arch. 2023;483(1):5–20.
13. McMahon MA, Haigh I, Chen Y, et al. Role of vacuum assisted excision in minimising overtreatment of ductal atypias. Eur J Radiol. 2020;131:109258.
14. Catanzariti F, Avendano D, Cicero G, et al. High-risk lesions of the breast: Concurrent diagnostic tools and management recommendations. Insights Imaging. 2021;12(1):63.
15. Rubio IT, Wyld L, Marotti L, et al. European guidelines for the diagnosis, treatment and follow-up of breast lesions with uncertain malignant potential (B3 lesions) developed jointly by EUSOMA, EUSOBI, ESP (BWG) and ESSO. Eur J Surg Oncol. 2023;50(1):107292.
16. Ahmed M, Rubio IT, Klaase JM, et al. Surgical treatment of nonpalpable primary invasive and in situ breast cancer. Nat Rev Clin Oncol. 2015;12(11):645–63.
17. Coopey SB, Mazzola E, Buckley JM, et al. The role of chemoprevention in modifying the risk of breast cancer in women with atypical breast lesions. Breast Cancer Res Treat. 2012;136(3):627–33.
18. Ropka ME, Keim J, Philbrick JT. Patient decisions about breast cancer chemoprevention: A systematic review and meta-analysis. J Clin Oncol. 2010;28(18):3090–5.
19. Danaei G, Vander Hoorn S, Lopez AD, et al; Comparative Risk Assessment Collaborating Group (Cancers). Causes of cancer in the world: Comparative risk assessment of nine behavioural and environmental risk factors. Lancet. 2005;366(9499):1784–93.
20. Tyrer J, Duffy SW, Cuzick J. A breast cancer prediction model incorporating familial and personal risk factors. Stat Med. 2004;23(7):1111–30.
21. Harrington L, diFlorio-Alexander R, Trinh K, et al. Prediction of atypical ductal hyperplasia upgrades through a machine learning approach to reduce unnecessary surgical excisions. JCO Clin Cancer Inform. 2018;2:1–11.
22. Berg WA, Zhang Z, Lehrer D, et al. Detection of breast cancer with addition of annual screening ultrasound or a single screening MRI to mammography in women with elevated breast cancer risk. JAMA. 2012;307(13):1394–404.
23. Shaaban AM, Sharma N. Management of B3 lesions—practical issues. Curr Breast Cancer Rep. 2019;11:83–8.
24. Royal College of Pathologists. Guidelines for non-operative diagnostic procedures and reporting in breast cancer screening [Internet]. 2021. Available at: https://www.rcpath.org/uploads/assets/4b16f19c-f7bd-456c-b212f557f8040f66/G150-Non-op-reporting-breast-cancer-screening.pdf.
25. Rageth CJ, Rubenov R, Bronz C, et al. Atypical ductal hyperplasia and the risk of underestimation: Tissue sampling method, multifocality, and associated calcification significantly influence the diagnostic upgrade rate based on subsequent surgical specimens. Breast Cancer. 2019;26(4):452–8.
26. Giannotti E, James JJ, Chen Y, et al. Effectiveness of percutaneous vacuum-assisted excision (VAE) of breast lesions of uncertain malignant potential (B3 lesions) as an alternative to open surgical biopsy. Eur Radiol. 2021;31(12):9540–7.
27. Nicosia L, Latronico A, Addante F, et al. Atypical ductal hyperplasia after vacuum-assisted breast biopsy: Can we reduce the upgrade to breast cancer to an acceptable rate? Diagnostics. 2021;11(6).
28. Schiaffino S, Calabrese M, Melani EF, et al. Upgrade rate of percutaneously diagnosed pure atypical ductal hyperplasia: Systematic review and meta-analysis of 6458 lesions. Radiology. 2020;294(1):76–86.
29. Solorzano S, Mesurolle B, Omeroglu A, et al. Flat epithelial atypia of the breast: Pathological-radiological correlation. AJR. 2011;197(3):740–6.
30. Pandey S, Kornstein MJ, Shank W, et al. Columnar cell lesions of the breast: Mammographic findings with histopathologic correlation. Radiographics. 2007;27(Suppl 1):S79–89.
31. Leibl S, Regitnig P, Moinfar F. Flat epithelial atypia (DIN 1a, atypical columnar change): An underdiagnosed entity very frequently coexisting with lobular neoplasia. Histopathology. 2007;50(7):859–65.
32. Wahab RA, Lee SJ, Mulligan ME, et al. Upgrade rate of pure flat epithelial atypia diagnosed at core needle biopsy: A systematic review and meta-analysis. Radiol Imaging Cancer. 2021;3(1):e200116.
33. Ferre R, Kuzmiak CM. Upgrade rate of percutaneously diagnosed pure flat epithelial atypia: Systematic review and meta-analysis of 1,924 lesions. J Osteopathic Med. 2022;122(5):253–62.
34. Rudin AV, Hoskin TL, Fahy A, et al. Flat epithelial atypia on core biopsy and upgrade to cancer: A systematic review and meta-analysis. Ann Surg Oncol. 2017;24(12):3549–58.
35. Grabenstetter A, Brennan S, Salagean ED, et al. Flat epithelial atypia in breast core needle biopsies with radiologic-pathologic concordance: Is excision necessary? Am J Surg Pathol. 2020;44(2): 182–90.
36. Lucioni M, Rossi C, Lomoro P, et al. Positive predictive value for malignancy of uncertain malignant potential (B3) breast lesions diagnosed on vacuum-assisted biopsy (VAB): Is surgical excision still recommended? Eur Radiol. 2021;31(2):920–7.
37. Mariscotti G, Durando M, Ruggirello I, et al. Lesions of uncertain malignant potential of the breast (B3) on vacuum-assisted biopsy for microcalcifications: Predictors of malignancy. Eur J Radiol. 2020;130:109194.
38. Arbeitsgemeinschaft Gynäkologische Onkologie. Empfehlungen gynäkologische Onkologie Kommission Mamma. 2022. Available at: https://www.ago-online.de/leitlinien-empfehlungen/leitlinien-empfehlungen/kommission-mamma.
39. Egyed Z, Péntek Z, Járay B, et al. Radial scar-significant diagnostic challenge. Pathol Oncol Res. 2008;14(2):123–9.
40. Lee E, Wylie E, Metcalf C. Ultrasound imaging features of radial scars of the breast. Australas Radiol. 2007;51(3):240–5.
41. Grunwald S, Heyer H, Kühl A, et al. Radial scar/complex sclerosing lesion of the breast—value of ultrasound. Ultraschall Med. 2007;28(2):206–11.
42. Choudhery S, Johnson MP, Larson NB, et al. Malignant outcomes of architectural distortion on tomosynthesis: A systematic review and meta-analysis. AJR. 2021;217(2):295–303.
43. Cohen MA, Newell MS. Radial scars of the breast encountered at core biopsy: Review of histologic, imaging, and management considerations. AJR. 2017;209(5):1168–77.
44. Hammersley JA, Partridge SC, Blitzer GC, et al. Management of high-risk breast lesions found on mammogram or ultrasound: The value of contrast-enhanced MRI to exclude malignancy. Clin Imaging. 2018;49:174–80.
45. Amitai Y, Scaranelo A, Menes TS, et al. Can breast MRI accurately exclude malignancy in mammographic architectural distortion? Eur Radiol. 2020;30(5):2751–60.
46. Alsharif S, Aldis A, Subahi A, et al. Breast MRI does not help differentiating radial scar with and without associated atypia or malignancy. Can Assoc Radiol J. 2021;72(4):759–66.
47. Rakha E, Beca F, D'Andrea M, et al. Outcome of radial scar/complex sclerosing lesion associated with epithelial proliferations with atypia diagnosed on breast core biopsy: Results from a multicentric UK-based study. J Clin Pathol. 2019;72(12):800–4.
48. Farshid G, Buckley E. Meta-analysis of upgrade rates in 3163 radial scars excised after needle core biopsy diagnosis. Breast Cancer Res Treat. 2019;174(1):165.

49. Kraft E, Limberg JN, Dodelzon K, et al. Radial scars and complex sclerosing lesions of the breast: Prevalence of malignancy and natural history under active surveillance. Ann Surg Oncol. 2021;28(9):5149–55.
50. Ferreira AI, Borges S, Sousa A, et al. Radial scar of the breast: Is it possible to avoid surgery? Eur J Surg Oncol. 2017;43(7):1265–72.
51. Groen EJ, Hudecek J, Mulder L, et al. Prognostic value of histopathological DCIS features in a large-scale international interrater reliability study. Breast Cancer Res Treat. 2020;183(3):759–70.
52. King TA, Pilewskie M, Muhsen S, et al. Lobular carcinoma in situ: A 29-year longitudinal experience evaluating clinicopathologic features and breast cancer risk. J Clin Oncol. 2015;33(33):3945–52.
53. Page DL, Schuyler PA, Dupont WD, et al. Atypical lobular hyperplasia as a unilateral predictor of breast cancer risk: A retrospective cohort study. Lancet. 2003;361(9352):125–9.
54. Brouwers MC, Kerkvliet K, Spithoff K. The AGREE Reporting Checklist: A tool to improve reporting of clinical practice guidelines. BMJ. 2016;352:i1152.
55. Carder P, Shaaban A. Pleomorphic lobular carcinoma in situ. Diag Histopathol. 2012;18(3):119–23.
56. Masannat YA, Husain E, Roylance R, et al. Pleomorphic LCIS what do we know? A UK multicenter audit of pleomorphic lobular carcinoma in situ. Breast. 2018;38:120–4.
57. Zhong E, Solomon JP, Cheng E, et al. Apocrine variant of pleomorphic lobular carcinoma in situ: Further clinical, histopathologic, immunohistochemical, and molecular characterization of an emerging entity. Am J Surg Pathol. 2020;44(8):1092–103.
58. Berx G, Cleton-Jansen AM, Strumane K, et al. E-cadherin is inactivated in a majority of invasive human lobular breast cancers by truncation mutations throughout its extracellular domain. Oncogene. 1996;13(9):1919–25.
59. Dabbs DJ, Bhargava R, Chivukula M. Lobular versus ductal breast neoplasms: The diagnostic utility of p120 catenin. Am J Surg Pathol. 2007;31(3):427–37.
60. Dabbs DJ, Schnitt SJ, Geyer FC, et al. Lobular neoplasia of the breast revisited with emphasis on the role of E-cadherin immunohistochemistry. Am J Surg Pathol. 2013;37(7):e1–11.
61. Hussain M, Cunnick GH. Management of lobular carcinoma in-situ and atypical lobular hyperplasia of the breast—a review. Eur J Surg Oncol. 2011;37(4):279–89.
62. Shehata MN, Rahbar H, Flanagan MR, et al. Risk for upgrade to malignancy after breast core needle biopsy diagnosis of lobular neoplasia: A systematic review and meta-analysis. J Am Coll Radiol. 2020;17(10):1207–19.
63. Foschini MP, Miglio R, Fiore R, et al. Pre-operative management of pleomorphic and florid lobular carcinoma in situ of the breast: Report of a large multi-institutional series and review of the literature. Eur J Surg Oncol. 2019;45(12):2279–86.
64. Morrow M, Schnitt SJ, Norton L. Current management of lesions associated with an increased risk of breast cancer. Nat Rev Clin Oncol. 2015;12(4):227–38.
65. Nakhlis F, Gilmore L, Gelman R, et al. Incidence of adjacent synchronous invasive carcinoma and/or ductal carcinoma in-situ in patients with lobular neoplasia on core biopsy: Results from a prospective multi-institutional registry (TBCRC 020). Ann Surg Oncol. 2016;23(3):722–8.
66. Brogi E. The morphologic spectrum of lobular carcinoma in situ (LCIS) observations on clinical significance, management implications and diagnostic pitfalls of classic, florid and pleomorphic LCIS. Virchows Archiv. 2022;481(6):823-37.
67. Cheng P, Huang Q, Shou J, et al. Treatment and survival outcomes of lobular carcinoma in situ of the breast: A SEER population based study. Oncotarget. 2017;8(61):103047–54.
68. van Maaren MC, Ávila AO, van Manen JG, et al. Trends in incidence, treatment, survival and subsequent breast cancer in lobular carcinoma in situ in the Netherlands: A population-based analysis. Breast. 2021;59:376–82.
69. Eiada R, Chong J, Kulkarni S, et al. Papillary lesions of the breast: MRI, ultrasound, and mammographic appearances. AJR Am J Roentgenol. 2012;198(2):264–71.
70. Kulka J, Madaras L, Floris G, et al. Papillary lesions of the breast. Virchows Arch. 2022;480(1):65–84.
71. Ginter PS, Hoda SA, Ozerdem U. Exuberant squamous metaplasia in an intraductal papilloma of breast. Int J Surg Pathol. 2015;23(2):125–6.
72. Guidelines Working Group of the UK National Coordinating Committee for Breast Pathology. Pathology reporting of breast disease in surgical excision specimens incorporating the dataset for histological reporting of breast cancer. The Royal College of Pathologists, 2016. Available at: https://www.rcpath.org/profession/guidelines/cancer-datasets-and-tissue-pathways.html (Accessed September 2022).
73. Jacobs TW, Connolly JL, Schnitt SJ. Nonmalignant lesions in breast core needle biopsies: To excise or not to excise? Am J Surg Pathol. 2002;26(9):1095–110.
74. Shouhed D, Amersi FF, Spurrier R, et al. Intraductal papillary lesions of the breast: Clinical and pathological correlation. Am Surgeon. 2012;78(10):1161–5.
75. Lin LH, Ozerdem U, Cotzia P, et al. Upgrade rate of intraductal papilloma diagnosed on core needle biopsy in a single institution. Human Pathol. 2021;110:43–9.
76. Khan S, Diaz A, Archer KJ, et al. Papillary lesions of the breast: To excise or observe? Breast J. 2018;24(3):350–5.
77. Zhang X, Liu W, Hai T, et al. Upgrade rate and predictive factors for breast benign intraductal papilloma diagnosed at biopsy: A meta-analysis. Ann Surg Oncol. 2021;28(13):8643–50.
78. Kuehner G, Darbinian J, Habel L, et al. Benign papillary breast mass lesions: Favorable outcomes with surgical excision or imaging surveillance. Ann Surg Oncol. 2019;26(6):1695–703.
79. Choi HY, Kim SM, Jang M, et al. Benign breast papilloma without atypia: Outcomes of surgical excision versus US-guided directional vacuum-assisted removal or US follow-up. Radiology. 2019;293(1):72–80.
80. Ditsch N, Wocke A, Untch M, et al. AGO recommendations for the diagnosis and treatment of patients with early breast cancer: Update 2022. Breast Care. 2022;17(4):403–20.
81. Houssami N, Ciatto S, Bilous M, et al. Borderline breast core needle histology: Predictive values for malignancy in lesions of uncertain malignant potential (B3). Br J Cancer. 2007;96(8):1253–7.
82. Mousa-Doust D, Dingee CK, Chen L, et al. Excision of breast fibroepithelial lesions: When is it still necessary?-A 10-year review of a regional centre. Breast Cancer Res Treat. 2022;194(2):307–14.
83. Monticciolo DL, Newell MS, Moy L, et al. Breast cancer screening in women at higher than average risk: Recommendations from the ACR. J Am Coll Radiol. 2018;15(3):408–14.
84. Clauser P, Marino MA, Baltzer PAT, et al. Management of atypical lobular hyperplasia, atypical ductal hyperplasia, and lobular carcinoma in situ. Expert Rev Anticancer Ther. 2016;16:335–46.
85. Shoker BS, Jarvis C, Clarke RB, et al. Estrogen receptor-positive proliferating cells in the normal and precancerous breast. Am J Pathol. 1999;155(6):1811–5.
86. Mao X, Qiao Z, Fan C, et al. Expression pattern and methylation of estrogen receptor α in breast intraductal proliferative lesions. Oncol Rep. 2016;36(4):1868–74.
87. Fisher B, Costantino JP, Wickerham DL, et al. Tamoxifen for prevention of breast cancer: Report of the National Surgical Adjuvant Breast and Bowel Project P-1 study. J Natl Cancer Inst. 1998;90(18):1371–88.
88. Fisher B, Costantino JP, Wickerham DL, et al. Tamoxifen for the prevention of breast cancer: Current status of the National Surgical Adjuvant Breast and Bowel Project P-1 study. J Natl Cancer Inst. 2005;97(22):1652–62.
89. Cuzick J, Sestak I, Forbes JF, et al. Use of anastrozole for breast cancer prevention (IBIS-II): long-term results of a randomised controlled trial. Lancet. 2020;395(10218):117–22.
90. Goss PE, Ingle JN, Ales-Martinez JE, et al. Exemestane for breast-cancer prevention in postmenopausal women. N Engl J Med. 2011;364(25):2381–91.
91. Owens DK, Davidson KW, Krist AH, et al. Medication use to reduce risk of breast cancer: US preventive services task force recommendation statement. JAMA. 2019;322(9):857–67.
92. Sessa C, Balmaña J, Bober SL, et al. Risk reduction and screening of cancer in hereditary breast-ovarian cancer syndromes: ESMO Clinical Practice Guideline. Ann Oncol. 2023;34(1):33–47.

6

Breast Pathology

Elena Provenzano

6.1 Introduction

Histopathology forms one of the cornerstones of the triple assessment for all breast lesions alongside clinical examination and radiological investigations, with the histopathologist a key member of the multidisciplinary team. Within the United Kingdom National Health Service Breast Screening Programme (NHS BSP), all breast core biopsies are placed into five categories: B1—normal breast tissue, B2—benign lesions, B3—lesions of uncertain malignant potential including radial scars and papillary lesions where there is a risk of associated carcinoma, B4—suspicious for malignancy, B5—malignant (5a in situ, 5b invasive) (1). This chapter describes some of the common entities in breast pathology.

6.2 Fibroepithelial Lesions

Fibroepithelial lesions have two components, a glandular and a fibrous stromal element. There are three main fibroepithelial lesions arising in the breast: hamartomas, fibroadenomas, and phyllodes tumours.

Hamartomas are circumscribed lesions composed of normal breast tissue components including glands, fibrous stroma, fat, and smooth muscle with a disorganised configuration. There is no association with malignancy.

Fibroadenomas are biphasic lesions composed of tubular or elongated compressed glands within a fibrous stromal background [Figure 6.1a]. They are well circumscribed, and the stromal component is usually hypocellular with no atypia and absent or rare mitoses. Cellular fibroadenomas show mild to moderately increased cellularity but lack cytological atypia and the leaf-like growth pattern seen in phyllodes tumours. Juvenile fibroadenomas arise in adolescent females and have a pericanalicular growth pattern with epithelial hyperplasia like that seen in gynaecomastia.

Phyllodes tumours are neoplastic lesions that show increased stromal cellularity and have a prominent intracanalicular growth pattern with leaf-like architecture. They are much less common than fibroadenomas, accounting for about 2.5% of fibroepithelial lesions (2). Phyllodes tumours form a spectrum from benign to malignant [Table 6.1]. Benign phyllodes tumours are circumscribed with mildly increased stromal cellularity and minimal atypia [Figure 6.1b], whereas malignant phyllodes tumours show markedly increased cellularity with stromal overgrowth and severe atypia and have the appearance and behaviour of sarcomas [Figure 6.1c]. Borderline phyllodes tumours have intermediate characteristics. Local recurrences typically occur within 3 years of initial diagnosis, with progression to a higher grade in approximately one third of cases (3). Re-excision of benign phyllodes tumours is no longer advocated if tumour is present at margins; however, borderline and malignant lesions should be completely excised with a clear margin. Metastases occur in approximately 2% of cases, almost exclusively following excision of malignant lesions (2).

6.3 Sclerosing Lesions

Sclerosing lesions are benign glandular proliferations with a lobular distribution where the glands are distorted by fibrosis. They can mimic carcinoma both clinically and histologically (4). Sclerosing adenosis comprises expanded lobular units with proliferation of small acini and tubules that are compressed and distorted by stromal collagen. A myoepithelial layer is preserved around the glands, which can be demonstrated by immunohistochemistry for markers such as p63 or smooth-muscle myosin to distinguish sclerosing adenosis from invasive carcinoma.

DOI: 10.1201/9781003394785-6

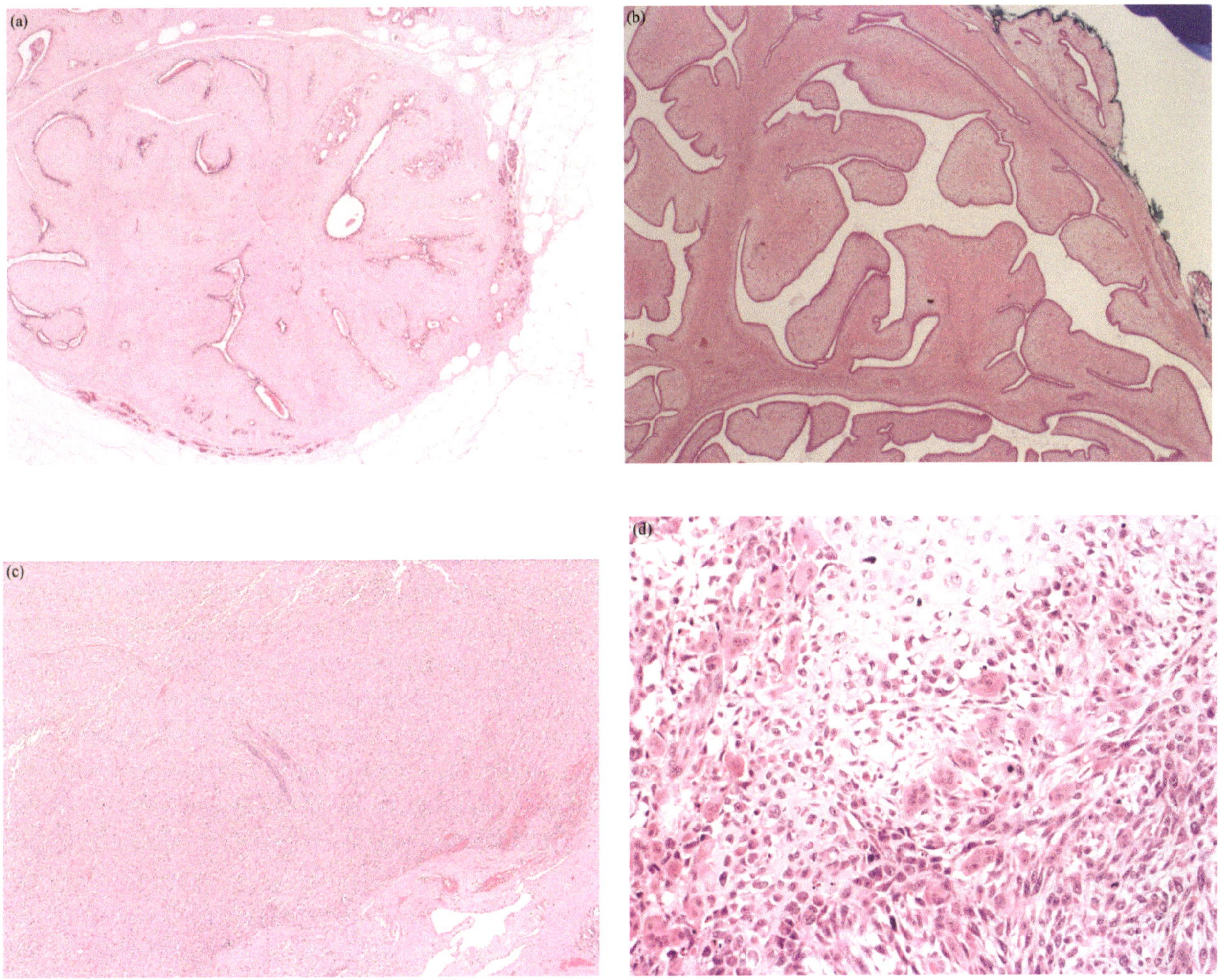

FIGURE 6.1
(a) Fibroadenoma. Circumscribed lesion with compressed, elongated glands within a hypocellular fibrous stroma. (b) Benign phyllodes tumour. Lesion shows glandular spaces with leaf-like architecture within mildly cellular stroma. There is condensation of the stromal cells beneath the epithelium. (c) Malignant phyllodes tumour. Lesion with markedly increased stromal cellularity and stromal overgrowth with rare residual glands. The stromal cells show marked atypia and frequent mitoses. (d) Malignant phyllodes tumour with heterologous osteosarcomatous differentiation including osteoclastic giant cells.

TABLE 6.1
Grading System for Phyllodes Tumours of the Breast, Adapted from (2)

	Benign	Borderline	Malignant
Tumour edge	Well defined	May be focally infiltrative	Infiltrative
Stromal cellularity	Mild, non-uniform or diffuse	Moderate, non-uniform or diffuse	Marked, typically diffuse
Stromal atypia	Mild	Moderate	Severe
Stromal overgrowth	Absent	Absent	Present
Malignant heterologous elements	Absent	Absent	May be present—sufficient to class tumour as malignant
Frequency	60–75%	15–25%	8–20%
Risk of recurrence	10–17%	14–25%	23–30%

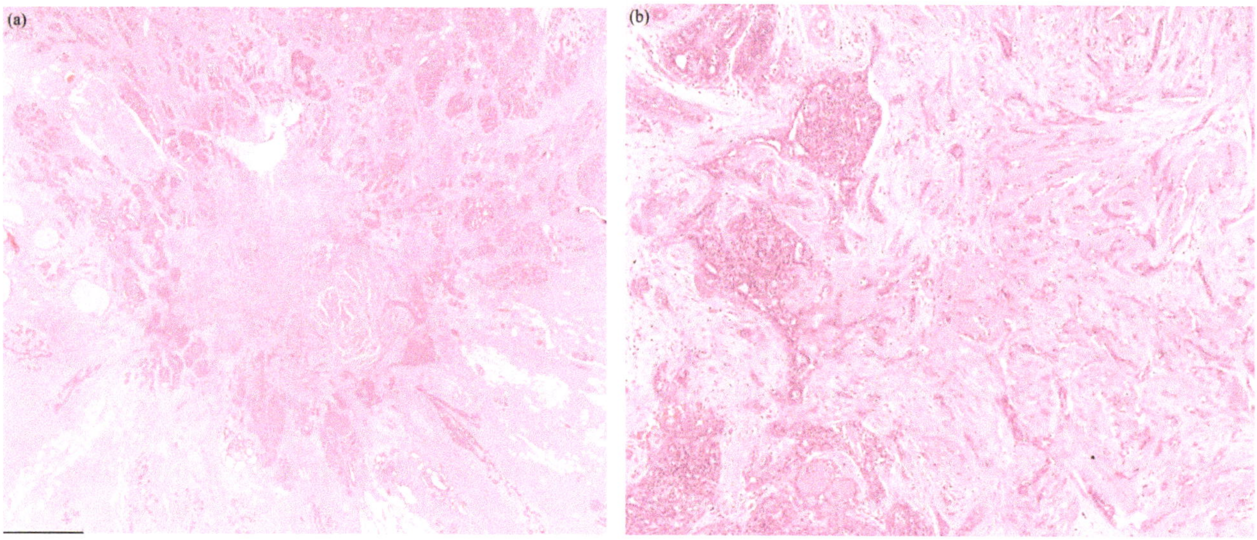

FIGURE 6.2
(a) Low-power view of a complex sclerosing lesion showing central fibroelastosis with entrapped glands and surrounding glandular proliferation with usual epithelial hyperplasia and fibrocystic change. (b) Higher-power view of central area with angulated glands distorted by fibrosis and more peripheral glands on the left with usual hyperplasia. The clear cells around the edge of the glands are myoepithelial cells.

Radial scars and complex sclerosing lesions (CSLs) have a central area of fibroelastosis with entrapped tubules surrounded by proliferative changes including usual epithelial hyperplasia and fibrocystic change [Figure 6.2]. Radial scars are small discrete lesions <1 cm in size, whereas CSLs are larger and more disorganised. In the NHS BSP, radial scars/CSLs are given a B3 classification as there is a risk of associated malignancy (1), usually in the form of grade 1 or 2 invasive carcinoma or low-grade DCIS (4). The risk of malignancy is related to the presence or absence of epithelial atypia; in cases without atypia, the upgrade rate is 4–6%, and as high as 44% when atypia is present (4). Hence, further tissue sampling with vacuum biopsy or open excision is recommended.

6.4 Papillary Lesions

Papillary lesions are characterised by fibrovascular cores lined by epithelial cells, often lying within a dilated duct or cystic space [Figure 6.3a]. The distinction between benign and malignant papillary lesions is based on the presence of epithelial atypia, and the presence or absence of a myoepithelial layer internally along the fibrovascular cores and/or externally in the surrounding cystic space (5). Benign papillomas have a preserved myoepithelial layer throughout and show no cytological atypia. Papillomas can become focally or entirely involved by ductal carcinoma in situ (DCIS), where the epithelial component shows cytological and/or architectural atypia such as the formation of cribriform spaces. In papillary DCIS, the fibrovascular cores are often delicate and have lost their internal myoepithelial layer although the external layer lining the cyst is retained. The epithelium shows mild to moderate atypia and may have a tall columnar appearance.

Papillary carcinomas (PC) represent 0.5–1% of breast carcinomas and typically present as a mass lesion in post-menopausal patients, with an average age of 70–73 years (6–8). Many are situated close to the nipple, where they may present with nipple discharge. Macroscopically they are often circumscribed with a friable texture and areas of haemorrhage. On microscopy, PCs are typically low to intermediate grade with mild to moderate atypia (7–9). Around 75% of cases have an adjacent component of DCIS.

PC can be divided into three types (6, 10):

1. Encapsulated PC is well circumscribed, comprising a cystic space with a fibrous capsule containing a delicate network of fibrovascular cores lined by neoplastic epithelial cells [Figure 6.3b]. There is no myoepithelial layer. Encapsulated PC is regarded as an indolent form of invasive carcinoma that has an excellent prognosis (7). Distant metastases are extremely rare. In the absence of a frank invasive component extending beyond the

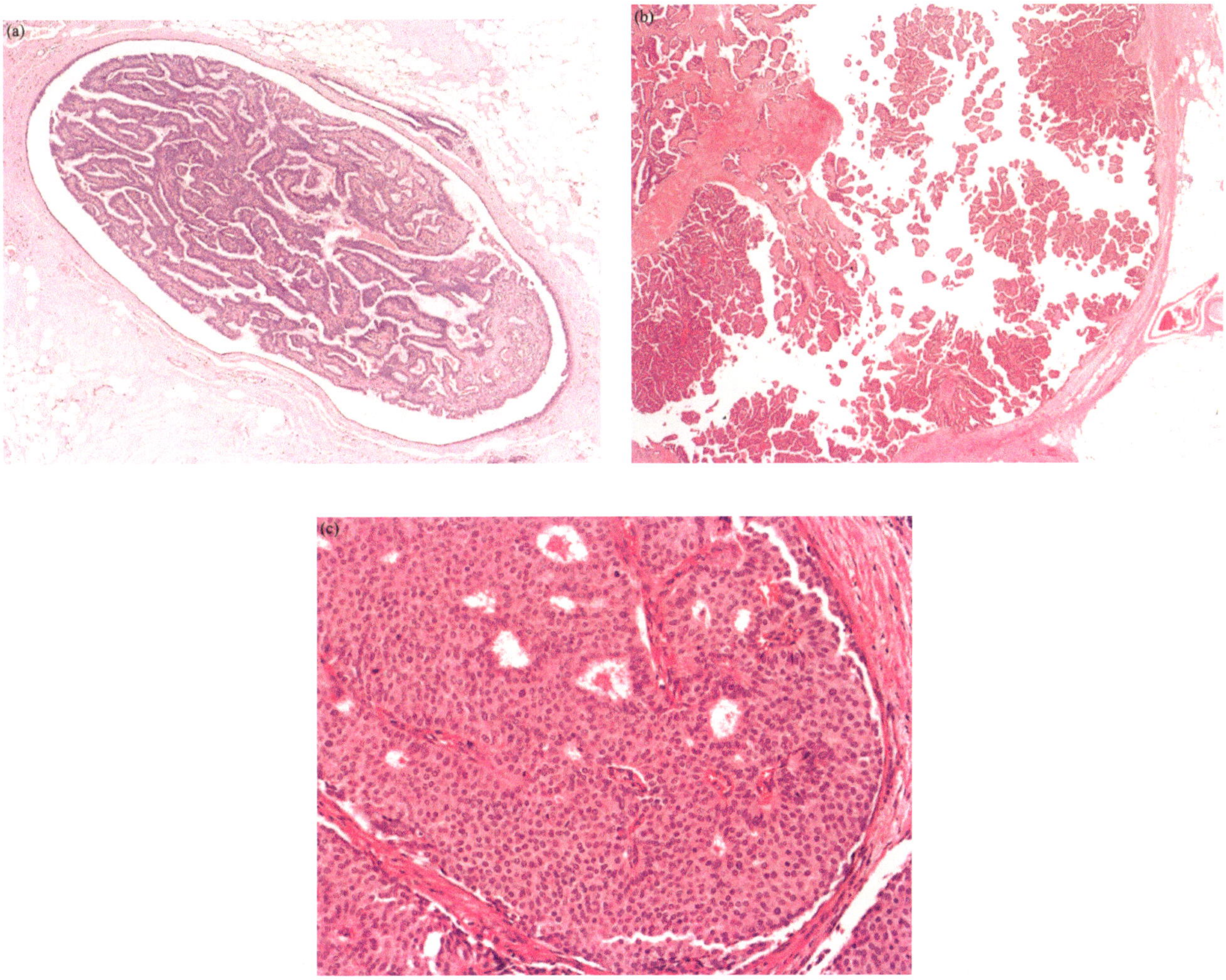

FIGURE 6.3
(a) Benign intraduct papilloma. Cystically dilated duct space containing a papillary lesion with fibrovascular cores lined by bland cuboidal to columnar cells. (b) Encapsulated papillary carcinoma. Cystic space with a thin fibrous capsule containing a complex network of fibrovascular cores lined by columnar cells with mild to moderate nuclear atypia (inset). (c) Solid papillary carcinoma in situ. Solid island of cells with a smooth outer contour that on closer inspection contains fibrovascular cores with polarisation of cells around the periphery.

capsule 3–6% have lymph node metastases, and they should be classified as in situ disease for TNM staging (7, 8, 11) and be managed in a similar fashion to DCIS (5, 7).

2. Solid PC comprises a well circumscribed or multinodular tumour formed by solid sheets of cells with delicate fibrovascular cores and may be in situ or invasive in nature [Figure 6.3c]. The cells may have a spindled or neuroendocrine appearance.
3. True invasive PCs are rare and consist of carcinoma with pure papillary morphology with an infiltrative growth pattern.

Nearly all PCs are oestrogen receptor (ER) and progesterone receptor (PR) positive and HER2 negative (8–10). They are of luminal A subtype and show similar genetic changes to low-grade NST carcinomas (10).

6.5 Carcinoma In Situ

Carcinoma in situ is a non-invasive proliferation of neoplastic cells confined to ducts and lobular acini. There are two forms of carcinoma in situ, ductal and lobular. Carcinoma in situ acts as a non-obligate precursor to invasive disease, although there is currently a lack of reliable markers to predict which lesions will progress.

Ductal carcinoma in situ (DCIS) is a proliferation of cohesive neoplastic epithelial cells typically confined to a single-duct system, although extension into lobules may occur. DCIS is heterogeneous with varying nuclear grade and architectural patterns [Figure 6.4] and different molecular subtypes akin to invasive breast cancer. Grading of DCIS is primarily on nuclear morphology, with low-grade DCIS having regular round nuclei 1.5–2 times the size of a red blood cell, whereas high-grade DCIS has large irregular nuclei >2.5 times the size of a red blood cell and can show other features such as necrosis (12). Intermediate-grade DCIS is in between. Architectural patterns include solid, cribriform, micropapillary, and flat. DCIS may be associated with microcalcification, which is commonly how it is identified mammographically, and DCIS represents approximately 20–25% of screen-detected cancers (13).

Lobular carcinoma in situ (LCIS) is a non-invasive proliferation of discohesive cells arising in the terminal duct lobular unit. There are three main types of LCIS: classical LCIS, florid LCIS, and pleomorphic LCIS (14). In classical LCIS, acini are expanded by small, uniform cells which may contain mucin vacuoles [Figure 6.5a]. Florid LCIS has cells like those in classical LCIS, but with marked distension of acini more than 40–50 cells across, forming a mass-like lesion. Pleomorphic LCIS is composed of cells with marked nuclear atypia like high-grade DCIS [Figure 6.5b]. The cells may have an apocrine appearance with abundant eosinophilic cytoplasm, and there may be associated central necrosis and coarse microcalcifications.

LCIS was initially described as a marker of bilateral increased risk of invasive breast carcinoma; however, it is now recognised to act as a non-obligate precursor of invasive lobular carcinoma. Classical LCIS is multicentric in the ipsilateral breast in as many as 80% of patients and bilateral in 30–67% and is given a B3 classification with recommendation for further tissue sampling followed by annual follow-up (1). Florid and pleomorphic LCIS tend to be focal lesions with a risk of coexistent invasive carcinoma of up to 33% so recommended management is complete excision with clear margins as for DCIS (14).

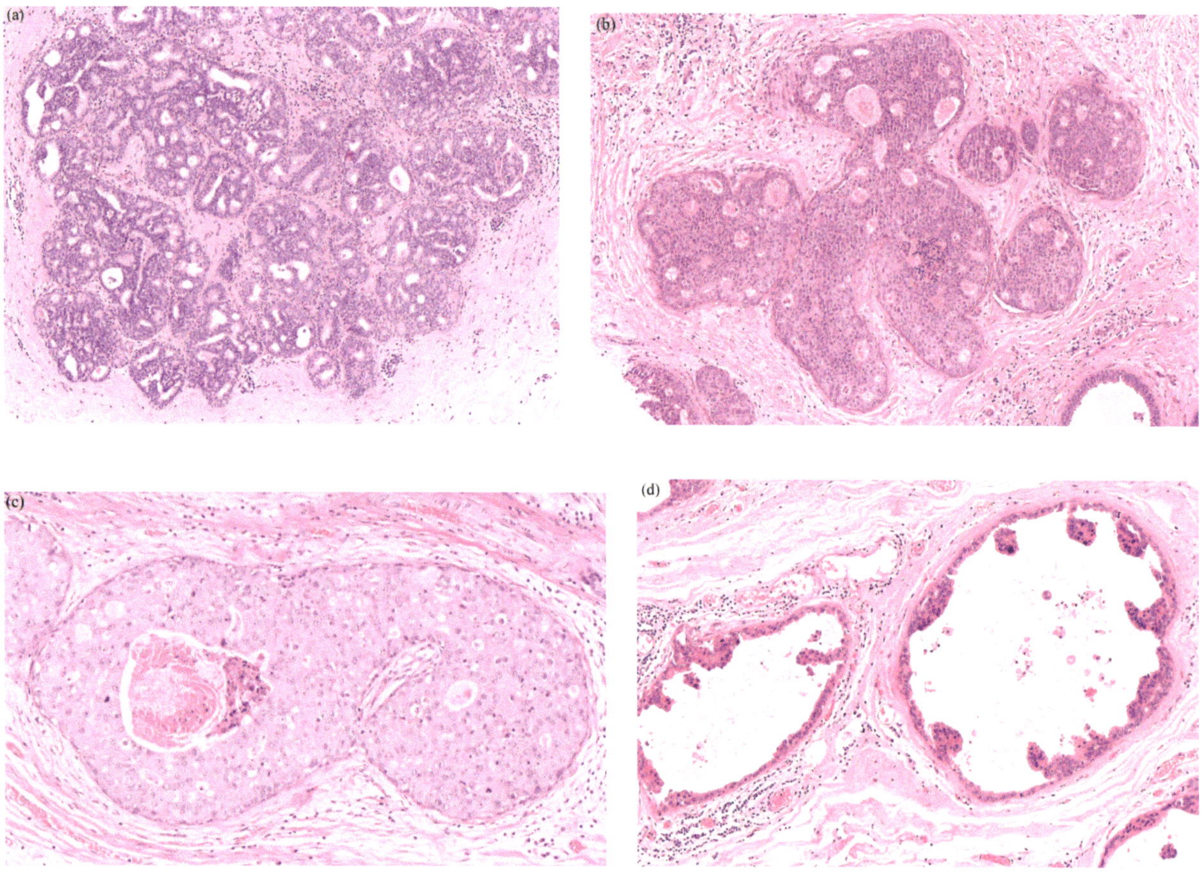

FIGURE 6.4
(a) Low-grade DCIS. The cells have regular small round nuclei and form a cribriform pattern with punched out glandular spaces. (b) Intermediate-grade DCIS. The cell nuclei are slightly larger with more variation in size and shape. There is focal necrosis in one of the ducts. c) High-grade solid DCIS. The cells show marked atypia with variation in size and shape. Central necrosis is present. d) High-grade DCIS with micropapillary architecture. There is marked nuclear atypia and mitotic figures can be seen.

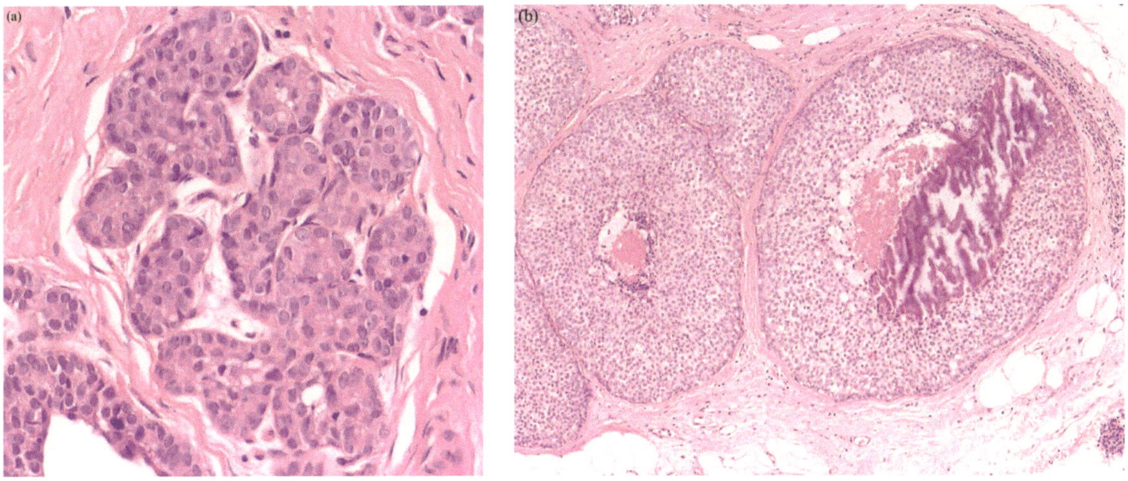

FIGURE 6.5
(a) Classical LCIS. Expansion of acini by a monomorphic population of cells with a discohesive pattern. Some of the cells have mucin vacuoles which appear as clear spaces within the cytoplasm. (b) Pleomorphic LCIS. Marked expansion of acini by cells with marked nuclear atypia like those seen in high-grade DCIS. The cells have a discohesive growth pattern. There is central necrosis and coarse calcification (granular purple material).

6.6 Microinvasive Carcinoma

Microinvasion is defined as one or more foci of invasive cancer <1 mm in size (15, 16). It is typically identified in the context of extensive high-grade DCIS, although more rarely it can be seen with low-grade DCIS or LCIS. Microinvasion often occurs in the setting of inflammation and a desmoplastic stromal reaction, and immunohistochemistry to confirm absence of a myoepithelial cell layer around the infiltrating tumour cells may be required for a definite diagnosis. If there is any doubt about the diagnosis, the lesion should be classified as in situ carcinoma. Microinvasive carcinoma has an excellent prognosis like that of pure in situ carcinoma, with a low incidence of axillary lymph node metastases (17).

6.7 Invasive Breast Cancer

Breast cancer is not one disease but a group of diseases with different underlying molecular drivers. Traditionally, breast cancers are classified by tumour grade and histological subtype, many of which are associated with distinct molecular profiles and clinical behaviour [Table 6.2] (18, 19). Alongside the increase in understanding of breast cancer biology, surgical and oncological management has become more sophisticated. Neoadjuvant treatment has become standard of care for high-risk breast cancer, particularly HER2-positive and triple-negative disease (20). As a result, the complexity of breast cancer specimens has increased. Pathological work up requires a team approach, and relevant clinical and radiological information must accompany the surgical specimen to ensure accurate histological interpretation (21).

6.7.1 Histological Grade

All breast cancers including special types should be graded using the Nottingham Grading System (22). Three features are evaluated—tubule formation, nuclear pleomorphism, and mitotic count [Figure 6.6], with each component given a score of 1–3 [Table 6.3]. Tubule or gland formation is assessed across the whole tumour at low magnification. Nuclear pleomorphism is assessed in the area showing the most severe atypia compared with normal epithelial nuclei. Mitotic count is also determined in the area with the highest number of mitoses, often at the tumour edge. Cut off values depend upon the x40 field diameter of the microscope. The three scores are then added up to give the final tumour grade.

6.7.2 Histological Subtypes

6.7.2.1 Invasive Carcinoma of No Special Type (NST)

The most common type of infiltrating breast carcinoma, accounting for up to 75% of all cancers (23). NST cancers are also referred to as invasive ductal carcinoma, from the historical concept that they arose from the ductal epithelium, in contrast to lobular

TABLE 6.2

Incidence, Molecular Subtype, and Prognosis of More Common Forms of Special-Type Breast Cancer

Special Type	Incidence	ER/HER2 Status	Molecular Subtype	Prognosis
Lobular—classical	5–15%	ER+, HER2−	Luminal A	Better or similar to NST; poor response to NACT
Lobular—pleomorphic		Up to 23% ER−, 14% HER2+	Luminal B, HER2E or molecular apocrine	Worse than classical lobular
Tubular	2%; 9–19% screen detected ca	ER+, HER2−	Luminal A	Excellent
Cribriform	1–3.5%	ER+, HER2−	Luminal A	Excellent
Mucinous	2–5%; more common in older women	ER+, HER2−	Luminal A	Pure form good prognosis in older women
Micropapillary	<2%, 6% mixed tumours	75–92% ER+, up to 33% HER2+	Luminal B	Worse prognosis, often N+
Apocrine	1%	ER−, up to 30% HER2+	Molecular apocrine, HER2E	Similar to NST; lower response to NACT
Metaplastic	<1%	Triple negative	Basal	Poor prognosis; lower response to NACT
Adenoid cystic	0.1%	Triple negative	Basal	Good prognosis
Secretory	<0.2%	Triple negative	Basal	Good prognosis

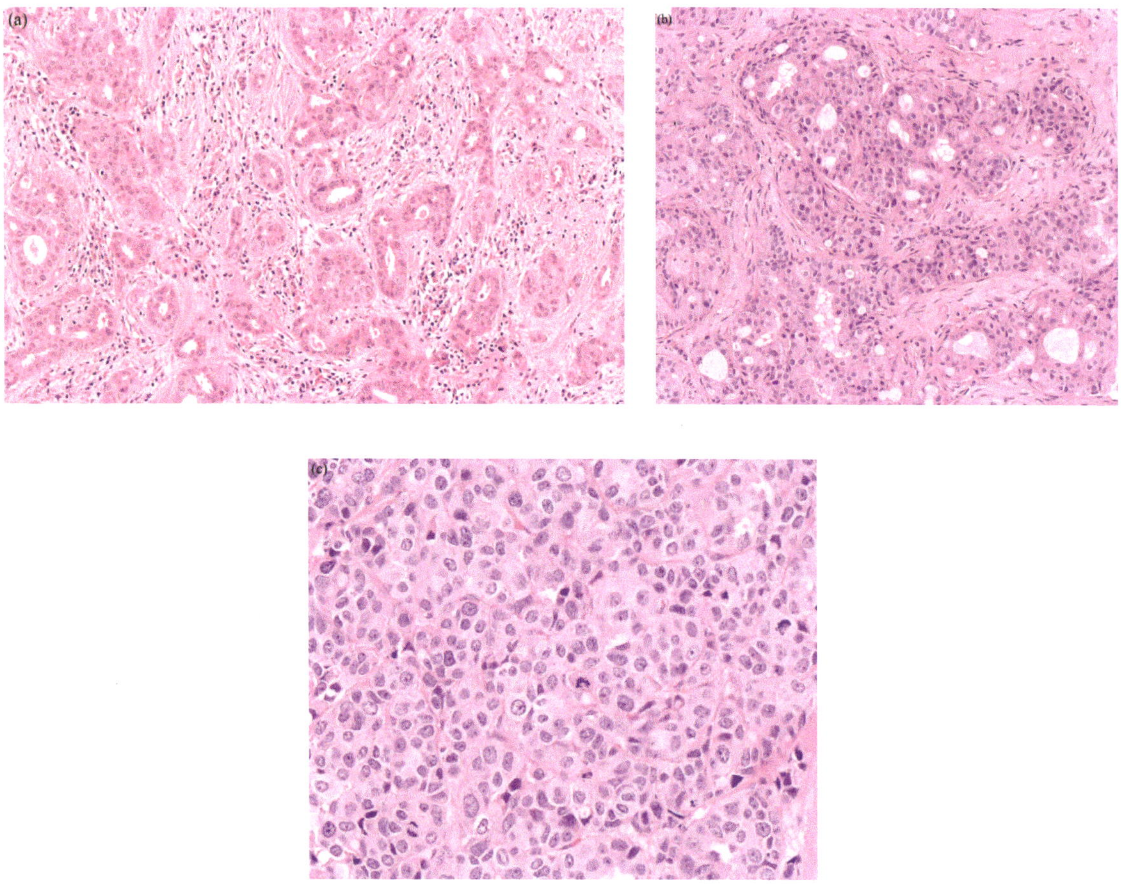

FIGURE 6.6
(a) Grade 1 invasive carcinoma with extensive tubule formation (score 1) and regular round nuclei (pleomorphism score 2). Mitoses are rare (score 1). (b) Grade 2 invasive carcinoma showing some tubule formation (score 2). The nuclei are larger with more variation in size and shape (score 3); however, mitoses are infrequent (score 1). (c) Grade 3 invasive carcinoma. There is no tubule formation (score 3). There is marked variation in nuclear size and shape (score 3) and mitoses are frequent (score 3). All these cancers lack features of any of the special types so are invasive carcinoma of no special type (NST).

TABLE 6.3

Nottingham Grading System for Determining Tumour Grade in Breast Cancer, High-Power Field (40× Objective), Modified from (22)

Feature		Score
Tubule/gland formation	>75%	1
	10–75%	2
	<10%	3
Nuclear pleomorphism	Small, regular round nuclei	1
	Moderate variation in size and shape	2
	Marked variation in size and shape	3
Mitoses	Count per 10 HPF, cut-offs dependent on field area	1–3
	Overall Grade	**Final Score**
	Grade 1	3–5
	Grade 2	6, 7
	Grade 3	8, 9

cancers that arose within the lobules. It is now known the site of origin of most breast cancers is the terminal duct lobular unit (24), where the mammary progenitor cells are believed to be located (25).

Invasive carcinoma NST lacks the histological features of one of the special types of cancer described later. If more than 10% of the tumour has a specialised pattern, the tumour is referred to as mixed NST and special type (26). NST cancers are very heterogeneous composed of tumour cells arranged in glands, clusters, trabeculae, or solid sheets set within a variable amount of fibrous stroma. There may be a prominent lymphoplasmacytic inflammatory infiltrate, called tumour infiltrating lymphocytes (TILS). NST cancers commonly appear macroscopically as moderately circumscribed firm grey-white masses with a stellate or rounded outline.

An associated component of DCIS may be present in up to 80% of cases (26), and the grade of the DCIS usually reflects that of the invasive cancer (27). The DCIS component may be confined to the invasive tumour or extend into the surrounding breast tissue. In the latter situation the entire lesion size including DCIS must be recorded as well as the invasive tumour size, and the distance of DCIS to excision margins measured (28).

Approximately 70–80% of NST cancers are ER positive (29, 30), and around 10–20% are HER2 positive (29, 31). Low-grade NST cancers tend to be of luminal subtype and are typically ER positive and HER2 negative, whilst high-grade cancers may be negative for ER and are more likely to be HER2 positive.

Prognosis is influenced by grade, size, lymph node status, and the presence of lymphovascular invasion, with grade and nodal involvement being the most important determinants of outcome (32, 33). ER and HER2 status are important predictive factors in determining the benefit of adjuvant hormonal and chemotherapy but also have prognostic value. Molecular studies highlight the great heterogeneity amongst NST tumours at the genetic level, leading to novel classification systems that subclassify NST tumours into groups with distinct clinical behaviour, discussed further in the next section (34).

6.7.2.2 *Invasive Carcinoma NST with Medullary Features*

In the most recent WHO classification of tumours of the breast, medullary carcinoma is now considered a subtype of NST cancers (26). Invasive carcinoma NST with medullary features are highly cellular tumours composed of sheets of markedly pleomorphic cells with a high mitotic rate, well-circumscribed 'pushing' margin, and a prominent lymphoplasmacytic infiltrate [Figure 6.7]. They tend to occur in younger women (35). As they are well circumscribed with a soft texture, they may be confused with benign lesions clinically and radiologically. There may be associated necrosis and haemorrhage.

Medullary-like carcinomas are typically triple negative (ER, PR, and HER2) and show positive staining for basal cytokeratins CK5 and CK14 (36). On gene expression array analysis, they belong with the basal group of breast cancers (19).

Carcinomas with medullary features are more frequently found in BRCA1 mutation carriers (37). Conversely, BRCA1 gene mutations have been identified in up to 11% of medullary cancers (38). In the absence of a somatic mutation, there is often downregulation of BRCA1 function by other mechanisms such as gene promoter methylation.

Despite the aggressive tumour characteristics, medullary-like carcinomas have been associated with a relatively favourable prognosis compared to grade matched NST cancers (35, 39). This is believed to be due to the presence of a florid host immune reaction with high TILS. The combination of deficient DNA repair with a high proliferation rate may confer increased sensitivity to chemotherapy (39).

6.7.2.3 *Invasive Lobular Carcinoma (ILC)*

The second most common type of invasive breast carcinoma (40). ILC has a distinctive growth pattern with discohesive round cells forming single files or cords [Figure 6.8]. The cells may have intracytoplasmic mucin vacuoles resulting in a signet-ring appearance. Up to 90% of cases are associated with LCIS (41). ILC

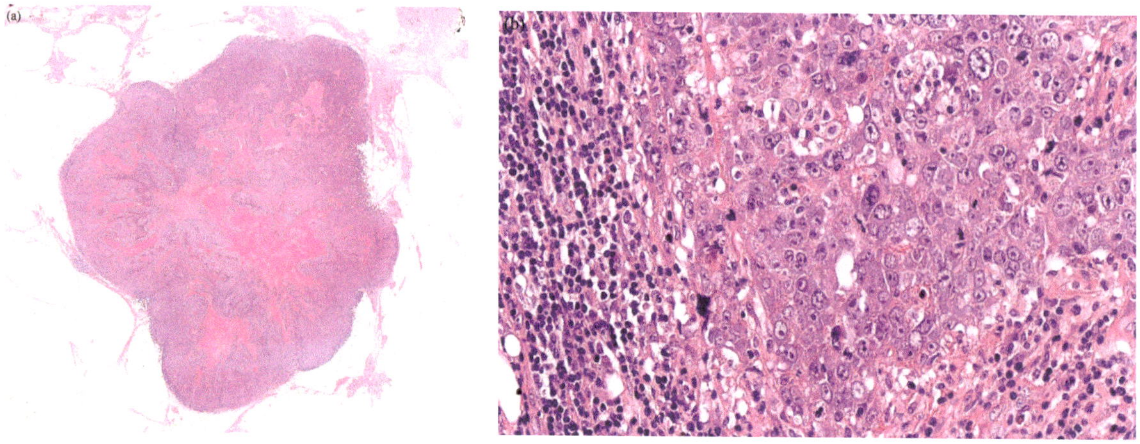

FIGURE 6.7
Invasive carcinoma NST with medullary features. (a) Low-power view showing a well-circumscribed tumour formed by sheets of cells with zones of necrosis. (b) High-power view showing pushing margin. The cells show marked nuclear atypia and mitoses are frequent. There is a dense lymphocytic infiltrate (small blue cells).

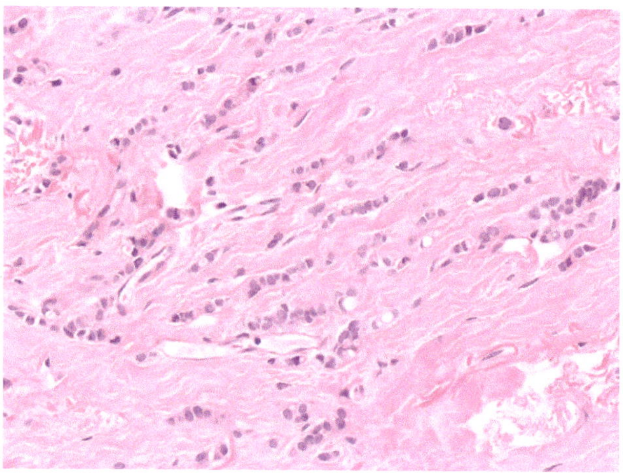

FIGURE 6.8
Invasive lobular carcinoma, classical type. Small uniform cells growing as cords and single files. Some of the cells contain mucin vacuoles giving them a signet ring appearance.

is more likely to be multifocal, and bilateral disease has been reported in 5–20% of cases (40). ILC typically grows around existing structures with little stromal reaction and therefore clinically present as ill-defined masses that may be radiologically occult or appear as asymmetric stromal density. Tumour extent is often underestimated radiologically, and MRI is a more accurate means of determining pre-operative size and detecting multifocal disease (42, 43).

Variants include solid and alveolar types, forming solid sheets and small globular aggregates of cells, respectively. The pleomorphic variant has a typical lobular growth pattern, but the cells show severe nuclear atypia and often have abundant eosinophilic cytoplasm giving them an apocrine appearance. Pleomorphic ILC is commonly associated with the pleomorphic variant of LCIS and is biologically more aggressive (44). ILC can appear macroscopically as a stellate white-grey lesion, although there may be no visible lesion with only a vague area of firmness on palpation. Tumour size may be significantly larger than the macroscopic lesion.

ILC is characterised by loss of E-cadherin expression, a protein involved in cell-to-cell adhesion and differentiation (45). However, 16–26% of phenotypically lobular cancers may show aberrant positive staining (46–48). The loss of cell adhesion gives ILC its discohesive appearance and typical growth pattern.

Some series report a slightly better prognosis for ILC than NST cancers, whilst others show similar or worse outcomes (35, 49, 50). The classical subtype of ILC has a better prognosis than the solid or alveolar variants, with pleomorphic ILC having the worst prognosis (51, 52). ILC has been associated with poor response to neoadjuvant chemotherapy (53). There is a tendency for late recurrence with a distinct pattern of metastatic spread to ovary, uterus, serosal surfaces, gastrointestinal tract, and meninges (49).

6.7.2.4 Tubular Cancer

Tubular carcinomas are well differentiated carcinomas where at least 90% of the tumour comprises angulated tubules lined by a single layer of bland cells [Figure 6.9] set in a desmoplastic stroma giving a spiculate appearance on mammography. Compared to NST tumours, they are more likely to be smaller and screen-detected (50, 54). Tubular carcinomas are commonly associated with a component of low-grade DCIS, typically of cribriform or micropapillary pattern. Lymph node metastases are rare with single node involvement.

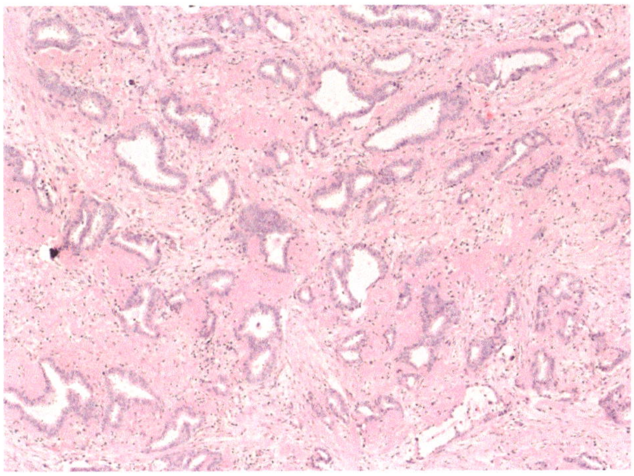

FIGURE 6.9
Invasive tubular carcinoma. Carcinoma formed almost entirely of irregular angulated tubular structures lying within a reactive stromal background. The nuclei are round and regular with minimal atypia and no mitoses.

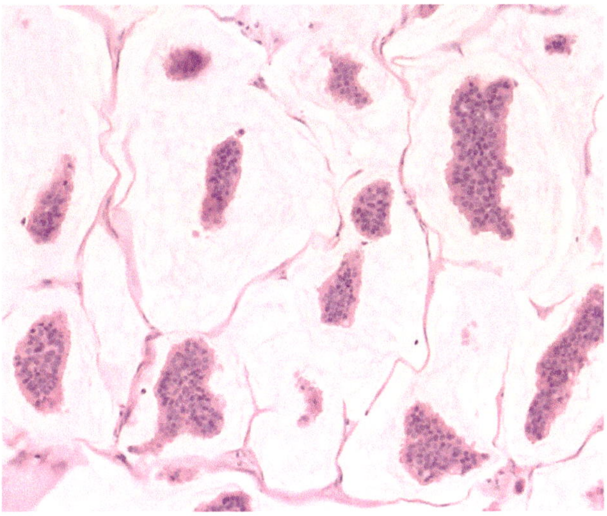

FIGURE 6.10
Invasive mucinous carcinoma. Islands of tumour cells with mild to moderate nuclear atypia floating in extracellular mucin (bluish-grey substance in the background).

6.7.2.5 Invasive Cribriform Carcinoma

Invasive carcinoma composed of irregular islands of cells with a cribriform growth pattern, like cribriform DCIS, in at least 90% of the tumour. Up to 80% of cases have an associated in situ component, most commonly low-grade cribriform DCIS (55). Cribriform carcinomas are usually screen-detected presenting as a stellate mass with associated microcalcifications.

6.7.2.6 Mucinous Carcinoma

Mucinous carcinomas consist of islands of tumour cells floating in pools of extracellular mucin [Figure 6.10]. Although these tumours are typically low-grade, high-grade cases with marked pleomorphism and mitoses can occur (56). They have a soft consistency with little fibrosis and a smooth or lobulated outline resulting in an indeterminate or benign appearance on imaging. Macroscopically, the tumours are well circumscribed with a glistening gelatinous appearance and soft consistency.

6.7.2.7 Invasive Micropapillary Carcinoma

Invasive micropapillary carcinomas consists of morule-like clusters of cells lying within stromal spaces [Figure 6.11]. The tumour cells are cuboidal to columnar with moderate to severe nuclear atypia. There may be a component of micropapillary or cribriform DCIS. Lymphovascular space invasion is common, and there is a high rate of axillary node metastases at presentation (>66%) (57).

6.7.2.8 Apocrine Carcinoma

Apocrine carcinomas show cytological features of apocrine cells with abundant granular eosinophilic cytoplasm and large nuclei with prominent nucleoli in over 90% of tumour cells [Figure 6.12] (58). Cells with apocrine differentiation can be found in NST, papillary, micropapillary, and pleomorphic lobular carcinomas.

Apocrine carcinomas are ER and PR negative, and up to 30% are HER2 positive. They express androgen receptor (58) and have a distinct gene expression profile with upregulation of androgen receptor signalling pathways (59).

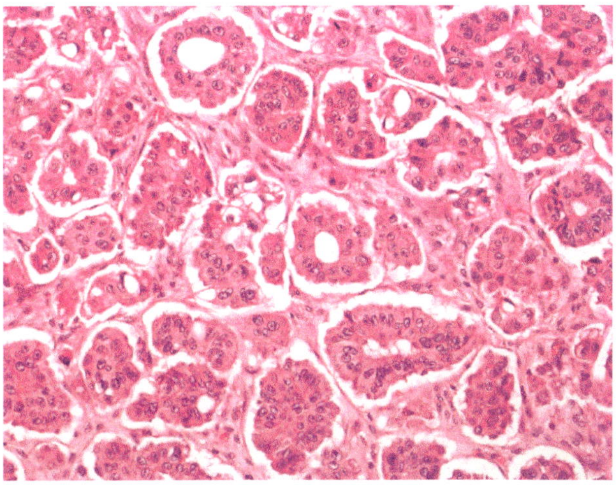

FIGURE 6.11
Invasive micropapillary carcinoma. Grape-like morular clusters and tubular structures lying within clear spaces. The cells show marked nuclear atypia and occasional mitoses can be seen.

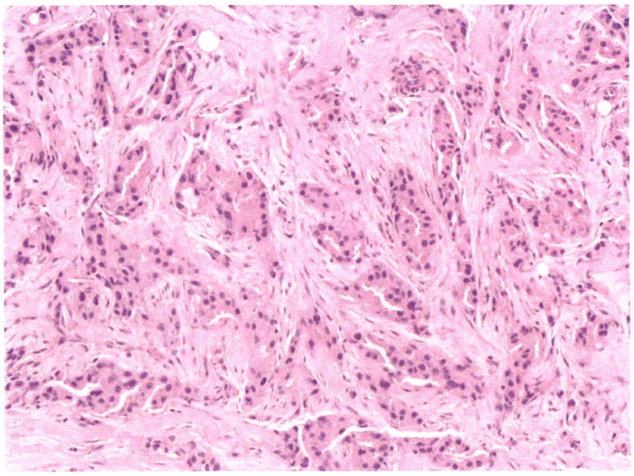

FIGURE 6.12
Invasive carcinoma with apocrine differentiation. The carcinoma consists of cells with abundant eosinophilic cytoplasm and round nuclei with prominent nucleoli.

6.7.2.9 Metaplastic Carcinoma

Metaplastic carcinomas are a group of tumours characterised by areas of spindle cell, squamous, and/or mesenchymal differentiation (60). Spindle cell carcinoma may resemble a sarcoma but show areas of epithelial differentiation and/or positive immunohistochemical staining for cytokeratins [Figure 6.13a]. Primary sarcomas of the breast are extremely rare, so a diagnosis of metaplastic carcinoma should be considered for all atypical spindle cell lesions of the breast. The epithelial component may be minimal and cytokeratin staining can be very focal, making diagnosis on core biopsy difficult (4). Pure squamous cell carcinomas of the breast are exceedingly rare [Figure 6.13b] and must be distinguished from metastatic carcinoma from other sites, particularly lung, cervix, or bladder, or primary skin cancers with extension into the breast (61).

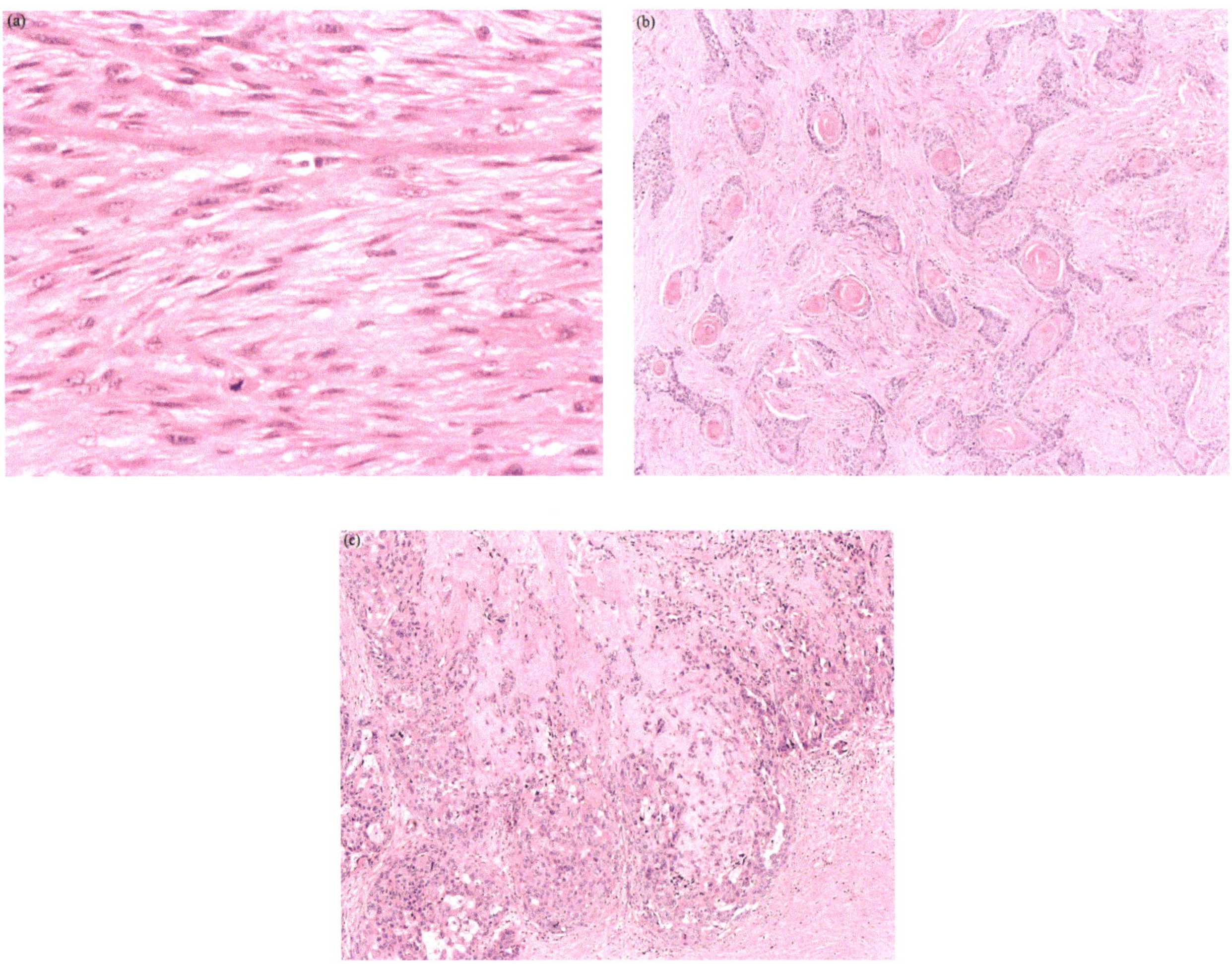

FIGURE 6.13
Metaplastic carcinoma. (a) Spindle cell carcinoma composed of elongated tapering cells with marked nuclear atypia and frequent mitoses mimicking a sarcoma. (b) Metaplastic squamous cell carcinoma showing focal keratinisation (dark pink material in some of the cell nests). Metastasis from a primary skin cancer was excluded in this case. (c) Metaplastic carcinoma with mesenchymal differentiation. The greyish pink material in the background is chondroid stroma.

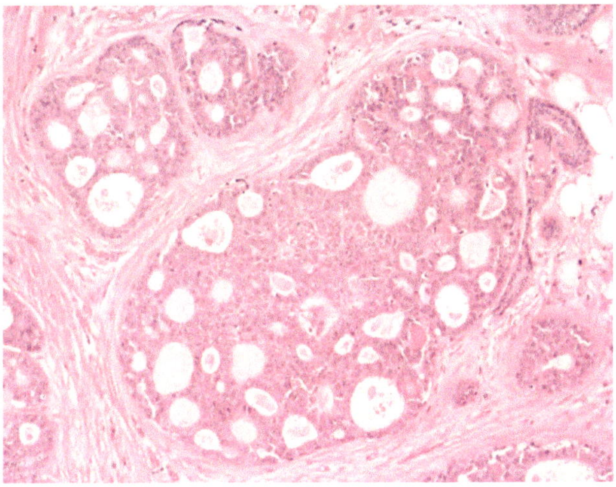

FIGURE 6.14
Adenoid cystic carcinoma. The tumour is composed of basaloid cells with cribriform architecture. Some of the spaces contain pink basement membrane material, whilst others contain bluish mucin.

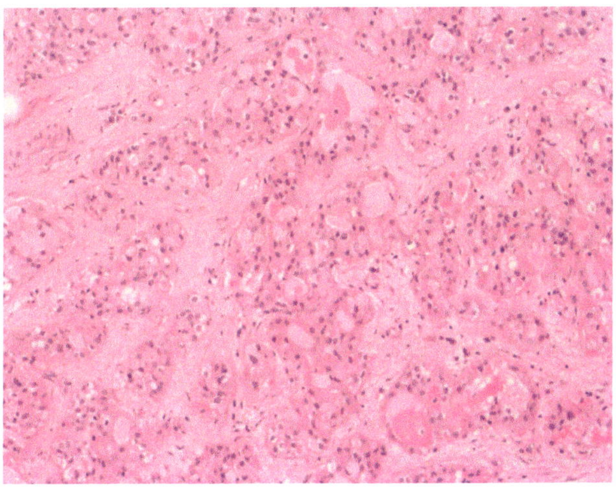

FIGURE 6.15
Secretory carcinoma. Carcinoma with microcystic spaces containing bright pink material that resembles colloid. There is mild to moderate nuclear pleomorphism.

Low-grade adenosquamous carcinoma composed of small glandular structures and nests of squamous cells in a cellular background stroma. The tendency is for local recurrence, with lymph node metastasis being extremely rare (62).

Metaplastic carcinoma with mesenchymal differentiation (previously called matrix-producing) are high-grade carcinomas with pleomorphic cells lying within a chondroid or osteoid matrix [Figure 6.13c].

Low-grade adenosquamous and fibromatosis-like cancers have a good prognosis with surgical excision alone and represent subtypes of triple-negative breast cancer where chemotherapy should be avoided. High-grade metaplastic cancers have a worse prognosis than NST cancers (35, 63) and are less responsive to neoadjuvant chemotherapy (53). They have a distinct molecular profile without the genetic instability of typical NST triple-negative breast cancers (64).

6.7.2.10 Adenoid Cystic Carcinoma

Adenoid cystic carcinomas (AdCC) of the breast share the histological features of their salivary gland counterpart. Histologically, they are composed of small basaloid cells with minimal cytoplasm with a solid, cribriform, or trabecular growth pattern with rounded spaces containing either mucin or pink basement-membrane material [Figure 6.14]. Lymph node metastases are extremely rare (0–2%), as are distant metastases (65). Complete resection is often curative. At the genetic level, AdCC are characterised by a translocation t(6;9) involving the MYB and NFIB genes (66) and display low levels of genomic instability.

Other salivary type tumours that rarely arise in the breast include acinic cell, oncocytic, and mucoepidermoid carcinomas (67).

6.7.2.11 Secretory Carcinoma

A rare form of carcinoma that often occurs in young patients with a median age of 25 years (68). Secretory carcinoma consists of cells with pale granular cytoplasm with prominent intracytoplasmic lumina, intra- and extracellular eosinophilic secretions, and variable architecture with microcystic, solid, or tubular patterns [Figure 6.15]. They are usually low-grade and may be associated with secretory or low-grade DCIS. Secretory carcinomas have a characteristic t(12;15) translocation involving the ETS variant 6 (ETV6) gene and the neurotrophic tyrosine kinase receptor 3 (NTKR3), also described in paediatric mesenchymal tumours, including congenital fibrosarcoma and congenital mesoblastic nephroma (69). Local recurrence in children is rare, although delayed recurrences have been described.

6.8 Therapy-Related Changes

Neoadjuvant chemotherapy and/or endocrine therapy is increasingly being used in the management of breast cancer and has been shown to be as effective as adjuvant therapy. Clinical indications for neoadjuvant treatment have moved beyond inflammatory breast cancer and downstaging of large tumours to convert inoperable to operable disease or allow breast conservation, and it is now standard of care for HER2-positive and triple-negative disease (20). Neoadjuvant therapy offers a unique opportunity to evaluate treatment response; pathological complete response (pCR), defined as absence of invasive cancer in the breast and axillary lymph nodes, acts as a surrogate marker of survival allowing more rapid evaluation of new chemotherapeutic agents. Serial evaluation of biomarkers may also be used to assess treatment response, with measurement of the Ki67 labelling index following two weeks of neoadjuvant endocrine therapy predictive of recurrence-free survival (70). There can be considerable changes in the macroscopic and microscopic appearances of a tumour post neoadjuvant therapy (71). The tumour may become ill-defined with no residual macroscopic lesion or only a vague area of fibrosis to indicate the tumour bed. In this setting, detailed clinical information regarding pre-treatment tumour location and size is vital to allow accurate pathological sampling. Placement of a marker clip to indicate the site of the tumour before commencement of treatment is very useful in the event of an excellent clinical response, and essential if breast-conserving surgery is being considered (21).

Response to neoadjuvant chemotherapy shows an association with prognosis, with pCR being a strong predictor of improved survival across all molecular subtypes. The residual cancer burden (RCB) derives a score based on tumour bed volume, average tumour cellularity, number of involved lymph nodes, and the size of the largest metastasis and relates to survival outcomes (72, 73). Traditional pTNM system using the prefix 'y' to indicate neoadjuvant treatment also retains prognostic value post chemotherapy (74).

6.9 Metastatic Carcinoma

Not all malignant tumours of the breast are of primary breast origin. Recognition of metastatic malignancy or lymphoma is important, as extensive local surgery is often inappropriate. A wide range of tumours can metastasise to the breast including lymphoma, melanoma, and carcinoma of lung, ovary, kidney, or stomach (75). Presentation is usually with a superficial, well-circumscribed, rapidly growing mass. The majority are solitary (85%), and there may be accompanying axillary lymphadenopathy (76). On microscopy, morphological features may suggest a metastatic lesion, such as pigment in melanoma [Figure 6.16]. However, around one-third of lesions do not show specific histological features and poorly differentiated carcinomas from other sites may resemble grade 3 breast carcinomas (75).

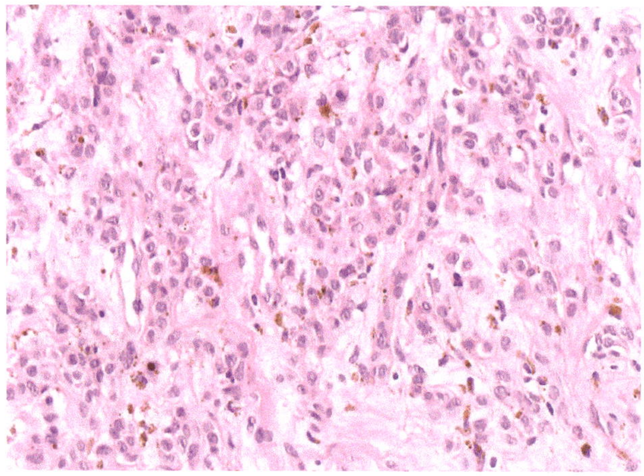

FIGURE 6.16
Metastatic melanoma. Core biopsy from a breast mass showing cells with clear cytoplasm and atypical nuclei with coarse brown pigment in keeping with melanin. The patient had a known history of melanoma.

In cases with no past history, immunohistochemistry can help identify the primary site. Strong, diffuse staining for ER is only seen in tumours of breast or gynaecological tract origin, although tumours from other sites can show weak, focal staining (75). Useful markers include GATA-3, which stains breast, salivary gland, and urothelial tumours; TTF1 for primary lung adenocarcinoma; WT1 and PAX 8 for ovarian cancer; and melanoma markers, such as melan A or HMB45.

6.10 Male Breast Cancer

Breast cancer is much rarer in men than in women and accounts for less than 1% of male cancers (77, 78). It is more prevalent in older men with an average age of 68 years, 5–10 years later than in women. In about 5% of cases there is a family history of breast cancer (79). Male breast cancer has been associated with BRCA2 gene mutations, with a 6% risk of developing the disease by age 70 compared with 0.1% in the general population (77).

The most common presentation is with a subareolar mass. Most male breast cancers are NST, with ILC being extremely rare in males. Papillary carcinomas are proportionally more common representing up to 12% of cases (6, 80). Grading and staging are the same as for female patients, and the tumours are typically grade 2 or 3. Male breast cancers are commonly ER positive (90–100%) (78, 80, 81). HER2 overexpression is rare, as are triple-negative breast cancers, representing only 2–4% of cases (78, 81).

When matched for grade and stage, the prognosis is similar to that of female breast cancer (78). Lymph node involvement is more common at presentation (40–55%) (77). Most patients are treated with mastectomy and axillary clearance, although sentinel lymph node biopsy (SLNB) has been shown to be successful in males (82).

6.11 Molecular Classification of Breast Cancer

Accurate prediction of tumour behaviour in an individual patient is essential to avoid overtreatment for good prognosis cancers and to identify poor prognosis cancers that require chemotherapy at the outset. Historically, these decisions have been based on traditional histological factors such as size, histological grade, nodal status, and hormone receptor and HER2 status, along with patient characteristics such as age and menopausal status. These clinical-pathological variables have been combined in algorithms such as the Nottingham Prognostic Index and Predict, which show a strong association with survival outcomes but are crude measures of risk for individual patients, resulting in overtreatment of many women with approximately 85% of patients not benefitting from cytotoxic chemotherapy, whilst 20% die despite cytotoxic therapy (83–85).

High-throughput genomic techniques have refined how we classify breast cancer and have the potential to improve patient management by more precise determination of patient prognosis based on tumour biology and targeted treatment directed at the molecular alterations driving tumour growth. Perou et al. used gene expression profiling to examine the genetic complexity of breast cancer, identifying four 'intrinsic' subtypes with different survival outcomes separated primarily by ER and HER2 status (34, 86).

Luminal breast cancers are enriched for ER positive tumours and form a continuous spectrum divided into two subgroups based on expression of proliferation-related genes. Luminal A tumours are typically low-grade with an excellent prognosis, characterised by ER and PR positivity and HER2 negativity, with high expression of ER-related genes and low expression of proliferation-related genes. In contrast, luminal B tumours are higher-grade, have a worse prognosis, and may be PR negative and/or HER2 positive, with high expression of proliferation-related genes.

ER-negative tumours comprise biologically distinct entities with different drivers divided into two main groups—HER2-enriched and basal-like. HER2-enriched tumours are driven by overexpression of HER2 and related pathways and had a poor prognosis before the advent of HER2-targeted therapies. Although many tumours within this subgroup (66%) show *HER2* gene amplification or HER2 protein overexpression on immunohistochemistry, not all clinically defined HER2-positive tumours fall into this subgroup; many ER-positive/HER2-positive tumours fall into the luminal B group mentioned earlier (87).

Basal-like breast cancers are ER, PR, and HER2 negative (triple negative) and are characterised by upregulation of genes expressed by basal/myoepithelial cells including high molecular weight cytokeratins (CK5 and 14). The basal-like group includes diverse histological types of breast cancer such as medullary-like

TABLE 6.4

Main Multigene Prognostic Tests for Breast Cancer, Modified from (93)

	Oncotype Dx	Prosigna (PAM 50)	EndoPredict	Mammaprint
Method	RT-PCR	RT-PCR	RT-PCR	DNA microarray
No. of genes	21	50	11	70
Tissue	FFPE	FFPE	FFPE	Frozen/FFPE
Scoring system	Recurrence score: low (<20), intermediate (21–30), high (>30)	Risk of recurrence score (0–100): low <24, intermediate 24–53, high >53; intrinsic subtype	EP score (0–15): low <5, high >5; EPclin including T and N	Genomic risk score: low (<0.4), high (>0.4)
Node negative	Yes—TAILORx trial	Yes	Yes	Yes
Node positive (1–3)	Yes—RxPONDER trial	No—OPTIMA trial in progress	No	No
Approval pN0	NCCN, ASCO, St Gallen, EGTM	ASCO, St Gallen, EGTM	ASCO, St Gallen, EGTM	St Gallen, EGTM
Approval pN1	NCCN, ASCO, St Gallen, EGTM	St Gallen, EGTM	St Gallen, EGTM	St Gallen, EGTM

cancers, metaplastic cancers, and rare special type cancers like AdCC which carry a good prognosis. Breast cancers arising in BRCA1 mutation carriers are typically basal-like, and BRCA1 dysfunction mediated by alternative mechanisms such as methylation has been identified in non-BRCA1 mutated basal-like tumours.

The separation into good- and poor-prognosis ER-positive, HER2-positive, and triple-negative groups is clinically relevant based on current therapeutic regimens centred on hormonal therapy, chemotherapy and HER2 targeted agents. Classification of cohorts of breast cancers into the intrinsic subtypes is robust; however, assignment of individual tumours to a subgroup shows only moderate reproducibility with the basal-like group being most reproducible, and the luminal B and HER2-enriched the most poorly reproducible (88, 89). Attempts to replicate these groups using immunohistochemistry-based panels, including ER, PR, HER2, and Ki67, show modest concordance with microarray defined intrinsic subtypes at best (90).

There are several commercially available multigene assays based on gene expression signatures that have been developed as predictors of prognosis or response to treatment (91–93). Most current gene-based tests are limited to use in ER-positive/HER2-negative early breast cancer patients with low nodal burden. Tumour size and nodal status retain independent prognostic value, and some of the assays incorporate these clinical variables when determining risk. The four main tests are summarised in Table 6.4.

References

1. Lee AHS, Ellis IO, Pinder SE, et al. Guidelines for non-operative diagnostic procedures and reporting in breast cancer screening. London: Royal College of Pathologists; 2021. G150-Non-op-reporting-breast-cancer-screening.pdf (Accessed 1 August 2023).
2. Tse G, Koo JS, Thike AA. Phyllodes tumour. In: WHO Classification of Tumours Editorial Board, ed. Breast Tumours, vol 2, 5th edn. Lyon: IARC; 2019: 172–76.
3. Tan PH, Thike AA, Tan WJ, et al. Predicting clinical behaviour of breast phyllodes tumours: A nomogram based on histological criteria and surgical margins. J Clin Pathol. 2012;65(1):69–76.
4. Provenzano E, Pinder SE. Pre-operative diagnosis of breast cancer in screening: Problems and pitfalls. Pathology. 2009;41(1):3–17.
5. Collins LC, Schnitt SJ. Papillary lesions of the breast: Selected diagnostic and management issues. Histopathology. 2008;52(1):20–9.
6. Pal SK, Lau SK, Kruper L, et al. Papillary carcinoma of the breast: An overview. Breast Cancer Res Treat. 2010;122(3):637–45.
7. Rakha EA, Gandhi N, Climent F, et al. Encapsulated papillary carcinoma of the breast: An invasive tumor with excellent prognosis. Am J Surg Pathol. 2011;35(8):1093–103.
8. Wynveen CA, Nehhozina T, Akram M, et al. Intracystic papillary carcinoma of the breast: An in situ or invasive tumor? Results of immunohistochemical analysis and clinical follow-up. Am J Surg Pathol. 2011;35(1):1–14.
9. Nassar H, Qureshi H, Adsay NV, et al. Clinicopathologic analysis of solid papillary carcinoma of the breast and associated invasive carcinomas. Am J Surg Pathol. 2006;30(4):501–7.
10. Duprez R, Wilkerson PM, Lacroix-Triki M, et al. Immunophenotypic and genomic characterization of papillary carcinomas of the breast. J Pathol. 2012;226(3):427–41.
11. Collins LC, Carlo VP, Hwang H, et al. Intracystic papillary carcinomas of the breast: A reevaluation using a panel of myoepithelial cell markers. Am J Surg Pathol. 2006;30(8):1002–7.
12. Pinder SE, Collins LC, Fox SB, et al. Ductal carcinoma in situ. In: WHO Classification of Tumours Editorial Board, eds. Breast Tumours, vol 2, 5th edn. Lyon: IARC; 2019: 76–81.
13. Pinder SE. Ductal carcinoma in situ (DCIS): Pathological features, differential diagnosis, prognostic factors and specimen evaluation. Mod Pathol. 2010;23(Suppl 2):S8–13.
14. Cope W, Provenzano E. The diagnosis and management of lobular carcinoma in situ. Diagn Histopathol. 2023;29(3):153–61.
15. Ellis IO, Lee AH, Elston CW, et al. Microinvasive carcinoma of the breast: Diagnostic criteria and clinical relevance. Histopathol. 1999;35(5):470–2.
16. Breast. In: Edge SB, Byrd DR, Compton CC, et al., eds. Cancer Staging Handbook from the AJCC Cancer Staging Manual, 7th edn. New York: Springer; 2010: 419–60.
17. Shaaban AM, Hilton B, Clements K, et al. The presentation, management and outcome of patients with ductal carcinoma in situ (DCIS) with microinvasion (invasion </=1 mm in size)-results from the UK Sloane Project. Br J Cancer. 2022;127(12):2125–32.
18. Reis-Filho JS, Lakhani SR. Breast cancer special types: Why bother? J Pathol. 2008;216(4):394–8.
19. Weigelt B, Horlings HM, Kreike B, et al. Refinement of breast cancer classification by molecular characterization of histological special types. J Pathol. 2008;216(2):141–50.
20. Provenzano E. Neoadjuvant chemotherapy for breast cancer: Moving beyond pathological complete response in the molecular age. Acta Med Acad. 2021;50(1):88–109.
21. Bossuyt V, Provenzano E, Symmans WF, et al. Recommendations for standardized pathological characterization of residual disease for neoadjuvant clinical trials of breast cancer by the BIG-NABCG collaboration. Ann Oncol. 2015;26(7):1280–91.
22. Rakha E, Allison KH, Ellis IO, et al. Invasive breast carcinoma: General overview. In: WHO Classification of Tumours Editorial Board, ed. Breast Tumours, vol 2, 5th edn. Lyon: IARC; 2019: 82–101.
23. Ellis IO, Collins LC, Ichihara S, et al. Invasive carcinoma of no special type. In: Lakhani SR, Ellis IO, Schnitt SJ, et al., eds. WHO Classification of Tumours of the Breast. Lyon: IARC; 2012: 34–8.
24. Wellings SR, Jensen HM, Marcum RG. An atlas of subgross pathology of the human breast with special reference to possible precancerous lesions. J Natl Cancer Inst. 1975;55(2):231–73.
25. Boecker W, Buerger H. Evidence of progenitor cells of glandular and myoepithelial cell lineages in the human adult female breast epithelium: A new progenitor (adult stem) cell concept. Cell Prolif. 2003;36(Suppl 1):73–84.
26. Rakha E, Allison KH, Bu H, et al. Invasive breast carcinoma of no special type. In: WHO Classification of Tumours Editorial Board, ed. Breast Tumours, vol. 2, 5th edn. Lyon: IARC; 2019: 102–9.
27. Gupta SK, Douglas-Jones AG, Fenn N, et al. The clinical behavior of breast carcinoma is probably determined at the preinvasive stage (ductal carcinoma in situ). Cancer. 1997;80(9):1740–5.
28. Ellis IO, Carder P, Hales S, et al. Pathology Reporting of Breast Disease in Surgical Excision Specimens Incorporating the Dataset for Histological Reporting of Breast Cancer. Sheffield: NHS Cancer Screening Programmes; 2016. G148_BreastDataset-lowres-Jun16.pdf (Accessed 1 August 2023).
29. Gown AM. Current issues in ER and HER2 testing by IHC in breast cancer. Mod Pathol. 2008;21(Suppl 2):S8–S15.

30. Diaz LK, Sneige N. Estrogen receptor analysis for breast cancer: Current issues and keys to increasing testing accuracy. Adv Anat Pathol. 2005;12(1):10–9.
31. Walker RA, Bartlett JM, Dowsett M, et al. HER2 testing in the UK: Further update to recommendations. J Clin Pathol. 2008;61(7):818–24.
32. Carter CL, Allen C, Henson DE. Relation of tumor size, lymph node status, and survival in 24,740 breast cancer cases. Cancer. 1989;63(1):181–7.
33. Rakha EA, Reis-Filho JS, Baehner F, et al. Breast cancer prognostic classification in the molecular era: The role of histological grade. Breast Cancer Res. 2010;12(4):207.
34. Sorlie T, Perou CM, Tibshirani R, et al. Gene expression patterns of breast carcinomas distinguish tumor subclasses with clinical implications. Proc Natl Acad Sci USA. 2001;98(19):10869–74.
35. Louwman MW, Vriezen M, van Beek MW, et al. Uncommon breast tumors in perspective: Incidence, treatment and survival in the Netherlands. Int J Cancer. 2007;121(1):127–35.
36. Jacquemier J, Padovani L, Rabayrol L, et al. Typical medullary breast carcinomas have a basal/myoepithelial phenotype. J Pathol. 2005;207(3):260–8.
37. Armes JE, Egan AJ, Southey MC, et al. The histologic phenotypes of breast carcinoma occurring before age 40 years in women with and without BRCA1 or BRCA2 germline mutations: A population-based study. Cancer. 1998;83(11):2335–45.
38. Eisinger F, Jacquemier J, Charpin C, et al. Mutations at BRCA1: The medullary breast carcinoma revisited. Cancer Res. 1998;58(8):1588–92.
39. Rakha EA, Aleskandarany M, El-Sayed ME, et al. The prognostic significance of inflammation and medullary histological type in invasive carcinoma of the breast. Eur J Cancer. 2009;45(10):1780–7.
40. Shin SJ, Desmedt C, Kristiansen G, et al. Invasive lobular carcinoma. In: WHO Classification of Tumours Editorial Board, ed. Breast Tumours, vol. 2, 5th edn. Lyon: IARC; 2019: 114–8.
41. Dixon JM, Anderson TJ, Page DL, et al. Infiltrating lobular carcinoma of the breast. Histopathology. 1982;6(2):149–61.
42. Mann RM, Hoogeveen YL, Blickman JG, et al. MRI compared to conventional diagnostic work-up in the detection and evaluation of invasive lobular carcinoma of the breast: A review of existing literature. Breast Cancer Res Treat. 2008;107(1):1–14.
43. Mann RM, Veltman J, Barentsz JO, et al. The value of MRI compared to mammography in the assessment of tumour extent in invasive lobular carcinoma of the breast. Eur J Surg Oncol. 2008;34(2):135–42.
44. Vargas AC, Lakhani SR, Simpson PT. Pleomorphic lobular carcinoma of the breast: Molecular pathology and clinical impact. Future Oncol. 2009;5(2):233–43.
45. Weigelt B, Geyer FC, Natrajan R, et al. The molecular underpinning of lobular histological growth pattern: A genome-wide transcriptomic analysis of invasive lobular carcinomas and grade- and molecular subtype-matched invasive ductal carcinomas of no special type. J Pathol. 2010;220(1):45–57.
46. Da Silva L, Parry S, Reid L, et al. Aberrant expression of E-cadherin in lobular carcinomas of the breast. Am J Surg Pathol. 2008;32(5):773–83.
47. Dabbs DJ, Kaplai M, Chivukula M, et al. The spectrum of morphomolecular abnormalities of the E-cadherin/catenin complex in pleomorphic lobular carcinoma of the breast. Appl Immunohistochem Mol Morphol. 2007;15(3):260–6.
48. Rakha EA, Patel A, Powe DG, et al. Clinical and biological significance of E-cadherin protein expression in invasive lobular carcinoma of the breast. Am J Surg Pathol. 2010;34(10):1472–9.
49. Arpino G, Bardou VJ, Clark GM, et al. Infiltrating lobular carcinoma of the breast: Tumor characteristics and clinical outcome. Breast Cancer Res. 2004;6(3):R149–56.
50. Colleoni M, Rotmensz N, Maisonneuve P, et al. Outcome of special types of luminal breast cancer. Ann Oncol. 2012;23(6):1428–36.
51. Middleton LP, Palacios DM, Bryant BR, et al. Pleomorphic lobular carcinoma: Morphology, immunohistochemistry, and molecular analysis. Am J Surg Pathol. 2000;24(12):1650–6.
52. Orvieto E, Maiorano E, Bottiglieri L, et al. Clinicopathologic characteristics of invasive lobular carcinoma of the breast: Results of an analysis of 530 cases from a single institution. Cancer. 2008;113(7):1511–20.
53. Nagao T, Kinoshita T, Hojo T, et al. The differences in the histological types of breast cancer and the response to neoadjuvant chemotherapy: The relationship between the outcome and the clinicopathological characteristics. Breast. 2012;21(3):289–95.
54. Rakha EA, Lee AH, Evans AJ, et al. Tubular carcinoma of the breast: Further evidence to support its excellent prognosis. J Clin Oncol. 2010;28(1):99–104.
55. Page DL, Dixon JM, Anderson TJ, et al. Invasive cribriform carcinoma of the breast. Histopathology. 1983;7(4):525–36.
56. Di Saverio S, Gutierrez J, Avisar E. A retrospective review with long term follow up of 11,400 cases of pure mucinous breast carcinoma. Breast Cancer Res Treat. 2008;111(3):541–7.
57. Marchio C, Horlings HM, Vincent-Salomon A. Invasive micropapillary carcinoma. In: WHO Classification of Tumours Editorial Board, ed. Breast Tumours, vol. 2, 5th edn. Lyon: IARC; 2019: 128–30.
58. Provenzano E, Gatalica Z, Vranic S. Carcinoma with apocrine differentiation. In: WHO Classification of Tumours Editorial Board, ed. Breast Tumours, vol. 2, 5th edn. Lyon: IARC; 2019: 131–3.
59. Farmer P, Bonnefoi H, Becette V, et al. Identification of molecular apocrine breast tumours by microarray analysis. Oncogene. 2005;24(29):4660–71.
60. Reis-Filho JS, Gobbi H, McCart Reed AE, et al. Metaplastic carcinoma. In: WHO Classification of Tumours Editorial Board, ed. Breast Tumours, vol. 2, 5th ed. Lyon: IARC; 2019: 134–8.
61. Rosen PP. Squamous Carcinoma. In: Rosen PP, ed. Rosen's Breast Pathology, 3rd ed. Philadelphia: Lippincott Williams & Wilkins; 2009: 506–14.
62. Van Hoeven KH, Drudis T, Cranor ML, et al. Low-grade adenosquamous carcinoma of the breast. A clinocopathologic study of 32 cases with ultrastructural analysis. Am J Surg Pathol. 1993;17(3):248–58.
63. Bae SY, Lee SK, Koo MY, et al. The prognoses of metaplastic breast cancer patients compared to those of triple-negative breast cancer patients. Breast Cancer Res Treat. 2100;126(2):471–8.
64. Weigelt B, Kreike B, Reis-Filho JS. Metaplastic breast carcinomas are basal-like breast cancers: A genomic profiling analysis. Breast Cancer Res Treat. 2009;117(2):273–80.
65. Boujelbene N, Khabir A, Jeanneret Sozzi W, et al. Clinical review—breast adenoid cystic carcinoma. Breast. 2012;21(2):124–7.
66. Wetterskog D, Lopez-Garcia MA, Lambros MB, et al. Adenoid cystic carcinomas constitute a genomically distinct subgroup of triple-negative and basal-like breast cancers. J Pathol. 2012;226(1):84–96.
67. Pia-Foschini M, Reis-Filho JS, Eusebi V, et al. Salivary gland-like tumours of the breast: Surgical and molecular pathology. J Clin Pathol. 2003;56(7):497–506.
68. Vasudev P, Onuma K. Secretory breast carcinoma: Unique, triple-negative carcinoma with a favorable prognosis and characteristic molecular expression. Arch Pathol Lab Med. 2011;135(12):1606–10.
69. Lae M, Freneaux P, Sastre-Garau X, et al. Secretory breast carcinomas with ETV6-NTRK3 fusion gene belong to the basal-like carcinoma spectrum. Mod Pathol. 2009;22(2):291–8.
70. Shaaban AM, Provenzano E. Receptor status after neoadjuvant therapy of breast cancer: Significance and implications. Pathobiol. 2022;89(5):297–308.
71. Pinder SE, Provenzano E, Earl H, et al. Laboratory handling and histology reporting of breast specimens from patients who have received neoadjuvant chemotherapy. Histopathol. 2007;50(4):409–17.
72. Symmans WF, Peintinger F, Hatzis C, et al. Measurement of residual breast cancer burden to predict survival after neoadjuvant chemotherapy. J Clin Oncol. 2007;25(28):4414–22.
73. Yau C, Osdoit M, van der Noordaa M, et al. Residual cancer burden after neoadjuvant chemotherapy and long-term survival outcomes in breast cancer: A multicentre pooled analysis of 5161 patients. Lancet Oncol. 2022;23(1):149–60.

74. Campbell JI, Yau C, Krass P, et al. Comparison of residual cancer burden, American Joint Committee on Cancer staging and pathologic complete response in breast cancer after neoadjuvant chemotherapy: Results from the I-SPY 1 TRIAL (CALGB 150007/150012; ACRIN 6657). Breast Cancer Res Treat. 2017;165(1):181–91.
75. Lee AH. The histological diagnosis of metastases to the breast from extramammary malignancies. J Clin Pathol. 2007;60(12):1333–41.
76. Lamovec J, Wotherspoon A, Jacquemier J. Malignant lymphoma and metastatic tumours. In: Tavassoli FA, Devilee P, eds. Pathology & Genetics Tumours of the Breast and Female Genital Organs. World Health Organization Classification of Tumours. Lyon: IARC; 2003: 107–9.
77. Reis LO, Dias FG, Castro MA, et al. Male breast cancer. Aging Male. 2011;14(2):99–109.
78. Shaaban AM, Ball GR, Brannan RA, et al. A comparative biomarker study of 514 matched cases of male and female breast cancer reveals gender-specific biological differences. Breast Cancer Res Treat. 2012;133(3):949–58.
79. Prechtel K, Levi F, La Vecchia C, et al. Tumours of the male breast. In: Tavassoli FA, Devilee P, eds. Pathology & Genetics Tumour of the Breast and Female Genital Organs. Lyon: IARC; 2003: 110–2.
80. Ge Y, Sneige N, Eltorky MA, et al. Immunohistochemical characterization of subtypes of male breast carcinoma. Breast Cancer Res. 2009;11(3):R28.
81. Kornegoor R, Verschuur-Maes AH, Buerger H, et al. Molecular subtyping of male breast cancer by immunohistochemistry. Mod Pathol. 2012;25(3)398–404.
82. Agrawal A, Ayantunde AA, Rampaul R, et al. Male breast cancer: A review of clinical management. Breast Cancer Res Treat. 2007;103(1):11–21.
83. Candido Dos Reis FJ, Wishart GC, Dicks EM, et al. An updated PREDICT breast cancer prognostication and treatment benefit prediction model with independent validation. Breast Cancer Res. 2017;19(1):58.
84. Early Breast Cancer Trialists' Collaborative Group, Peto R, Davies C, et al. Comparisons between different polychemotherapy regimens for early breast cancer: Meta-analyses of long-term outcome among 100,000 women in 123 randomised trials. Lancet. 2012;379(9814):432–44.
85. Todd JH, Dowle C, Williams MR, et al. Confirmation of a prognostic index in primary breast cancer. Br J Cancer. 1987;56(4):489–92.
86. Perou CM, Sorlie T, Eisen MB, et al. Molecular portraits of human breast tumours. Nature. 2000;406(6797):747–52.
87. Prat A, Perou CM. Deconstructing the molecular portraits of breast cancer. Molec Oncol. 2011;5(1):5–23.
88. Zhao X, Rodland EA, Sorlie T, et al. Systematic assessment of prognostic gene signatures for breast cancer shows distinct influence of time and ER status. BMC Cancer. 2014;14:211.
89. Weigelt B, Mackay A, A'Hern R, et al. Breast cancer molecular profiling with single sample predictors: A retrospective analysis. Lancet Oncol. 2010;11(4):339–49.
90. Prat A, Pineda E, Adamo B, et al. Clinical implications of the intrinsic molecular subtypes of breast cancer. Breast. 2015;24(Suppl 2):S26–35.
91. Barbi M, Makower D, Sparano JA. The clinical utility of gene expression assays in breast cancer patients with 0–3 involved lymph nodes. Ther Adv Med Oncol. 2021;13.
92. Curigliano G, Dent R, Llombart-Cussac A, et al. Incorporating clinicopathological and molecular risk prediction tools to improve outcomes in early HR+/HER2- breast cancer. NPJ Breast Cancer. 2023;9(1):56.
93. Zeng C, Zhang J. A narrative review of five multigenetic assays in breast cancer. Transl Cancer Res. 2022;11(4):897–907.

7

Fibrocystic Changes, Fibroadenoma, Papillary Lesions, and Duct Ectasia

Sue Down

7.1 Introduction

Benign breast conditions represent 95% of symptomatic breast cases seen by clinicians in primary care (1). Presenting symptoms can range from painful nodularity and discrete mobile lumps to more worrying masses, breast distortion, and nipple bleeding.

Breast screening programmes also detect a significant number of incidental benign or indeterminate lesions, which are often asymptomatic but cause anxiety to women when recalled for further assessment.

The cornerstone of management is to undertake a detailed triple assessment of each case. A full clinical history will reveal the duration of symptoms, any family history of breast disease, relationship of symptoms to the woman's menstrual cycle, and any potential precipitating factors such as trauma to the breast or underlying health conditions. Thorough physical examination of both breasts and axillae, including assessment of the underlying chest wall musculature, will assist in making a differential diagnosis. Nipple discharge should be expressed by the patient and tested using a urinalysis dipstick for the presence of blood.

Imaging will be indicated in the presence of a focal clinical abnormality and will usually include mammography for women aged over 40 and men aged over 50. Ultrasound is appropriate for younger patients and for further assessment of any focal lesions identified on mammography or clinical assessment. MRI may be indicated when there is a discrepancy and lack of concordance between the clinical and radiological findings.

Biopsies should be undertaken under imaging guidance to ensure accurate targeting of a lesion and to reduce the false negative rate. Core biopsy is preferable to fine-needle aspiration cytology, as it allows the pathologist to diagnose invasion by assessment of cellular interactions and lesion architecture. In cases where there is no radiological abnormality evident, but a clinically indeterminate mass is palpable, a clinical core biopsy may be acceptable.

All biopsy results should be reviewed by a senior clinician to determine whether the clinical findings correlate with the pathological results. If there is concordance, management should follow the local guidelines for the relevant condition. If there is discordance, the patient should be re-examined by an experienced breast clinician and the biopsy repeated if indicated. Complex benign breast cases may benefit from discussion in a breast multidisciplinary team meeting to determine optimal management.

Benign breast lesions are classified histologically as non-proliferative, proliferative without atypia, and proliferative with atypia. The degree of atypia is associated with the subsequent risk of breast cancer development (Table 7.1).

True benign breast disease will be classified as a B2 result on biopsy. B1 results indicate normal breast tissue; this may not represent the true pathology if a lesion can clearly be seen on imaging. A repeat biopsy may therefore be indicated on the assumption of a targeting error. B3 results indicate a benign lesion of uncertain malignant potential which may include features of atypia. B3 lesions are usually excised surgically (diagnostic excision biopsy) or radiologically (VAE) to provide further tissue sampling.

Benign breast symptoms and incidental screening findings can cause great anxiety for patients. Assessment should be timely, and a full explanation given for their symptoms, along with advice on regular breast self-examination. Patient information leaflets are useful sources of further patient education and reassurance.

The following sections will discuss a variety of benign breast conditions, contextualised by examples of relevant case scenarios and imaging findings. The approach to the diagnosis and management of complex benign breast disease can involve a wide multidisciplinary approach (breast clinician, general surgeon, gynaecologist, radiologist, pathologist, plastic surgeon, etc.), so local pathways should be in place to support this.

DOI: 10.1201/9781003394785-7

7.2 Section I: Breast Lumps

7.2.1 Fibrocystic Changes

CLINICAL CASE

A 53-year-old lady presents to your practice with a lump above her right nipple which has been present for the last six days.

Clinically there is a 2 cm firm smooth lump, which is slightly tender. There is no nipple discharge.

Mammographic and ultrasound images are shown in Figures 7.1 and 7.2.

Fibrocystic disease includes a spectrum of normal changes within the mammary tissue. This may include simple cysts, which are not associated with an increased risk of malignancy, through to more complex cysts, which should be biopsied due to a potential associated risk of malignancy of approximately 30% (1).

Breast cysts affect approximately 10% of peri-menopausal women and usually regress following the menopause. Breast involution occurs during the peri-menopausal period as female hormone levels fluctuate, coinciding with the development of breast cysts. The use of hormone replacement therapy (HRT) may therefore be associated with cyst development in older women.

Cysts usually present as a discrete lump, often associated with discomfort. They are also commonly present on screening mammograms. Multiple cysts may be present bilaterally. When symptomatic, the patient may describe a lump which developed rapidly and is associated with the onset of the menstrual cycle. Examination will reveal a mobile smooth lump, or focal nodularity in the presence of multiple smaller cysts.

Differential diagnoses should include a galactocele (if the patient was recently breastfeeding), high-grade carcinoma (if the lump is very firm and non-tender), or an oil cyst due to fat necrosis (if there is a history of trauma to the area).

Women over 40 should undergo both mammography and ultrasound, whilst women under 40 should undergo ultrasound only in the first instance.

Ultrasound should demonstrate a thin-walled, well-defined, fluid-filled (hypoechoic) lesion, either in isolation or in the presence of similar adjacent structures.

Simple symptomatic cysts can be aspirated to dryness under ultrasound control. Asymptomatic simple cysts do not require aspiration unless requested by

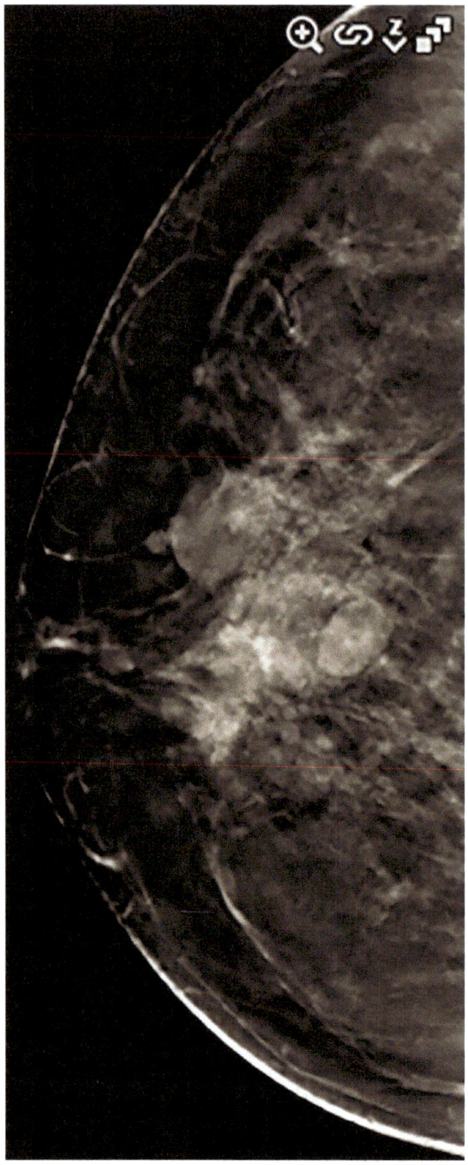

FIGURE 7.1
Right mammogram: Two distinct opacities are seen behind the nipple in this craniocaudal view.

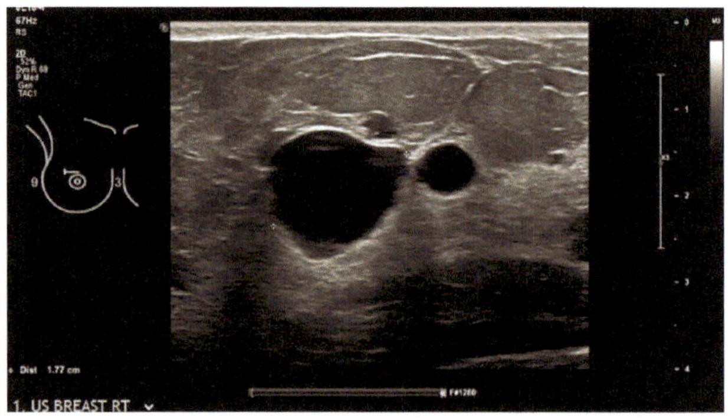

FIGURE 7.2
Ultrasound of the right breast: One large and one adjacent small hypoechoic well-defined lesion are seen.

TABLE 7.1

Cancer Risk Associated with Benign Breast Biopsy

Non-proliferative disease/normal pathology (B1/B2)
Lesions with no association with increased breast cancer risk:
Fibrosis
Cysts
Apocrine metaplasia
Simple fibroadenoma
Proliferative disease without atypia (B2/B3)
Lesions with potential increased breast cancer risk:
Epithelial hyperplasia without atypia
Columnar cell hyperplasia without atypia
Complex fibroadenoma without atypia
Sclerosing adenosis
Radial scar
Papilloma
Proliferative disease with atypia (B3)
Lesions associated with moderately increased breast cancer risk:
Atypical ductal hyperplasia
Atypical lobular hyperplasia
Atypical columnar hyperplasia
Complex fibroadenoma with atypia

Source: Adapted from ref. 4.

the patient. Yellow, green, brown, and black cyst fluid is normal, but bloodstained fluid should be sent for urgent cytology to exclude an intra-cystic cancer.

Radiological features suggestive of possible malignancy include a thickened cyst wall, or complex internal echoes. Complex and indeterminate cysts should be biopsied under radiological guidance, and a marker clip placed. The results should then be discussed in a multidisciplinary breast team meeting.

Women with simple cysts can be reassured but made aware about the possibility of developing further cysts in the future. Symptomatic cysts associated with persistent breast pain can be aspirated. There is some interest in the potential use of metformin to control symptoms related to breast pain due to inhibition of oestrogen, and trials are ongoing (2).

Women with a history of recurrent cysts may be provided direct access to breast imaging if they develop further lumps. Simple cysts that recur can be repeatedly aspirated but should be assessed radiologically on each occasion to exclude cyst wall thickening or other changes which would mandate biopsy (3). See also Table 7.1.

Management summary: Mammograms showed two oval densities measuring approximately 20 mm in diameter in the upper outer quadrant of the right breast close to the 12 o'clock position.

Ultrasound confirmed a 20 mm benign-looking cyst, which was completely aspirated. A second deeper cyst measuring approximately 22 mm in diameter was also aspirated. Yellow aspirate was noted for both lesions. Numerous other tiny, small cysts were scattered in the upper/central right breast.

The patient was reassured and advised that cysts may refill or recur. She was told to reattend for assessment if further lumps were detected on breast self-examination.

7.2.2 Fibroadenoma

CLINICAL CASE

A 35-year-old woman with a strong family history of breast cancer presents with a two-week history of a lump in the lateral aspect of her lateral right breast.

Clinically, this is smooth and mobile, and there is no tenderness.

Due to her family history, she undergoes mammography and ultrasound assessment (Figures 7.3 and 7.4).

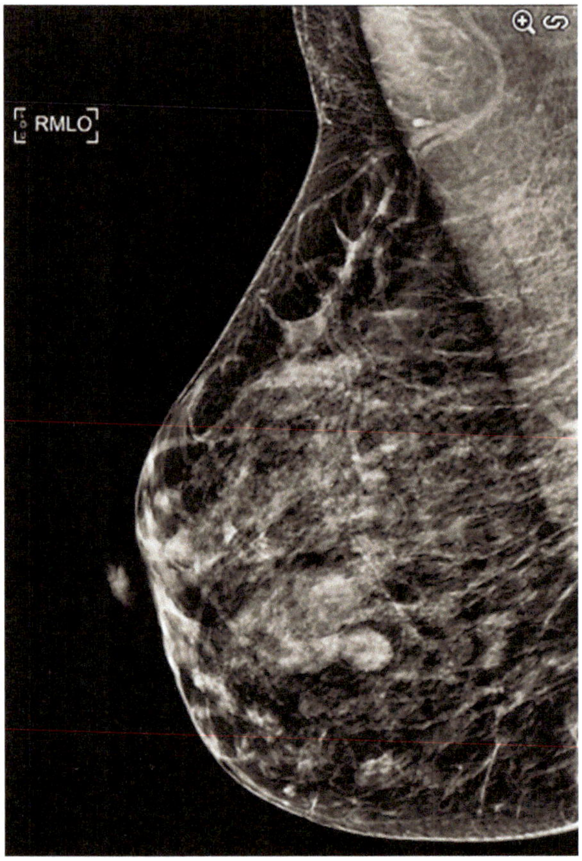

FIGURE 7.3
Right mammogram: a well-defined lesion is present below the level of the nipple in this mediolateral oblique view.

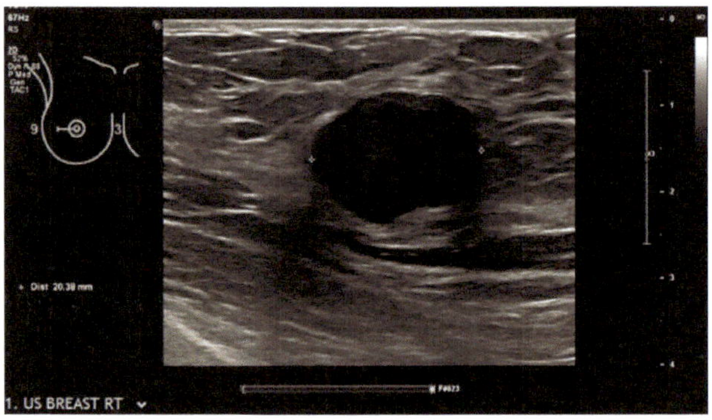

FIGURE 7.4
Right breast ultrasound: a smooth homogenous mass measuring 20 mm is visualised.

Fibroadenomas are the most common benign breast 'tumour', representing 25% of breast lumps (1). They develop within a breast lobule due to hormonal stimulation and therefore usually present during the period of breast lobule development from late teens into the 20s.

They usually present as a discrete, extremely mobile lump within the breast tissue (being otherwise termed a 'breast mouse'). They may measure up to 3 cm in size and, although usually painless, can be associated with discomfort which may be cyclical.

Giant fibroadenomas are over 5 cm in size or weigh over 500 g and present in patients less than 20 years of age. They are rare and represent less than 1% of fibroadenoma cases (Sosin 2015). Due to their rapidly increasing size, they can compress the normal surrounding breast tissue. Between 10 and 59% of giant fibroadenomas will regress spontaneously, but they cause embarrassment and anxiety in this young subset of patients.

Fibroadenomas in peri- or post-menopausal women are less common. Long-standing asymptomatic lesions may be detected on routine screening mammograms, associated with popcorn calcification appearances.

Women over 40 presenting with a discrete lump should undergo both mammography and ultrasound. Women under 40 should undergo initial ultrasound.

For women aged under 25, ultrasound assessment incorporates the Stavros criteria to determine whether the appearances are benign and if a biopsy is required; if the lesion is wider then tall, well defined, with fewer than four gentle lobulations, a smooth edge and thin capsule, biopsy is not warranted in this age group (4).

For all women aged 25 and over presenting with a solid lump, an ultrasound-guided core biopsy should be undertaken.

Simple fibroadenomas consist of stromal proliferation of low cellularity and regular cytology. They must, however, be distinguished from phyllodes tumours, which have a spectrum of stromal hypercellularity and may be associated with degrees of atypia.

Asymptomatic simple fibroadenomas not associated with atypia do not require excision. These patients can be reassured and advised that the majority of fibroadenomas remain static in size and that approximately one third will shrink or resolve over a two-year period. Approximately 10% will enlarge and patients should be asked to reattend for further assessment if this occurs, as excision via surgical enucleation may be considered. Pregnancy can occasionally result in rapid growth of fibroadenomas due to hormonal changes.

Giant fibroadenomas can be surgically enucleated, preserving the surrounding breast parenchyma which re-expands to fill the space previously occupied by the fibroadenoma. In younger patients, surgical excision biopsy may be preferable to core biopsy due to the psychological impact and discomfort of undertaking procedures under local anaesthesia (5).

Complex fibroadenomas with atypia and phyllodes tumours are classified pathologically as B3 and require excision. Phyllodes tumours are described in more detail in the following section.

> Management summary: Imaging confirms a well-defined solid lesion measuring 20 mm in the lateral right breast. A core biopsy confirms a benign fibroadenoma.
>
> She is reassured and discharged, with advice to reattend if the lump increases significantly in size, or if she detects any new lumps on self-examination.

7.2.3 Phyllodes Tumour

> **CLINICAL CASE**
>
> A 19-year-old student presents with a lump in the left breast that had grown rapidly growing lump over the preceding four weeks. There is no relevant family history.
>
> Clinically there is a large smooth mass present in her lower left breast measuring over 10 cm. Axillary examination is normal.
>
> Ultrasound images are shown in Figures 7.5 and 7.6.

Phyllodes tumours are uncommon but may appear similar to fibroadenomas on initial clinical examination and ultrasound imaging. They are often larger than fibroadenomas on presentation, with a history of rapid enlargement. The diagnosis is made histologically as they display a characteristic leaf-like appearance with stromal hypercellularity, increased mitotic count, and potential atypia (6).

Phyllodes tumours range from benign lesions (60–75%) through to borderline (15–20%) and malignant (10–20%) tumours based on the histological appearances (7). Benign variants can resemble cellular fibroadenomas histologically, and malignant variants may resemble sarcoma or metaplastic breast cancer. Therefore, all potential phyllodes tumours should be excised.

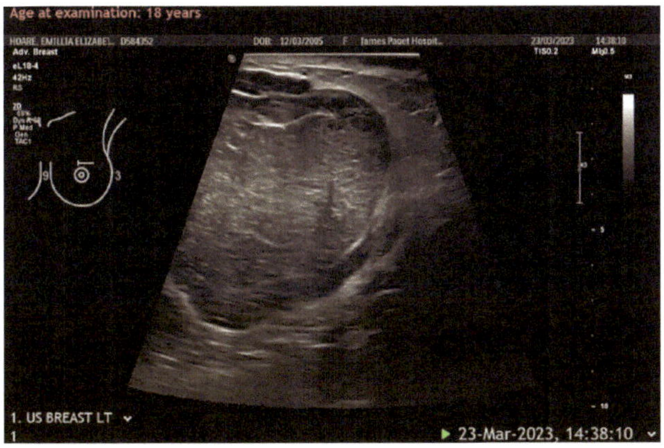

FIGURE 7.5
Ultrasound of the left breast showing a lobulated mass with well-defined edges.

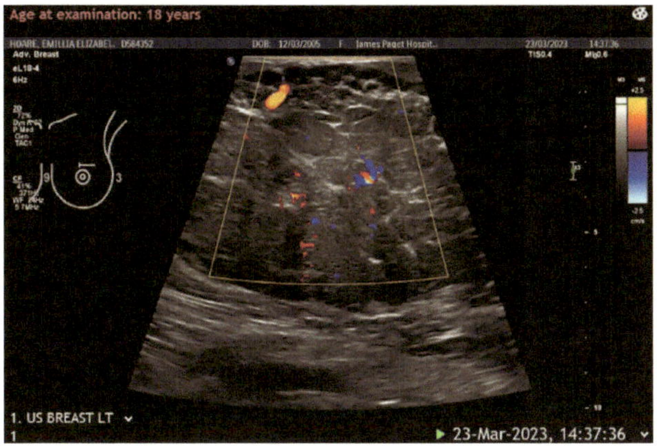

FIGURE 7.6
Ultrasound of the left breast showing blood flow within the mass.

Phyllodes tumours should be excised with a surrounding margin of at least 10 mm of macroscopically normal breast tissue as there is a high rate of recurrence for all lesion types (approximately 20%), and a potential for distant metastasis ranging from approximately 2% in benign tumours to 27% in malignant tumours (6). There is no role for axillary staging.

Following adequate excision, discussion at the breast multidisciplinary meeting should include the option of radiotherapy for malignant phyllodes tumours.

> Management summary: Ultrasound shows a 150 mm abnormal mass in the left lower breast. A core biopsy confirms a borderline phyllodes tumour.
>
> She requires surgery with a minimum margin of 5 mm healthy tissue. Depending on her breast size, this could be either a wide local excision or a mastectomy.

7.2.4 Other Common Benign Breast Lumps

7.2.4.1 Hamartoma

Hamartomas usually present as a painless well-defined mass in women over the age of 35.

They are formed by proliferation of normal breast tissue elements including glandular, fibrous, and fatty tissue with a connective tissue capsule. Normal tissue components are typically present in the wrong proportion. Although they are benign, they may enlarge progressively. As hamartomas do not have distinctive histopathological features, diagnosis requires biopsy and correlation between the clinical, radiological, and pathological findings (8).

Multiple hamartomas may be related to Cowden syndrome (PTEN mutation), which carries an increased risk of developing breast cancer and other malignancies, namely, thyroid cancer. Patients presenting with breast haematomas, fibrocystic disease, or papillary changes in association with skin lesions or thyroid disorders should be referred for genetic assessment (9).

Excision can be offered for large lesions or symptomatic cases and should include a narrow margin of breast tissue, although local recurrence is rare.

7.2.4.2 Granulomatous Mastitis

Granulomatous mastitis represents a rare, benign, inflammatory condition of the breast. The condition presents most commonly in women in their 30s and 40s and may be associated with recent pregnancy and lactation.

Multiple potential causes have been suggested including *Corynebacterium* infection, tuberculosis, sarcoidosis, foreign body reaction, and parasitic or fungal infections. However, in most cases, no cause is found, and the condition is described as idiopathic granulomatous mastitis (10).

Granulomatous mastitis typically presents with a painful mass and may be associated with overlying skin changes such as erythema and skin ulceration. Regional lymph nodes may also be enlarged, raising the possibility of a cancer diagnosis.

Clinical history should include recent pregnancies and breastfeeding, any history of autoimmune conditions or diabetes, and recent travel or potential exposure to infectious diseases.

Mammograms show focal asymmetric density and distortion of the breast parenchyma. Ultrasound examination may show focal enhancing masses and abscess formation.

Diagnosis is made by core biopsy showing granulomas associated with multinucleated giant cells and micro-abscesses. Biopsies should also undergo culture and staining to identify any potential causative organisms such as tuberculosis or *Corynebacterium*.

The condition should be distinguished from diabetic mastopathy, which affects younger women with type one diabetes. Core biopsy will differentiate these conditions, as diabetic mastopathy typically involves lymphocytic lobulitis and dense fibrosis (11).

As granulomatous mastitis represents a spectrum of diseases, treatment should be targeted at the underlying cause if identified. Smaller lesions may be managed conservatively.

Abscesses should be drained under ultrasound guidance. Prolonged courses of antibiotics are indicated for symptomatic lesions in the presence of proven pathogens. For idiopathic symptomatic cases, a trial of steroid treatment or immunosuppression may be effective (1). However, if the lesion is symptomatic, and persists or enlarges, wide excision may be considered. However, disease recurrence and wound complications following surgery are significant issues (10).

7.2.4.3 Pseudoangiomatous Stromal Hyperplasia (PASH)

Pseudoangiomatous stromal hyperplasia (PASH) is a benign condition, hypothesised to be associated with hormonal stimulation (12).

PASH generally occurs in younger women, presenting as a discrete painless breast lump. PASH may also be detected incidentally during breast screening in older women, particularly those taking hormonal replacement therapy, or associated with cases of gynaecomastia.

Radiological appearances are non-specific. Some lesions may appear similar to fibroadenomas, consisting of a hypoechoic mass with a well-circumscribed edge, but in dense breast tissue, the lesion may not be sonographically visible and MRI may be required.

Diagnosis is made by ultrasound-guided or clinical core biopsy. In cases of clinical and radiological discrepancy, or if the lesion is progressively enlarging, surgery may be required with clear margins to reduce recurrence (1). Otherwise, conservative management is recommended.

7.2.4.4 Lipoma

CLINICAL CASE

A 28-year-old cleaner presents with a painful lump in the upper outer left breast. She has a relatively high BMI and a large cup size. Examination reveals no discrete breast mass.

Ultrasound findings are shown in Figure 7.7.

Breast lipomas present as soft mobile masses, which may be tender on palpation. There may be a history of other lipomata in different body sites.

Clinically, the lump is compressible and large lesions may be fluctuant. On imaging this has the typical appearance of a smooth rounded isoechoic lesion containing adipose tissue which is similar in echogenicity to the surrounding mammary fat.

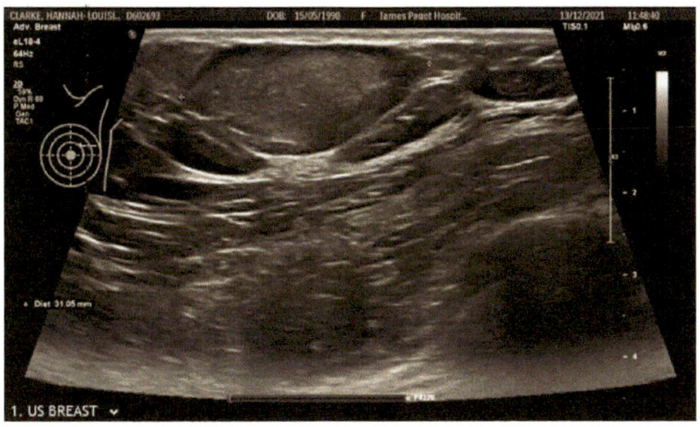

FIGURE 7.7
A well-defined 3 cm lesion was noted in the left upper outer quadrant, isoechoic with the surrounding fat.

Breast lipomas are benign and do not require surveillance or removal unless symptomatic and over 5 cm in size.

> Management summary: Ultrasound confirms a 3 cm lipoma in the left axillary tail. Core biopsy is not required to confirm the diagnosis. She is reassured and reassessed in clinic several weeks later.
>
> Her pain persists, and she undergoes image-guided surgical excision of the lesion which confirms a 5 cm lipoma.

7.2.4.5 Fat Necrosis

> **CLINICAL CASE**
>
> A 51-year-old woman who previously underwent right therapeutic mammoplasty for breast cancer presents with a painful lump in the inner aspect of the right breast 14 months following surgery. She is concerned about cancer recurrence.
>
> On clinical examination there is an ill-defined but firm lump in the medial right breast with no palpable axillary lymphadenopathy.
>
> Mammograms and ultrasound findings are shown in Figures 7.8 and 7.9.

Fat necrosis represents saponification of adipose tissue with an associated inflammatory response. It can occur due to trauma, surgery, radiotherapy, anti-coagulation, and breast infection, especially in fatty breast tissue. It is most prevalent in peri-menopausal women.

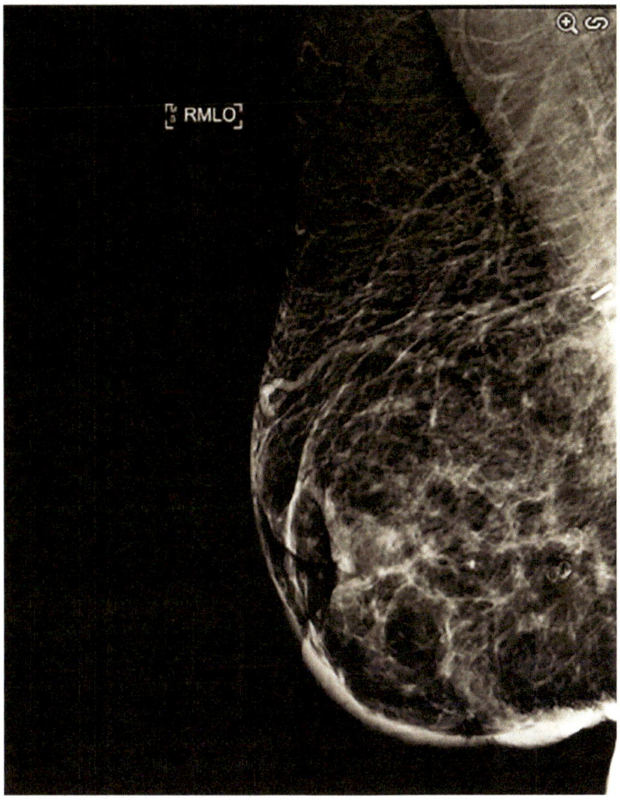

FIGURE 7.8
Right breast mediolateral oblique mammogram demonstrated skin thickening and post-surgical fibrotic changes with no mass lesion apparent.

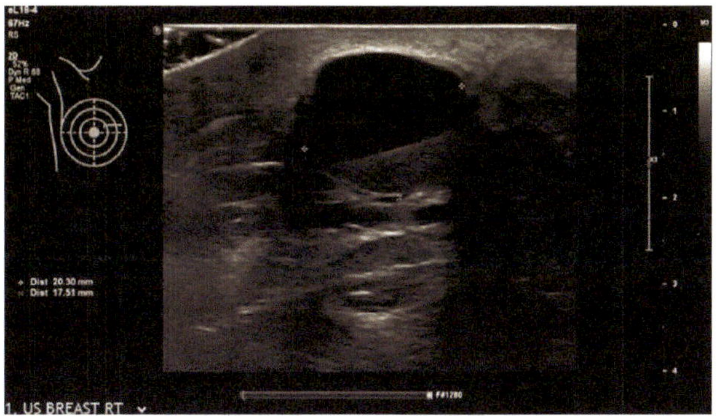

FIGURE 7.9
Ultrasound of the medial right breast demonstrated extensive areas of increased echogenicity surrounding a cystic structure with wall nodularity and a visible fluid level.

Fat necrosis usually presents as a firm, tender lump. A careful history should be taken to identify any previous episode of trauma or extensive bruising to the breast, such as may be sustained by a seatbelt injury. Initially, there may be a local inflammatory response present, causing erythema or skin thickening. Subsequent scarring may cause parenchymal distortion or nipple retraction, mimicking cancer (13).

Mammograms may show a focal mass or spiculations associated with dystrophic calcifications, skin thickening, and parenchymal distortion. Ultrasound may show nodules with increased tissue echogenicity and cystic structures.

Core biopsy should be undertaken to exclude carcinoma if there is radiological uncertainty, or a lack of correlation between clinical and radiological findings.

If treated conservatively, the lump will usually soften and reduce in size. If the lump persists or enlarges, and remains symptomatic, surgical excision can be considered.

> Management summary: Ultrasound demonstrates a 20 mm oil cyst with extensive surrounding fat necrosis, U2. The contents are aspirated, yielding a milky fluid.
>
> The patient is treated conservatively, with gradual resolution of the lump and discomfort over a period of 12 months.

7.3 Section II: Nipple Discharge

7.3.1 Duct Ectasia

> **CLINICAL CASE**
>
> A 49-year-old woman presents with spontaneous yellowish discharge from her right nipple. She has noticed blood on one occasion. On examination there is no associated lump, and it is possible to express a milky yellow fluid, which tests negative for blood on urinalysis dipstick.
>
> Ultrasound findings are shown in Figure 7.10.

Duct ectasia is a normal involutional process whereby the sub-areolar ducts become dilated and tortuous. It most often presents in the peri-menopausal period as physiological nipple discharge which may vary in colour from yellow through to green or black and may either be spontaneous or elicited with direct pressure. It may be associated with hypothyroidism or medication side effects (14). Nipple inversion may be a feature due to duct fibrosis and shortening.

Clinical examination should assess for any breast lumps and an attempt made to elicit the discharge. It should be noted if it is unilateral or bilateral and whether

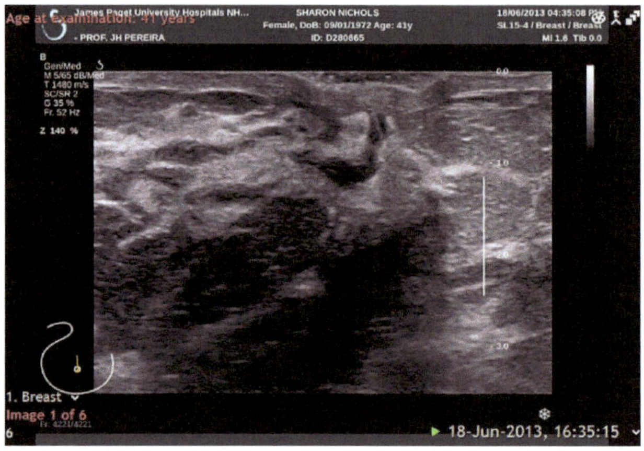

FIGURE 7.10
Ultrasound shows dilated retro-areolar ducts with thick contents.

it is produced from several ducts (physiological) or a single duct (pathological). The discharge should be tested for the presence of blood using a urinalysis dipstick. If blood is identified, this must be further investigated to exclude a papilloma or breast carcinoma as only 25–25% of cases of nipple bleeding are due to duct ectasia.

Nipple discharge is not routinely sent for cytology due to the high false negative rate (14).

Mammography is usually non-specific, but ultrasound will demonstrate widened ectatic ducts behind the nipple (over 3 mm in diameter) and may confirm the presence of duct contents. If there is any evidence of an intraductal lesion, a core biopsy should be undertaken.

Periductal mastitis is an associated condition involving inflammation of the ducts and is associated with smoking. This may progress into abscess formation and development of fistulae. Patients should be strongly encouraged to stop smoking (or use nicotine products), and cultures of the discharge should be obtained to guide appropriate anti-microbial treatment. Abscesses should be initially drained radiologically, whenever possible, to avoid extensive scarring and prolonged wound healing (15).

> Management summary: Ultrasound confirms mild duct ectasia behind the nipple areola complex on the right. The ducts appeared to have content within them—thick inspissated secretions or a papilloma. In view of this core biopsies were taken, which confirmed duct ectasia.
>
> The patient was reassured but asked to reattend the event of further bleeding from the nipple occurred as further investigations such as MRI would be required.

7.3.2 Papillary Lesions

> **CLINICAL CASE**
>
> A 49-year-old teacher presents with a painless lump in the lower aspect of the right breast. She describes discharge from the right nipple when she presses directly on the lump.
>
> Clinically there is a small nodule immediately inferior to the right areola, with clear discharge from a single duct, which tests positive for blood on urinalysis dipstick.
>
> Ultrasound images are shown in Figure 7.11.

7.3.2.1 Solitary Intraductal Papilloma

Papillary lesions of the breast are common and range from benign intraductal papillomas through papillary DCIS to invasive papillary carcinomas (16, 17). They may be located centrally within the breast (solitary intraductal papillomas) or peripherally (multiple papillomatosis; described in more detail below).

Solitary intraductal papillomas typically present with unilateral nipple discharge, which may be clear, serous, or bloodstained. On clinical examination, a small lump may be palpable in the retro-areolar space. However, the definitive finding is discharge from a single duct, which tests positive for blood on urinalysis dipstick.

Most papillomas are mammographically occult but may be visualised as a 2–3 mm rounded mass within 5 cm of the nipple on ultrasound. MRI may be useful if conventional imaging is non-specific (14) but has a high false positive rate, especially in younger and dense breasts, potentially leading to unnecessary additional biopsies.

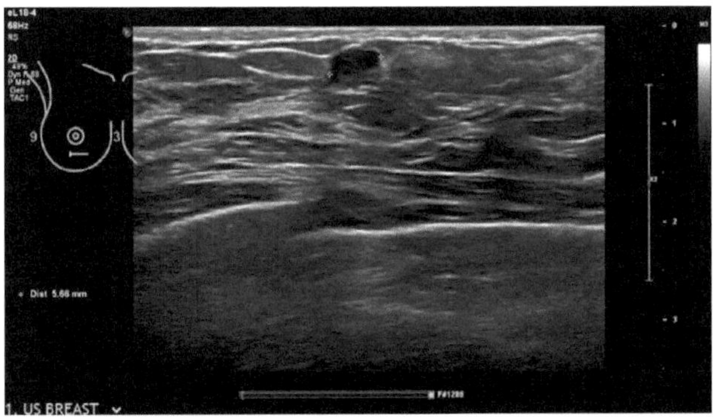

FIGURE 7.11
Ultrasound demonstrates a 5 mm indeterminate nodule in the lower right breast.

If a lesion is visualised within the duct, a core biopsy should be undertaken to determine the diagnosis. Intraductal papillomas without atypia are classified as B3 lesions, and although they have a low upgrade rate of 2.3%, they should be excised in their entirety either using vacuum excision or open image-guided surgical biopsy to ensure thorough sampling (18).

If no lesion is demonstrated on breast imaging, but there is persisting single-duct bloodstained discharge, a surgical microdochectomy or total duct excision should be undertaken. The affected duct is cannulated and removed in entirety for histological examination.

> Management summary: Ultrasound shows a 5 mm indeterminate U3 nodule in the subcutaneous space. Core biopsy confirms a benign intraductal papilloma (B3).
>
> The lesion is removed using ultrasound-guided vacuum excision. Final histology confirms a benign papilloma with no atypia. No additional treatment or surveillance is required.

7.3.2.2 Multiple Papillomatosis

Multiple papillomatosis (the presence of more than five papillomas within one breast) accounts for approximately 10% of papilloma cases and is associated with a threefold increased risk of breast cancer (16, 17).

Multiple-duct papillomas are less likely to be associated with nipple discharge as they are located more peripherally in the breast tissue. They may present symptomatically with a lump or be detected incidentally on screening mammograms. Ultrasound can demonstrate multiple hypoechoic masses with well circumscribed edges. MRI is the most sensitive imaging modality, although upgrade of papillary lesions to invasive disease may not easily be identified.

Due to the increased association with breast cancer, and the technical issues in removing all visualised lesions, patients should undergo regular surveillance monitoring and biopsies undertaken if indicated by any interval changes that are detected on serial imaging.

7.3.2.3 Conclusion

Benign breast conditions represent a spectrum of aberrations within normal breast tissue and may present in women of all ages. The underlying mechanisms differ, but most are believed to be linked to the influence of hormonal fluctuations on breast development or involution.

The term ANDI (aberrations in the normal development and involution of the breast) reflects how benign changes are not pathological per se but represent a normal response of breast tissue to aging (19). However, certain benign breast conditions, especially when associated with atypia, can be linked to a moderately increased risk of developing subsequent breast cancer (20).

Therefore, all women presenting with symptoms of benign breast disease should undergo a thorough clinical history, physical examination, and appropriate breast imaging. Core or vacuum biopsy of any focal lesions is indicated in the majority of cases except for those which fulfil specific exclusion criteria, such as non-complex fibroadenomas in young women, simple cysts, and lipomas.

Where there is discordance between clinical and radiological findings, further imaging should be undertaken (e.g. MRI), and surgical intervention contemplated when appropriate.

References

1 Stachs A, Stubert J, Reimer T, et al. Benign breast disease in women. Dtsch Arztebl Int. 2019;116(33–34):565–74.

2 Alipour S, Rastad H, Saberi A, et al. Metformin in the management of fibrocystic breast disease: A placebo-controlled randomized clinical trial. Daru. 2021;29(2):389–96.

3 Quinn CM, D'Arcy C, Wells C. Apocrine lesions of the breast. Virchows Arch. 2022;480(1):177–89.

4 Stavros AT, Thickman D, Rapp CL, et al. Solid breast nodules: Use of sonography to distinguish between benign and malignant lesions. Radiology. 1995;196(1):123–34.

5 Sosin M, Pulcrano M, Feldman ED, et al. Giant juvenile fibroadenoma: A systematic review with diagnostic and treatment recommendations. Gland Surg. 2015;4(4):312–21.

6 Tan BY, Acs G, Apple SK, et al. Phyllodes tumours of the breast: A consensus review. Histopathology. 2016;68(1):5–21.

7 Krings G, Bean GR, Chen YY. Fibroepithelial lesions; The WHO spectrum. Sem Diagn Pathol. 2017;34(5):438–52.

8 Tazeoğlu D, Dağ A, Arslan B, et al. Breast hamartoma: Clinical, radiological, and histopathological evaluation. Eur J Breast Health. 2021;17(4):328–32.

9 Carter C, Sciallis A. Benign breast disease in patients with Cowden syndrome. Am J Clin Pathol. 2016;146(Suppl_1):288.

10 Benson JR, Dumitru D. Idiopathic granulomatous mastitis: Presentation, investigation and management. Future Oncol. 2016;12(11):1381–94.

11 Leroux-Stewart J, Rabasa-Lhoret R. Diabetic mastopathy: Case report and summary of literature. Can J Diabetes. 2014;38(5):305–6.

12 Speer ME, Yoon EC, Berg WA et al. Pseudoangiomatous stromal hyperplasia: Radiologic-pathologic correlation. J Breast Imag. 2023;5(1):67–72.

13 Tan PH, Lai LM, Carrington EV, et al. Fat necrosis of the breast—a review. Breast. 2006;15(3):313–8.

14 Panzironi G, Pediconi F, Sardanelli F. Nipple discharge: The state of the art. BJR Open. 2018;1(1):20180016.

15 Hamzi MW, Winters R. Mammary duct ectasia. In: StatPearls [Internet]. Treasure Island, FL: StatPearls Publishing; 2023.

16 Kulka J, Madaras L, Floris G, et al. Papillary lesions of the breast. Virchows Arch. 2022;480(1):65–84.

17 Rella R, Romanucci G, Arciuolo D, et al. Multiple papillomas of the breast: A review of current evidence and challenges. J Imaging. 2022;8(7):198.

18 Elfgen C, Leo C, Kubik-Huch RA, et al. Third International Consensus Conference on lesions of uncertain malignant potential in the breast (B3 lesions). Virchows Arch. 2023;483(1):5–20.

19 Hughes LE. Classification of benign breast disorders. The ANDI classification based on physiological processes within the normal breast. Br Med Bull. 1991;47(2):251–7.

20 Kabat GC, Jones JG, Olson N, et al. A multi-center prospective cohort study of benign breast disease and risk of subsequent breast cancer. Cancer Causes Control. 2010;21(6):821–8.

8

Breast Pain

Sam Leinster

8.1 Clinical Features

Breast pain, otherwise known as mastalgia or mastodynia, is a common problem affecting up to 70% of women at some time in their life.[1–3] It accounts for 40–50% of referrals to specialist breast clinics.[4] Nevertheless, most women who experience breast pain do not seek medical advice. Breast pain can be classified into three aetiological categories—hormonal, non-hormonal, and extra-mammary. The three types can be distinguished from each other by careful history taking and clinical examination.

8.1.1 Hormonal Breast Pain

Hormonal breast pain is often labelled cyclical breast pain, but this can be a misnomer. Typically, hormonal pain occurs during the luteal phase of the menstrual cycle. Many women recognise this and regard it as normal and expected. The pain is often accompanied by tenderness and nodularity, particularly in the upper, outer quadrant of each breast. It starts up to 7 days before the next period is due and disappears with the onset of menstruation. For some women, the pain may become severe enough to begin to impact on their quality of life. In this group of women, the duration of pain may increase until it is present throughout the whole menstrual cycle. The pain then is hormonal but not cyclical. Careful history taking will elicit the presence of cyclical pain prior to the presenting continuous pain. Hormonal breast pain, by definition, ceases with the onset of the menopause.

The diagnostic features of hormonal pain are its location, character, and radiation. Hormonal breast pain is diffuse and poorly localised, often, but not exclusively in the upper, outer quadrant of the breast. The patient describes it as throbbing, aching, or heavy. If it radiates, it does so to the ipsilateral axilla. On clinical examination, there may be nodularity and tenderness, most frequently in the upper outer quadrant, but it is not unusual to find no palpable abnormality.

A wide range of drugs prescribed for non-mammary conditions can give rise to hormonal-type pain in the breast (Table 8.1). Their mode of action is possibly related to their effects on the endocrine system. The symptoms and signs they give rise to is indistinguishable from idiopathic hormonal pain, so in all cases it is important to take a careful drug history.

8.1.2 Non-Hormonal Breast Pain

Non-hormonal breast pain includes several distinct entities.[5] Persistent breast pain may occur as a long-term sequela of breast lump excision. It is largely unrecognised as a potential complication of breast surgery, but the literature suggests that it occurs in 20–30% of cases.[6] The pain is in the region of the scar and quite localised. There may or may not be associated tenderness. Patients should be warned of the possibility when giving informed consent for the surgical procedure. In rare cases, if there has been axillary surgery with injury to a nerve in the axilla the patient may develop causalgia (Complex Regional Pain Syndrome Type 2).

Breast cancer may present with pain.[7] Reports suggest that pain is present in 2–7% of breast cancers, but the pain is usually associated with the presence of a lump.[8] It is very rare for pain to be due to cancer in the absence of any palpable abnormality but incidental cancers, often in the contralateral breast may be found on imaging of patients with mastalgia.[9] Painful, rapidly growing lumps are more likely to be cysts than cancers.

TABLE 8.1

Drugs That May Cause Breast Pain

Oral contraceptive pill
Hormone replacement therapy
Chlorpromazine
Selective serotonin reuptake inhibitors
Metoclopramide
Spironolactone

DOI: 10.1201/9781003394785-8

Most cases of non-hormonal breast pain will not be associated with a lump but will have a localised area of tenderness on palpation, often known as a *trigger spot*. When this is within the breast mound, especially if it is close to the nipple, it is most likely due to duct ectasia and its complications. The pain is often described as sharp or burning. If the pain is located near the lateral edge of the breast, it has been designated *lateral chest wall pain*.[10] The patient usually describes it as sharp. This perhaps should be included under the extra-mammary category as its aetiology is obscure.

Non-hormonal pain is often described as burning or stabbing. If it radiates, it tends to do so towards the nipple and areola.

8.1.3 Extra-Mammary Pain

A wide range of unrelated conditions may present as breast pain including musculo-skeletal problems in the neck or upper limbs, cardiac problems, and gastro-oesophageal or biliary problems. One of the commonest presentations in the breast clinic is costochondritis or Tietze's syndrome. The patient presents with unilateral pain on the medial aspect of the breast. On examination, the pain is obviously arising from the chest wall beneath the breast. There is tenderness which is localised to a costochondral junction which may be swollen. The breast itself has no palpable abnormality.

8.2 Aetiology of Hormonal Breast Pain

No histological differences have been found between breast biopsies from patients with hormonal mastalgia and normal controls, suggesting that the difference between the two is functional rather than structural.[11] The structure of the breast changes across the menstrual cycle. Vogel et al. recognised five phases in the normal cycle (Table 8.2).[12] The presence of oedema in the stroma during the later luteal phase is consistent with the finding that the normal breast increases in volume by 30–40% in the second half of the menstrual cycle.[13] More recent studies using MRI have confirmed that the breast does retain water during the luteal phase of the cycle but there is no difference between patients with mastalgia and normal controls.[14]

The relationship of hormonal breast pain to the menstrual cycle, and the fact that it stops at the menopause is the presumptive evidence for labelling it hormonal. However, attempts to elucidate the exact hormonal disturbance that gives rise to the pain have been singularly unsuccessful in reaching a consensus. In part, this may be because the studies to date have focused on circulating hormone levels. Murrow et al.[15] have elegantly shown that the effect of hormones on the breast is mediated at a cellular level by paracrine and cell-to-cell signalling. The studies did not consider breast pain as a variable, but it is possible that the aetiology of hormonal mastalgia is related to changes at the cellular level within the breast rather than changes in the patient's hormonal profile. Nevertheless, many of the therapies that have been tried are based on assumptions about the hormonal aetiology of mastalgia, so it is worthwhile reviewing some of the suggested mechanisms.

8.2.1 Oestrogen/Progesterone Imbalance

An early candidate for the aetiological role was an imbalance between oestrogen and progesterone levels in the luteal phase of the menstrual cycle. This was postulated to be due to inadequate corpus luteum function related to ovulatory malfunction.[16] It was suggested that the resulting high oestrogen to progesterone ratio led to changes in the breast that caused mastalgia. Subsequent studies have failed to confirm a deficiency in progesterone.[17,18]

8.2.2 Dynamic Release of FSH/LH

Some investigators have shown differences in FSH and LH between women with cyclical mastalgia and controls at all stages of the menstrual cycle.[19] Other

TABLE 8.2

Changes in the Histology of the Breast During the Menstrual Cycle

Day	Menstrual Phase	Functional Phase	Histological Appearance
3–7	Follicular	Proliferative	Mitotic figures in acinar cells
8–14	Follicular	Differentiation	Basal cells and luminal cells visible in addition to acinar cells
15–20	Luteal	Differentiation	Ballooning of basal cells; lumen enlarges
21–27	Luteal	Secretory	True apocrine secretion into distended lumen; mantle tissue becomes oedematous.
28–2	Menstruation		Cells regress; oedema resolves

Note: Adapted from ref. 12.

investigators have found no absolute differences in levels but noted an increased pulse frequency with lowered amplitude in cases compared to controls.[20]

8.2.3 Dynamic Release of Prolactin

Women with hormonal mastalgia have been shown to have resting levels of prolactin which are higher than pain-free controls, but still fell within the normal range.[21] However, women with mastalgia show an abnormal release of prolactin in response to stimulation by thyroid-releasing factor. This response was not present in women who had breast nodularity without pain.[22] The effect is found in a subset of women with mastalgia and predicts response to hormone treatment.[23,24]

8.2.4 Psychological Factors

The failure to find unequivocal hormonal mechanisms to account for mastalgia led some workers to propose that underlying psychopathology accounted for women presenting with breast pain. This notion has a long history. Hedley Atkins writing in 1938[25] endorsed the view of Sir Astley Cooper, who wrote in 1829 that women with breast pain were of an irritable or nervous disposition.[26] Patey thought that *pain syndrome* (as he called it) was either due to fear of cancer or due to psychosexual problems.[27] This view was challenged by Preece, Mansel, and Hughes,[28] who found no difference in the incidence of psychological disorder between the patients with mastalgia and those with varicose veins. They concluded that psychopathology was not a factor in the aetiology of breast pain.

Rameriz et al. found that women with severe mastalgia had raised levels of anxiety compared to those with mastalgia that was classified as non-severe.[29] Downey and Leinster compared three groups of women—those with mastalgia who did not request treatment after receiving reassurance; those who, despite reassurance, still requested treatment; and normal controls.[30] Patients with mastalgia had higher levels of anxiety than controls. However, while those not seeking treatment showed no change in anxiety levels between the follicular and luteal phases, those seeking treatment showed a marked increase in anxiety levels in the luteal phase, coinciding with the occurrence of pain. A subsequent study from the same unit found that patients with breast pain were more anxious and depressed than patients presenting to the clinic with breast lumps. Trait anxiety was particularly high in those women who continued to complain of pain despite six months or more of treatment.[31] More recent studies have confirmed a relationship between anxiety and mastalgia in a range of countries including Turkey,[32] India,[33] and Iran.[34]

The link between mastalgia and measurable psychological distress has led several authors to suggest that psychological treatments may be benefit for women who are not relieved by simple reassurance. However, there have been few studies of the effectiveness of this approach. Although relaxation therapy[35] and a 'psychoeducation' session were said to be effective in reducing breast pain,[36] there is no well-validated psychological approach that has gained widespread acceptance.

8.3 Aetiology of Non-Hormonal Breast Pain

Non-hormonal breast pain is often associated with duct ectasia and periductal mastitis. Dilatation of the milk ducts is a natural occurrence with ageing, but the process is exacerbated and accelerated by smoking. Mastalgia is associated with dilatation of the milk ducts. Pain levels are correlated with the degree of dilatation and focal pain is localised to the areas of dilatation observed on ultrasound imaging.[37] Unlike hormonal pain, it does not resolve at menopause.

The aetiology and pathogenesis of lateral wall chest pain is unknown. Trigger pain within the breast mound is most likely the result of duct ectasia.

8.4 Management of a Patient with Mastalgia

Patients with breast pain present for a variety of reasons. One study in the USA found that women with mastalgia were more likely to be afraid that they had breast cancer than other women attending a breast clinic (40% v 25% $p < 0.0001$).[38] This is particularly the case if the pain is of recent onset or if it is non-cyclical. Alternatively, the pain may be severe enough to be having a significant negative effect on a woman's daily life.

8.4.1 Excluding Cancer

It is important to note that an isolated complaint of pain is very unlikely to be due to cancer; however, it is necessary to exclude cancer to set the patient's mind at rest. This does not necessarily mean extensive investigations. The first stage in the management is taking a careful history. The history should include a full obstetric and gynaecological history with explicit enquiry about any premenstrual symptoms at any stage since menarche. Any family history of breast cancer should also be noted. Careful systematic enquiry can help to exclude extra-mammary causes for the pain.

Whatever the history, a relevant clinical examination must be conducted. In all cases, this will include a full examination of the breasts with other systems being examined as indicated by the history.

The decision on whether further investigation is necessary is based on the history and clinical findings (Table 8.3). For those women who are experiencing typical hormonal mastalgia in the absence of physical signs within the breast no further investigation is needed, particularly if the pain is bilateral. In women under 40, with localised pain, an ultrasound should be performed. The American College of Radiology would advocate the addition of mammography in women between 30, but this seems over-investigation as the pick-up rate of cancers in this group is around 0.2%.[39] The UK Royal College of Radiologists recommend reserving mammography in this age group for women who are found to have an abnormality on ultrasound.[40] Focal, non-cyclical pain in women over 40 warrants mammography and ultrasound examination, especially if it is of recent onset.

8.4.2 Reassurance

For those women in whom no evidence of cancer is found, reassurance that the pain is not due to any serious disease is often sufficient and further intervention is unnecessary. Reassurance needs time and a careful explanation of what the symptoms are due to. It begins with a recognition of the significance of the pain to the patient followed by a careful explanation.

1. Explain that the symptoms that she is suffering from are common and that as clinicians we are used to dealing with them.
2. Explain the cause of the symptoms in terms that are appropriate to that patient's level of knowledge and understanding.
3. Explain that there are several treatments that are available should she feel the need to proceed to treatment.

8.4.3 Lifestyle Advice

In addition to offering reassurance, it has been common practice to offer lifestyle and dietary advice to women with mastalgia. A frequent piece of advice is the wearing of a well-fitting bra. The advice is plausible but there is little empirical evidence to support it.

At one stage, it was believed that reducing caffeine intake was effective, but randomised controlled trials have failed to show any benefit.[41] Another dietary intervention that has been reported as being effective is a low-fat diet.[42] One of the difficulties in showing benefit from such long-term interventions is tendency of the condition to resolve spontaneously.

Evening primrose oil (EPO) is recommended for mastalgia on several health websites, but systematic review of studies of EPO have shown it to be no better than placebo.[43] Other alternative therapies recommended on the internet include vitex agnus-castus, flaxseed, vitamin B6, iodine, and fish oil. The evidence for the effectiveness of any of these treatments is weak, and this should be pointed out to the patient. It is, nevertheless, the case that some patients want to take active steps and may see these treatments as a preferable alternative to drug treatment.

Advising patients to give up smoking is, of course, good general health advice but is particularly important for patients with non-hormonal breast pain where the underlying pathology is often duct ectasia, which is exacerbated by smoking.

Overall, while most women will be satisfied with the knowledge that there is no serious pathology to account for their symptoms and will be content to follow lifestyle advice, there is a small minority who will find the pain so disruptive of their normal life that they will continue to ask for treatment.

TABLE 8.3

Indications for Imaging in Women Presenting with Breast Pain

Age	Clinical Presentation	Imaging
<40	Cyclical pain with no palpable abnormality	None indicated
>40	Cyclical pain with no palpable abnormality	May offer screening mammogram
<40	Focal pain and tenderness	Ultrasound scan
>40	Focal pain and tenderness	Mammogram and ultrasound scan
<40	Focal nodularity or discrete lump	Ultrasound scan followed by mammogram if USS suspicious of malignancy
>40	Focal nodularity or discrete lump	Mammogram and ultrasound scan

8.5 Treatment of a Patient with Non-Hormonal Mastalgia

Patients with lateral chest wall pain or trigger spot pain often benefit from the injection of local anaesthetic and steroid.[44] If the pain is more diffuse, or the patient is reluctant to have an injection, topical non-steroidal gel is the treatment of choice.[45]

8.6 Treatment of a Patient with Hormonal Mastalgia

8.6.1 Further Assessment

Before commencing treatment, it is worthwhile to take time to fully assess the mastalgia and, in particular, confirm its relationship to the menstrual cycle. A useful tool for this purpose is a Breast Pain Chart (Figure 8.1).

The patient is given a chart and asked to complete it each day for three months according to the instructions on the chart. At the end of the three months, she is reviewed with the chart. If the chart confirms the cyclical nature of the pain and she is still requesting treatment, there are several options that have been shown to be effective in randomised, controlled clinical trials.

8.7 Drug Treatment of Hormonal Mastalgia

Since the 1970s, a range of drugs has been used to treat hormonal mastalgia. The choice of these drugs has been based on the understanding of the aetiology of mastalgia current at the time.

8.7.1 Medroxyprogesterone Acetate

The hypothesis that hormonal mastalgia was the result of a deficiency of progesterone in the luteal phase of the cycle led to the prescription of medroxyprogesterone acetate (MPA) from day 14 of the cycle till menstruation. Early trials suggested that this was effective but systematic review of all the trials of MPA fails to show any benefit.[47]

8.7.2 Bromocriptine

Bromocriptine is a dopamine agonist which inhibits the secretion of prolactin. It is given in a dose of 1.25–5 mg b.d. throughout the month for six months. A systematic review of trials carried out between 1978 and 1989 confirmed that it was highly effective in relieving breast pain.[21] However, there was a high incidence of troublesome side effects mainly relating to the GI tract, and it is no longer used as first-line therapy.[48] It can be considered for use in cases of mastalgia that are resistant to other forms of treatment, especially if they can be shown to have abnormalities of prolactin secretion.

8.7.3 Danazol

Danazol is an anti-gonadotropic agent, suppressing the release of gonadotrophins from the anterior pituitary. It also has anti-oestrogenic and androgenic effects, the latter contributing to its side effects. It is given in a dose of 100 mg b.d. throughout the month. It is usual to prescribe it for three months and then review the patient to assess its effectiveness. If has proved effective it is continued for a further 3 months

Name ______________________

Record the amount of breast pain you experience each day by shading in each box as illustrated

Severe pain

Mild pain

No pain

For example: if you get severe breast pain on the fifth of the month, then shade in completely the square under 5. Please note the day you period starts each month with the letter 'P'

Please bring this card with you on each visit

Month	1	2	3	4	5	6	7	8	9	10	11	12	13	14	15	16	17	18	19	20	21	22	23	24	25	26	27	28	29	30	31

FIGURE 8.1
Breast pain chart.

Source: **Adapted from the Cardiff Breast Pain Chart.**[46]

and then stopped. It has been widely used in the treatment of hormonal mastalgia and systematic review confirms its effectiveness.[21]

The main disadvantage of danazol is the side effects, which are mainly related to its androgenic effects and occur in up to 45% of women. Weight gain is extremely common, as is menstrual cycle irregularity and vaginal dryness and irritation. Some patients find the increased hirsutism and deepening of the voice more distressing. Despite these side effects, women who experience significant relief of their symptoms may be happy to continue the drug, especially if it relieves other premenstrual symptoms as well.

8.7.4 Selective Oestrogen Receptor Modulators (SERMs)

The putative link between oestrogen and mastalgia has led to the trialling of SERMs as a treatment. This group of drugs have anti-oestrogenic effects on the breast with weak oestrogenic effects on the endometrium.

8.7.5 Tamoxifen

Tamoxifen is effective in a dose of 10 mg daily throughout the month.[49] It has fewer side effects than bromocriptine or danazol, the main issues being menstrual irregularity and hot flushes. Once again, it should be given for three months, and the patient should then be reviewed. If it is effective, it should be continued for a further three months. Treatment for longer than six months should only be considered in exceptional circumstances because of the long-term side effects of tamoxifen, such as osteoporosis or endometrial cancer. Tamoxifen is currently the drug of first choice for hormonal mastalgia in the UK.

8.7.6 Ormeloxifene

Ormeloxifene has been widely used in South Asia since the 1990s as a contraceptive. Because of its availability it has been extensively trialled in South Asia for the treatment of mastalgia.[50–52] It is at least as effective as tamoxifen and more effective than danazol in randomised trials. Most series report a lower incidence of side effects than tamoxifen. A single series reports the reverse, but atypically that study reported no side effects in the tamoxifen group.[53] The usual regimen is 30 mg daily for three months. A prolonged residual effect has been noted. It is not clear why the drug has not been used in Western practice.

8.7.7 Toremifene

Two small studies have looked at the utility of toremifene in the treatment of mastalgia.[54,55] While both studies found it to be effective, Hamed et al. rejected it as a viable option for the treatment of mastalgia because of a high incidence of side effects.

8.7.8 Goserelin

Goserelin is a synthetic luteinising releasing hormone analogue which produces rapid-onset, reversible ovarian suppression that is given as a once-a-month depot injection. It is effective in improving mastalgia but is associated with the expected side effects of oestrogen depletion, such as vaginal dryness, hot flushes, decreased libido, and oily skin. In the European multicentre trial over 40% of the treatment group withdrew because the side effects were unacceptable.[56] Goserelin should, therefore, only be used in those patients who are refractory to other forms of treatment.

8.7.9 Summary

Once the decision has been taken that a woman should be started on drug treatment, the initial management should be a selective oestrogen receptor modulator. The drug of first choice in the UK is tamoxifen, but ormeloxifene is an effective alternative. The decision as to which to use should be based on the relative cost and availability in each setting.[52] Treatment should be reviewed at three months. If it is effective, it can be continued for up to six months, but it should then be stopped because of the potential long-term side effects. Around 60% of patients will not experience a recurrence of their symptoms requiring further treatment. If the pain recurs, a repeat course of tamoxifen can be tried, or the patient can be prescribed a second-line drug.

If the pain has not been relieved at the three-month review danazol is the next drug of choice. If danazol is ineffective, the options are bromocriptine or goserelin. Both have significant side effects, but patients who reach this stage will usually opt for treatment despite being warned of the side effects.

8.8 Refractory Hormonal Mastalgia

In a very small number of patients, all drug treatment options will prove ineffective. In the past, mastectomy with or without reconstruction has been recommended. These cases are so rare that it is impossible to get robust trial evidence of the effectiveness of this approach. Those few patients in whom I have carried out mastectomy for hormonal mastalgia have continued to experience phantom pain and I have abandoned the procedure. If the pain persists despite medical oophorectomy with goserelin, it seems very likely that the pain is not hormonal in origin. Referral for psychiatric or psychological assessment should be considered.

References

1. Leinster SJ, Whitehouse GH, Walsh PV. Cyclical mastalgia: Clinical and mammographic observations in a screened population. Br J Surg. 1987 Mar;74(3):220–2.
2. Ader DN, Browne MW. Prevalence and impact of cyclic mastalgia in a United States clinic-based sample. Am J Obstet Gynecol. 1997 Jul 1;177(1):126–32.
3. Scurr J, Hedger W, Morris P, Brown N. The prevalence, severity, and impact of breast pain in the general population. Breast J. 2014 Sep;20(5):508–13.
4. Hafiz SP, Barnes NL, Kirwan CC. Clinical management of idiopathic mastalgia: A systematic review. J Primary Health Care. 2018 Dec 19;10(4):312–23.
5. Maddox PR, Harrison BJ, Mansel RE, Hughes LE. Non-cyclical mastalgia: An improved classification and treatment. Br J Surg. 1989 Sep;76(9):901–4.
6. Spivey TL, Gutowski ED, Zinboonyahgoon N, et al. Chronic pain after breast surgery: A prospective, observational study. Ann Surg Oncol. 2018 Oct;25:2917–24.
7. Preece PE, Baum M, Mansel RE, et al. Importance of mastalgia in operable breast cancer. Br Med J (Clin Res Ed). 1982 May 1;284(6325):1299–300.
8. Eren T, Aslan A, Ozemir IA, et al. Factors effecting mastalgia. Breast Care. 2016 Mar 29;11(3):188–93.
9. Cook N, Batt J, Fowler C. Symptomatic breast cancers and why breast pain may not always need clinical review. Eur J Breast Health. 2020 Oct;16(4):267.
10. Khan HN, Rampaul R, Blamey RW. Local anaesthetic and steroid combined injection therapy in the management of non-cyclical mastalgia. Breast. 2004 Apr 1;13(2):129–32.
11. Jørgensen J, Watt-Boolsen S. Cyclical mastalgia and breast pathology. Acta Chir Scand. 1985;151(4):319–21.
12. Vogel PM, Georgiade NG, Fetter BF, et al. The correlation of histologic changes in the human breast with the menstrual cycle. Am J Pathol. 1981 Jul;104(1):23.
13. Milligan D, Drife JO, Short RV. Changes in breast volume during normal menstrual cycle and after oral contraceptives. Br Med J. 1975 Nov 29;4(5995):494–6.
14. Hussain Z, Brooks J, Percy D. Menstrual variation of breast volume and T2 relaxation times in cyclical mastalgia. Radiography. 2008 Feb 1;14(1):8–16.
15. Murrow LM, Weber RJ, Caruso JA, et al. Mapping hormone-regulated cell-cell interaction networks in the human breast at single-cell resolution. Cell Syst. 2022 Aug 17;13(8):644–64.
16. Sitruk-Ware R, Sterkers N, Mowszowicz I, Mauvais-Jarvis P. Inadequate corpus luteum function in women with benign breast disease. J Clin Endocrinol Metable. 1977;44:771–4.
17. Walsh PV, Bulbrook RD, Stell PM, et al. Serum progesterone concentration during the luteal phase in women with benign breast disease. Eur J Cancer Clin Oncol. 1984 Nov 1;20(11):1339–43.
18. Kumar S, Mansel RE, Wilson DW, et al. Daily salivary progesterone levels in cyclical mastalgia patients and their controls. Br J Surg. 1986;73:260–3.
19. Ecochard R, Marret H, Rabilloud M, et al. Gonadotropin level abnormalities in women with cyclic mastalgia. Eur J Obstet Gynecol Reprod Biol. 2001 Jan 1;94(1):92–6.
20. Facchinetti F, Genazzani AD, Martignoni EM, et al. Neuroendocrine changes in luteal function in patients with premenstrual syndrome. J Clin Endocrinol Metabol. 1993 May 1;76(5):1123–7.
21. Watt-Boolsen S, Andersen AN, Blichert-Toft M. Serum prolactin and oestradiol levels in women with cyclical mastalgia. Horm Metabol Res. 1981 Dec;13(12):700–2.
22. Ayers JW, Gidwani GP. The "luteal breast": Hormonal and sonographic investigation of benign breast disease in patients with cyclic mastalgia. Fertil Steril. 1983 Dec 1;40(6):779–84.
23. Kumar S, Mansel RE, Hughes LE, et al. Prediction of response to endocrine therapy in pronounced cyclical mastalgia using dynamic tests of prolactin release. Clin Endocrinol. 1985 Dec;23(6):699–704.
24. Rea N, Bove F, Gentile A, Parmeggiani U. Prolactin response to thyrotropin-releasing hormone as a guideline for cyclical mastalgia treatment. Minerva Med. 1997 Nov 1;88(11):479–87.
25. Atkins HJ. Chronic mastitis. Lancet. 1938 Mar 26;231(5978):707–12.
26. Cooper A. Illustrations of Diseases of the Breast—Part 1 1829: 78–9. Available at: https://archive.org/details/b21913249/page/78/mode/2up
27. Patey DH. Two non-malignant conditions of breast. Br Med J. 1949 Jan 1;1(4593):96.
28. Preece PE, Mansel RE, Hughes LE. Mastalgia: Psychoneurosis or organic disease? Br Med J. 1978 Jan 7;1(6104):29–30.
29. Ramirez AJ, Jarrett SR, Hamed H, et al. Psychosocial adjustment of women with mastalgia. Breast. 1995 Mar 1;4(1):48–51.
30. Downey H, Leinster S. Mood changes—an explanation why women request treatment for cyclical mastalgia. InRecent developments. In: The Study of Benign Breast Disease. The Proceedings of the 5th International Symposim of Benign Breast Disease. Parthenon Publishing Group, 1993:117–32.
31. Colegrave S, Holcombe C, Salmon P. Psychological characteristics of women presenting with breast pain. J Psychosomatic Res. 2001 Jun 1;50(6):303–7.
32. Kağan Katar M, Başer M, Katar MK. Relationship between mastalgia and anxiety-depression: An observational study. Cureus. 2021 Jan 16;13(1).
33. Kanat BH, Atmaca M, Girgin M, et al. Effects of mastalgia in young women on quality of life, depression, and anxiety levels. Ind J Surg. 2016 Apr;78:96–9.
34. Mirghafourvand M, Ahmadpour P, Rahi P, Salehiniya H. Relationship between depression and anxiety with the severity and length of cyclic mastalgia in women. Iran J Obstet Gynecol Infertil. 2016 Jan 21;18(179):1–7.
35. Fox H, Walker LG, Heys SD, et al. Are patients with mastalgia anxious, and does relaxation therapy help? Breast. 1997 Jun 1;6(3):138–42.
36. Öztürk AB, Özenlı Y, Öztürk SB, et al. The effect of psychoeducation on anxiety and pain in patients with mastalgia. Nordic J Psychiatr. 2015 Jul 4;69(5):380–5.
37. Peters F, Diemer P, Mecks O. Severity of mastalgia in relation to milk duct dilatation. Obstetr Gynecol. 2003 Jan 1;101(1):54–60.
38. Komenaka IK, Nodora J, Martinez ME, et al. Mastalgia is not an indication for mammogram. J Am Board Family Med. 2022 Oct 18;35(5):998–1006.
39. Chetlen AL, Kapoor MM, Watts MR. Mastalgia: Imaging work-up appropriateness. Acad Radiol. 2017 Mar 1;24(3):345–9.
40. The Royal College of Radiologists. Guidance on Screening and Symptomatic Breast Imaging, 4th edition. London: The Royal College of Radiologists, 2019: 7.
41. Ader DN, South-Paul J, Adera T, Deuster PA. Cyclical mastalgia: Prevalence and associated health and behavioral factors. J Psychosom Obstetr Gynecol. 2001 Jan 1;22(2):71–6.
42. Iddon J, Dixon JM. Mastalgia. Br Med J. 2013 Dec 13;347.
43. Srivastava A, Mansel RE, Arvind N, et al. Evidence-based management of Mastalgia: A meta-analysis of randomised trials. Breast. 2007 Oct 1;16(5):503–12.
44. Khan HN, Rampaul R, Blamey RW. Local anaesthetic and steroid combined injection therapy in the management of non-cyclical mastalgia. Breast. 2004 Apr 1;13(2):129–32.

45. Irving AD, Morrison SL. Effectiveness of topical non-steroidal anti-inflammatory drugs in the management of breast pain. J Royal Coll Surg Edin. 1998 Jun 1;43(3):158–9.
46. Gateley CA, Miers M, Mansel RE, Hughes LE. Drug treatments for mastalgia: 17 years experience in the Cardiff Mastalgia Clinic. J Royal Soc Med. 1992 Jan;85(1):12–5.
47. Maddox PR, Harrison BJ, Horobin JM, et al. A randomised controlled trial of medroxyprogesterone acetate in mastalgia. Ann Royal Coll Surg Engl. 1990 Mar;72(2):71.
48. Kataria K, Dhar A, Srivastava A, et al. A systematic review of current understanding and management of mastalgia. Indian J Surg. 2014 Jun;76:217–22.
49. Fentiman IS, Brame K, Caleffi M, et al. Double-blind controlled trial of tamoxifen therapy for mastalgia. Lancet. 1986 Feb 8;327(8476):287–8.
50. Tejwani PL, Srivastava A, Nerkar H, et al. Centchroman regresses mastalgia: A randomized comparison with danazol. Indian J Surg. 2011 Jun;73:199–205.
51. Brahmachari S, Bhagat V, Patil P, Vasuniya V. Evaluating the effect of ormeloxifene on multiple fibroadenomas and mastalgia. J Pharmacy Bioallied Sci. 2021 Nov;13(Suppl 2):S1386.
52. Jain BK, Bansal A, Choudhary D, et al. Centchroman vs tamoxifen for regression of mastalgia: A randomized controlled trial. Int J Surg. 2015 Mar 1;15:11–6.
53. Khadka S, Adhikary S, Rajbanshi S, et al. Effective regression of mastalgia with centchroman and tamoxifen: A randomised comparison. Indian J Surg. 2019 Jun 1;81:271–6.
54. Oksa S, Luukkaala T, Mäenpää J. Toremifene for premenstrual mastalgia: A randomised, placebo-controlled crossover study. BJOG. 2006 Jun;113(6):713–8.
55. Hamed H, Kotheri A, Beechey-Newman N, Fentiman IS. Toremifene, a new agent for treatment of mastalgia: An open study. Int J Fertil Women's Med. 2004 Nov 1;49(6):278–80.
56. Mansel RE, Goyal A, Preece P, et al. European randomized, multicenter study of goserelin (Zoladex) in the management of mastalgia. Am J Obstet Gynecol. 2004 Dec 1;191(6):1942–9.

9

Nipple Discharge

Natasha E. Jiwa

9.1 Introduction

Nipple discharge is the result of fluid emanating from the ductal system and egressing onto the surface of one or both nipples and makes up 3–7% of referrals to a breast unit (1). It is a symptom that affects both men and women, and although its aetiology is often physiological, benign, and harmless, it may be indicative of underlying conditions that require further evaluation and management, with up to 20% caused by underlying malignant disease (2). In the normal physiological state, the nipple orifice of non-lactating women is blocked by keratin plugs, which prevents spontaneous leakage of duct contents. Nipple aspirate fluid (NAF) is the physiological fluid that lines the ductal epithelial cells of all women and can either flow spontaneously from or be expressed from mammary ducts (3, 4). It is constantly turning over but does not usually discharge spontaneously and is considered to be representative of the microenvironment of any developing pathology (5). There is significant growth of the ductal system in response to the hormones of pregnancy (progesterone, oestrogen, prolactin) in preparation for lactation. The suckling reflex triggered through breastfeeding ensures continuation of milk production via a mechanism of positive feedback for an appropriate length of time relating to the desired duration of lactation. These hormones which promote and sustain breastfeeding can also contribute to physiological nipple discharge in non-lactating women. By contrast, non-physiological spontaneous nipple discharge, is a consequence of pathological proliferation of the mammary ductal epithelial lining, leading to a variety of pathological conditions discussed in the following sections. This chapter will explore the various causes of nipple discharge, the diagnostic processes, and treatment options.

9.2 Characteristics, Aetiology, and Incidence

Nipple discharge can be of various types, and its physical characteristics or presentation often provide clues about the underlying cause (Figure 9.1). Nipple discharge can be either unilateral or bilateral, single-duct or multi-duct, and clear or coloured. In terms of the latter feature, different colours may be an important indicator of the potential underlying pathology. For example, clear or serous nipple discharge is typically associated with benign causes, such as hormonal changes or side effects of medication (6). Classically, yellow or greenish discharge is associated with infection, inflammation of the breast, such as mastitis or abscess, or duct ectasia (7). However, it is important to note that malignancy or high-risk lesions cannot be ruled out on the basis of discharge colour alone (8). Milky discharge, also known as galactorrhoea (Figure 9.2), is most commonly related to hormonal imbalance and can affect both sexes (9). Underlying causes may be attributable to medication, thyroid dysfunction, or pituitary gland issues (6). The presence of bloodstained nipple discharge can be alarming and result from either benign causes, such as nipple trauma or more serious conditions, including an underlying malignancy. A systematic review by Chen et al. (10) reported that bloodstained discharge is more likely to arise from a cancer than non-bloodstained discharge that contains no blood elements on routine testing (10). A recent systematic review calculated a malignancy rate of 0.57 for bloodstained discharge on cytology, which therefore requires further investigation or follow-up (11).

9.3 Diagnostic Evaluation

History and examination: The clinical presentation of nipple discharge should prompt referral to a breast

DOI: 10.1201/9781003394785-9

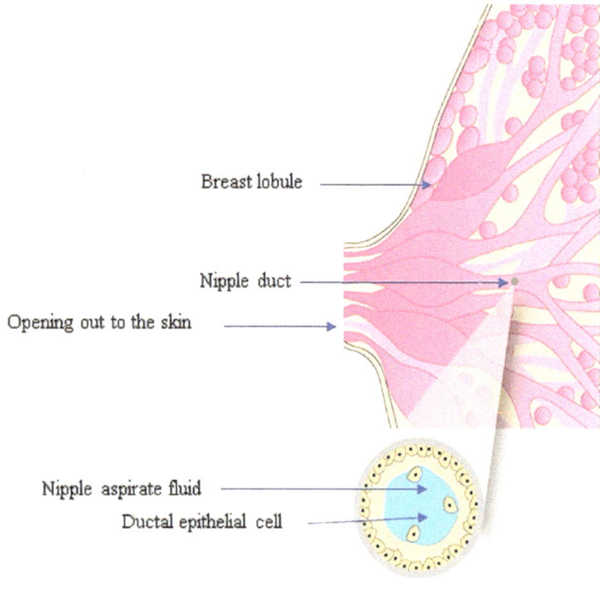

FIGURE 9.1
Spontaneous flow of discharge onto the nipple orifice.

clinic for further evaluation. Nipple discharge represents the third most common presenting breast symptom after the two most common symptoms of breast pain and a palpable breast mass (12). Assessment of nipple discharge involves a thorough clinical history, including careful documentation of the characteristics of the discharge, its duration, and any associated symptoms, such as a mass or palpable lymph nodes. Important features to establish include whether the discharge is single-duct or multi-duct, coloured or bloodstained, spontaneous, and/or unilateral or bilateral. A history of any recent breastfeeding should be noted (13). In addition, it is important to clarify whether the discharge is spontaneous or only occurs on deliberate expression/squeezing. See Table 9.1.

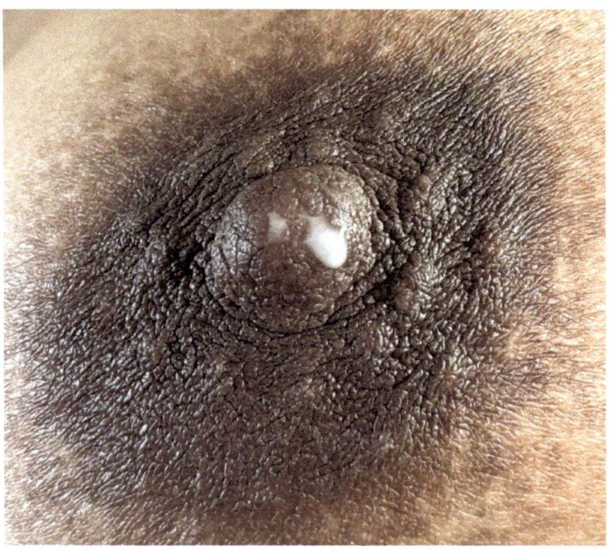

FIGURE 9.2
Milky multi-duct discharge typical of galactorrhoea.

A thorough physical examination should be undertaken following a detailed history and this should focus on the breast and nipples, with identification of any signs of infection or inflammation (i.e. tenderness, fluctuant breast tissue, skin erythema, or breast skin that is warm to touch). Examination should also detect any asymmetry of the breasts or nipples and clinically assess any palpable breast lumps or axillary lymph nodes.

Cytology and occult blood: During this physical examination, it is usually appropriate and opportune to acquire a sample of the discharge fluid for cytology (Figure 9.3). This should be performed in the presence of a chaperone and the patient placed on the examination couch at 45 degrees. The surface of the nipple is cleaned with an alcohol wipe and a gentle attempt made to express fluid; this can be achieved either by asking the patient to squeeze the nipple-areola complex themselves, or the clinician can apply digital pressure to acquire a sample. Any droplet(s) of fluid are then either transferred directly onto a cytology slide or the fluid is aspirated from the surface of the skin using a needle and syringe and thereafter placed on a cytology slide (14). Once the nipple smear sample is collected, a second slide is placed on top of the collection slide and swept across the surface to create a smear. The slide is then fixed by air-drying for 1–2 minutes and stained with May–Grünwald–Giemsa. Alternatively, the material can be fixed in alcohol, or sprayed with a lacquer and Papanicolaou stained (15). The labelled slide containing a patient's identifiable data is examined microscopically by a dedicated breast cytopathologist. Nipple aspirate cytology has been shown to have low sensitivity for detection of cancer and a low negative predictive value (11, 16) and is therefore not used routinely in many centres (17). Nonetheless, it remains a key diagnostic procedure and a means for identifying whether there are either red blood cells within the smear sample or evidence

TABLE 9.1
Differences between physiological and pathological nipple discharge

Physiological	Pathological
Bilateral	Unilateral
Multi-duct	Single-duct
Expressed	Spontaneous
Variable Frequency	Persistent
Colours: dark/green/yellow/grey	Colours: Clear/serous or blood-stained

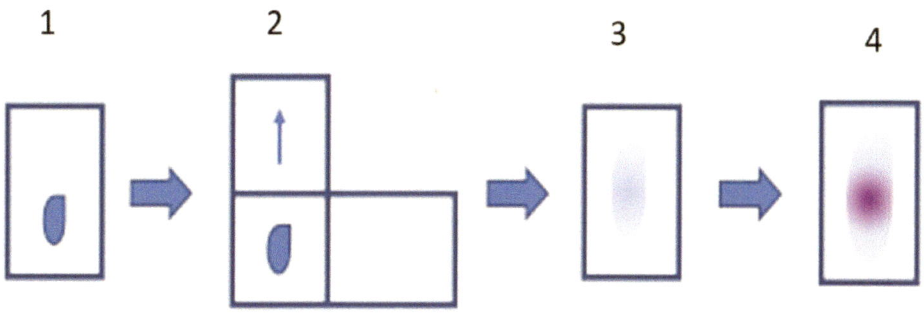

FIGURE 9.3
Nipple smear cytology: (1) a droplet of nipple discharge fluid placed onto slide; (2) a second slide is placed on top and swiped across to produce (3) a nipple smear, which is (4) air-dried for a minute and stained, ready for interpretation by the cytopathologist.

of abnormal/atypical cells, both of which require further clinical assessment.

Imaging: Patients attending a breast clinic will undergo routine imaging that may include mammography and/or a breast ultrasound scan as part of their initial diagnostic assessment. Mammography captures both breasts and is used to screen for any underlying lesions in women over the age of 40 years (18). Ultrasound can be used to interrogate the retro-areolar region of the breast and in particular to identify whether a lesion is solid or cystic. It is often complementary to mammography and can further characterise size, shape, and composition of a lesion found on a mammogram. Furthermore, if a suspicious lesion is identified that requires percutaneous needle biopsy, ultrasound is used to guide needle placement and minimise any targeting error. Ultrasound can evaluate ductal abnormalities including duct dilatation and thickening (e.g. duct ectasia) or discrete masses (e.g. papillomas) that might be causative factors for nipple discharge (18, 19). Core biopsies are performed under image guidance for suspicious radiological findings with surgical intervention reserved for cases where imaging is normal but there is persistent pathological nipple discharge (20).

In some cases, MRI is requested for further evaluation. Indications for use of this modality include inconclusive findings on conventional imaging (21), especially in patients with dense breast tissue or where multifocal or multicentric disease foci are identified. MRI will clarify the extent of disease prior to any treatment intervention. MRI is especially helpful in assessment of ductal abnormalities and has a high sensitivity for diagnosis of papillomas. MRI is increasingly being employed for evaluation of nipple discharge and is typically based on an individual patient's clinical history, the characteristics of discharge, and findings on mammography and/or ultrasound (22, 23).

Mammary ductography: Other specialist imaging modalities used to evaluate the ductal system include ductography. The latter is a contrast X-ray of the breast that specifically delineates the duct and is performed by insertion of a blunt-tip needle into the offending duct and infiltrating a small volume of water-soluble contrast to delineate the ductal system. Although useful as a means of localising pathology pre-operatively (24), it has a high false-negative rate and therefore should not be used as a sole method for deciding whether to proceed to surgical management (25). Similarly, ductoscopy uses an instrument called a ductoscope; a thin flexible tube with a light source and camera at the tip (Figure 9.4). Ductoscopy allows for real-time direct visualisation of the of the ducts through the nipple orifice and can therefore diagnose any abnormal pathology, from intraductal papillomas to DCIS or invasive cancers. Concurrently, it allows for targeted procedures, such as taking biopsies of suspicious areas or performing ductal lavage, whereby the duct is flushed with normal saline to collect a sample of cells for further interrogation. Ductal

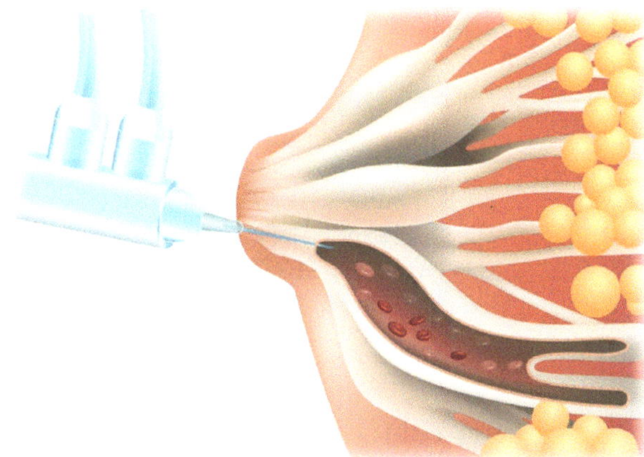

FIGURE 9.4
Nipple ductoscopy, involving cannulation of the nipple orifice with a thin flexible tube and infiltration with normal saline. It can be used for the collection of fluid as well as the localisation of pathology.

lavage is performed either with the patient under general anaesthetic or in the outpatient setting with the aid of local anaesthetic with or without sedation. It is one of the most consistent ways of retrieving nipple fluid samples and more cells are retrieved by ductal lavage than nipple fluid expression (26, 27). However, limitations of this method are that it is more invasive and time-consuming in the outpatient setting compared to direct nipple fluid expression and cytological evaluation. Potential complications, although uncommon include pain, inflammation, infection, and duct perforation. In addition, there is an inability to visualise or access many or all of the ducts, the length and outer diameter of the scope may limit access to the ductal system and many of the patients will have lesions beyond the reach of the scope (28). Moreover, ductoscopy, like other endoscopic techniques, is user dependent. In addition, there remains a high rate of inadequate cellular material for cytological diagnosis (29).

Supplementary tests: Other diagnostic tests that may be useful in the evaluation of nipple discharge include laboratory tests; if the history of the presenting complaint is relevant, blood tests may be conducted to assess hormone levels, such as prolactin, and rule out systematic causes such as thyroid function.

9.4 Management Options

The management of nipple discharge depends on its underlying cause and understanding potential causes is essential for accurate diagnosis and treatment. The following are the most common causes for presentation of nipple discharge:

9.4.1 Non-Pathological Nipple Discharge

1. Hormonal changes are a principal cause of physiological discharge that is related to the menstrual cycle, pregnancy, or breastfeeding (i.e. milk production). This type of discharge is typically clear or milky and more likely to be bilateral and multi-duct at presentation.
2. Lactation starts towards the end of pregnancy and last up to two years after delivery or cessation of breastfeeding.
3. Galactorrhoea is bilateral multiduct milky discharge but this is not attributed to any of the aforementioned physiological changes. It is usually caused by hyperprolactinaemia secondary to endocrine tumours, such as pituitary adenomas, thyroid disease, medications, or stress.
4. Medications that are responsible for nipple discharge include oral contraceptives, antipsychotics, and certain hypertension medications, which can lead to nipple discharge as a side effect (30). See Table 9.2 for a summary of the causes of galactorrhoea. Other causes of galactorrhoea may include frequent or vigorous stimulation of the nipples, such as through sexual activity or constant friction (31). In some cases, the cause of galactorrhoea may not be identified (idiopathic galactorrhoea). This may occur in the absence of obvious hormonal or medical issues.

9.4.2 Pathological Nipple Discharge

Pathological nipple discharge (PND) is defined as single-duct, spontaneous, persistent (at least twice a week) discharge which can be clear or bloodstained in nature or even pus-containing (32). Causes (Table 9.3) include the following:

1. Periductal mastitis presents more commonly in smokers with muti-coloured, thick, or sticky discharge. Assessment involves ultrasound-guided aspiration of any drainable collections of pus alongside antibiotics with gram-positive cover to eliminate the most common culprits, including *Staphylococcus aureus*, *Streptococcus*, and *Enterococcus*. Surgical management, where necessary, can be either minimally invasive (small incision and drainage or ductal irrigation), minor excision (with wound packing or primary closure), major excision (requiring a circumareolar or radial incision), or in the worst cases, plastic reconstruction (33, 34).
2. Mammary duct ectasia is a benign, non-proliferative process, where loss of duct wall elastin, leads to abnormally dilated and tortuous lactiferous ducts with associated periductal inflammation and fibrosis (35). Typically presenting in a very similar way to periductal mastitis, it is more common in peri-menopausal women (36) and caused by plugging of the ductal system. Clinically, it may be difficult to differentiate from periductal mastitis and a definitive diagnosis is reliant on histology.
3. Papillomas are benign centrally located tumours of the ductal system and can occur alone as single papillomas or be multiple (papillomatosis). They often present with bloodstained single-duct discharge with or without

TABLE 9.2

Summary of Causes of Galactorrhoea

Causes of Galactorrhoea
• Medication-induced – Antidepressants (e.g. TCAs, monoamine oxidase inhibitors) – Benzodiazepines e.g. diazepam – Anti-emetics e.g. metoclopramide, sulpiride – Antipsychotics e.g. Clozapine – Anti hypertensives e.g. Verapamil, Methyldopa, Reserpine – H2 receptor antagonists e.g. Cimetidine – Oral contraceptives, oestrogens, progestins, androgens – Anaesthetics • Opioid use e.g. cocaine, morphine • Herbal supplements e.g. Fennel, Aniseed or Fenugreek seed • Tumors – Pituitary (prolactinoma) – Hypothalamic – Craniopharyngioma, Meningiomas – Ectopic Prolactin e.g. bronchogenic carcinoma • Metabolic e.g. hypothyroidism, chronic kidney disease, Cushing's disease • Acromegaly • Chest wall abnormalities: nerve damage to the chest wall from chest surgery, burns or other chest injuries, Herpes zoster or spinal cord injuries of tumors • Stress • Physiological – post lactational and excessive breast stimulation e.g. with sexual activity, frequent breast self-exams with nipple manipulation or prolonged clothing friction • Idiopathic

TABLE 9.3

Causes of pathological nipple discharge (PND)

Causes of PND
Papilloma (up to 20% associated with occult DCIS)
Papillomatosis
Ductal epithelial hyperplasia
Ductal carcinoma in situ (DCIS)
Invasive ductal carcinoma (IDC)
Papillary cancer (IPC)

an accompanying palpable lump. Triple assessment including thorough examination of the nipple areolar complex, ultrasound, and biopsy can confirm a diagnosis. Papillomas visualised on ultrasound can be diagnosed and simultaneously removed using vacuum-assisted needle biopsy techniques—vacuum-assisted excision (VAE). Alternatively, these papillomas can be surgically excised with either a microdochectomy or a total duct excision (especially if superficial and close to the skin). It should be noted that in patients for whom only papillomatous disease is found, this is upgraded to DCIS in 30% of patients on surgical excision (23). Any patient with biopsy proven DCIS or invasive cancer will be discussed in a breast multidisciplinary team meeting attended by a radiologist, pathologist, surgeon, and oncologist to formulate an appropriate management plan. Treatment will then encompass surgery of the breast (with or without axillary surgery), radiotherapy to the breast or chest wall, and systemic therapies (chemotherapy, hormone therapy, and biological therapies) depending on the type and stage of cancer. A study by Chung et al. evaluating imaging for nipple discharge revealed that invasive cancer presented with nipple discharge as the sole symptom, in the absence of a mass in two-thirds of nipple discharge patients diagnosed with a malignancy (37). The decision for nipple-sparing versus nipple sacrificing surgery in these cases is dependent on several factors including size of the lesion, distance from the nipple-areola complex (i.e. no less than 1–2 cm from the nipple-areola complex) and the presence of multifocal-disease. Moreover, this is a surgical issue upon which patients often express a strong preference (namely, for nipple preservation).

9.5 Surgical Treatment

In terms of the management of those cases of nipple discharge where a cause is not found, patients with persistent and spontaneous single-duct discharge undergo diagnostic surgery to determine the underlying cause. A systematic review by Makineli et al. (38) reported that the malignancy rate in patients with PND without clinical or radiological abnormalities was only 8.1%, and therefore, the majority of these open surgical procedures are to confirm a benign aetiology (38). Microdochectomy involves the removal of a single duct in women presenting with single-duct discharge. This more limited duct surgery is indicated in cases where there is obvious discharge confined to a single offending duct which can be readily localised both pre- and intra-operatively. This avoids blind removal of a group of ducts with the patient under anaesthetic. The operation is performed through either a radial or circumareolar incision, using a lacrimal probe to cannulate the duct whilst simultaneously squeezing the offending duct to localise it. The probe serves two purposes; the first is to isolate the duct responsible for the single-duct discharge and the second is to aid dissection of this duct from surrounding tissues. A length of at least 2–3 cm of duct should be excised, and if possible, the duct should be opened to identify any cause of discharge. Moreover, the residual portion of a duct can be carefully examined to ensure the pathological area of duct tissue has been removed. A disadvantage of microdochectomy is that the probe inadvertently enters the incorrect distal portion of a duct due to bifurcation. It is therefore it is important to ensure that an appropriate length of the correct duct is excised to prevent recurrence of symptoms. Prior to closing the wound, it is prudent to apply pressure to the undersurface of the nipple-areola complex to ensure there is no residual discharge and the relevant duct(s) has been excised. The key to a successful microdochectomy is avoiding disruption of neighbouring ducts and maintaining the ability to breastfeed in the future. Microdochectomy is therefore the procedure of choice in women of childbearing age, where surgical intervention is deemed necessary to remove a suspected pathological lesion (Figure 9.5).

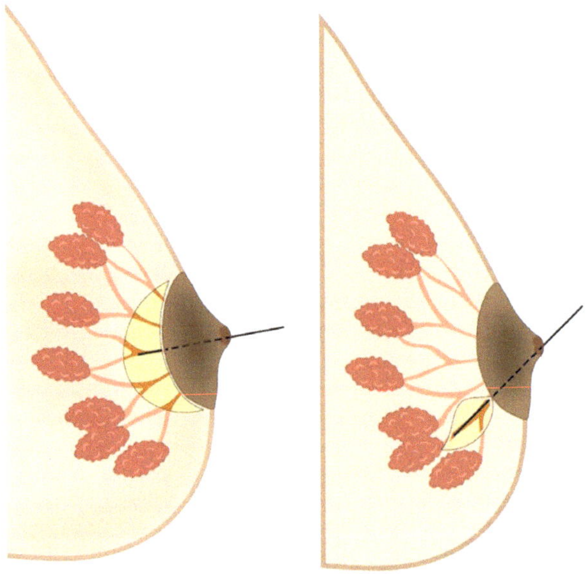

FIGURE 9.5
Two incisional approaches to a microdochectomy: (left) circumareolar incision; (right) radial incision.

Conversely, a total duct excision or Hadfield's procedure, is the operation of choice in post-menopausal women or where the ability to breastfeed in the future is not a consideration. A total duct excision is used for both single-duct discharge, where it may be more likely to yield a specific diagnosis, as well as for persistent multi-duct discharge associated with soiling of undergarments/nightclothes that adversely affects a patient's quality of life. The operation is performed through a circumareolar incision and aims to disconnect all ducts from beneath the nipple-areola complex, removing a cuff of tissue (approximately to a depth of 2 cm) (Figure 9.6). There are risks associated with both procedures including loss of sensation to the nipple, necrosis of the nipple tip (more common in total duct excision than microdochectomy), and nipple inversion. Necrotic complications are more common for total duct excision than micro-dochectomy.

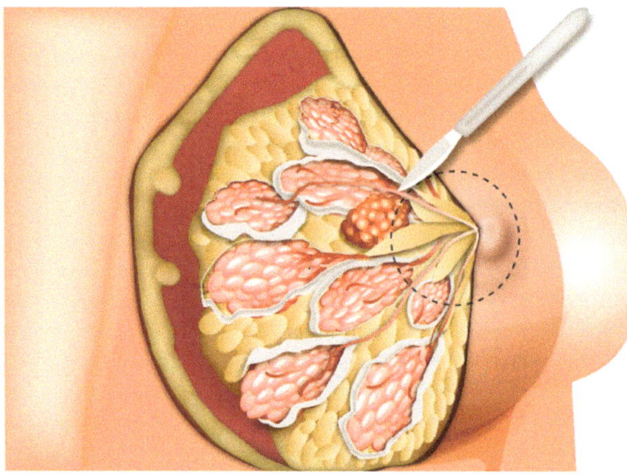

FIGURE 9.6
Total duct excision, with a circumareolar incision to disconnect and excise the central portion of ducts.

References

1 Richards T, Hunt A, Courtney S, Umeh H. Nipple discharge: a sign of breast cancer? The Annals of the Royal College of Surgeons of England. 2007;89(2):124–6.

2 Ostojic SB, Grbanovic L, Tonklin A, et al. Diagnostic performance of digital breast tomosynthesis in female patients with nipple discharge. Cancer Reports. 2022;5(10):e1602.
3 Armstrong AC, Evans GDJB. Management of women at high risk of breast cancer. BMJ. 2014;348:g2756.
4 Yaffe MJ, Mainprize JGJR. Risk of radiation-induced breast cancer from mammographic screening. Radiology. 2011;258(1):98–105.
5 Djuric Z, Chen G, Ren JV, et al. Effects of high fruit-vegetable and/or low-fat intervention on breast nipple aspirate fluid micronutrient levels. Cancer Epidemiology, Biomarkers & Prevention. 2007;16(7):1393–9.
6 Leis HP. Management of nipple discharge. World Journal of Surgery. 1989;13(6):736–42.
7 Lewis EC. The signficance of discharge from the nipple in breast lesions. The Lancet. 1922;199(5153):1093–5.
8 Clark S, Agrawal A, Laws S, et al. The investigation and management of unilateral nipple discharge. Annals of the Royal College of Surgeons of England. 2020;102(5):369–74.
9 Besser G, Edwards C. Galactorrhoea. British Medical Journal. 1972;2(5808):280.
10 Chen L, Zhou W-B, Zhao Y, et al. Bloody nipple discharge is a predictor of breast cancer risk: a meta-analysis. Breast Cancer Research and Treatment. 2012;132(1):9–14.
11 Jiwa N, Kumar S, Gandhewar R, et al. Diagnostic accuracy of nipple discharge fluid cytology: a meta-analysis and systematic review of the literature. Annals of Surgical Oncology. 2021;29(3):1774–86.
12 Panzironi G, Pediconi F, Sardanelli F. Nipple discharge: the state of the art. BJR Open. 2018;1:20180016.
13 Dixon JM. Breast Surgery: Companion to Specialist Surgical Practice. Elsevier Health Sciences; 2013.
14 Gandhewar R, Jiwa N, Leff D, et al. Improving confidence and technique when preparing nipple smears for cytology. British Journal of Surgery. 2021;108(Suppl 7):znab311.076.
15 Lippa N, Hurtevent-Labrot G, Ferron S, et al. Nipple discharge: the role of imaging. Diagnostic and Interventional Imaging. 2015;96(10):1017–32.
16 Montroni I, Santini D, Zucchini G, et al. Nipple discharge: is its significance as a risk factor for breast cancer fully understood? Observational study including 915 consecutive patients who underwent selective duct excision. Breast Cancer Research and Treatment. 2010;123(3):895–900.
17 Patel BK, Falcon S, Drukteinis J. Management of nipple discharge and the associated imaging findings. American Journal of Medicine. 2015;128(4):353–60.
18 Sanford MF, Slanetz PJ, Lewin AA, et al. ACR appropriateness criteria® evaluation of nipple discharge: 2022 update. Journal of the American College of Radiology. 2022;19(11):S304–18.
19 Gupta D, Mendelson EB, Karst I. Nipple discharge: current clinical and imaging evaluation. The American Journal of Roentgenology. 2021;216(2):330–9.
20 Vargas HI, Vargas MP, Eldrageely K, Gonzalez KD, Khalkhali I. Outcomes of clinical and surgical assessment of women with pathological nipple discharge. The American Surgeon. 2006;72(2):124–8.
21 Mann RM, Balleyguier C, Baltzer PA, et al. Breast MRI: EUSOBI recommendations for women's information. European Radiology. 2015;25(12):3669–78.
22 Bahl M, Baker JA, Greenup RA, Ghate SV. Evaluation of pathologic nipple discharge: what is the added diagnostic value of MRI? Annals of Surgical Oncology. 2015;22:435–41.
23 Zacharioudakis K, Kontoulis T, Vella JX, et al. Can we see what is invisible? The role of MRI in the evaluation and management of patients with pathological nipple discharge. Breast Cancer Research and Treatment. 2019;178(1):115–20.
24 Bagnera S, Comello EG, Berrino C, et al. Ductography and galactomosynthesis in the 21st century: role of imaging in identifying endoductal breast lesions and in pre-surgical planning. Open Journal of Radiology. 2021;11(3):55–69.
25 Yamamoto D, Shoji T, Kawanishi H, et al. A utility of ductography and fiberoptic ductoscopy for patients with nipple discharge. Breast Cancer Research and Treatment. 2001;70(2):103–8.
26 Dooley WC, Ljung B-M, Veronesi U, et al. Ductal lavage for detection of cellular atypia in women at high risk for breast cancer. Journal of National Cancer Institute. 2001;93(21):1624–32.
27 Twelves D, Nerurkar A, Osin P, et al. The feasibility of nipple aspiration and duct lavage to evaluate the breast duct epithelium of women with increased breast cancer risk. European Journal of Cancer. 2013;49(1):65–71.
28 Shen K-W, Wu J, Lu J-S, et al. Fiberoptic ductoscopy for breast cancer patients with nipple discharge. Surgical Endoscopy. 2001;15(11):1340–5.
29 Visvanathan K, Santor D, Ali SZ, et al. The reliability of nipple aspirate and ductal lavage in women at increased risk for breast cancer: a potential tool for breast cancer risk assessment and biomarker evaluation. Cancer Epidemiology, Biomarkers & Prevention. 2007;16(5):950–5.
30 Atluri S, Sarathi V, Goel A, et al. Etiological profile of galactorrhoea. Indian Journal of Endocrinology and Metabolism. 2018;22(4):489.
31 Jatoi I, Kaufmann M. Management of Breast Diseases. Springer; 2010.
32 Filipe MD, Patuleia SI, de Jong VM, et al. A network meta-analysis for the diagnostic approach to pathological nipple discharge. Clinical Breast Cancer. 2020;20(6):e723–e48.
33 Xu H, Liu R, Lv Y, et al. Treatments for periductal mastitis: systematic review and meta-analysis. Breast Care. 2022;17(1):55–62.
34 Zhang Y, Zhou Y, Mao F, et al. Clinical characteristics, classification and surgical treatment of periductal mastitis. Journal of Thoracic Diseases. 2018;10(4):2420.
35 Dixon J, Anderson T, Lumsden AB, et al. Mammary duct ectasia. British Journal of Surgery. 1983;70(10):601–3.
36 Sweeney D, Wylie E. Mammographic appearances of mammary duct ectasia that mimic carcinoma in a screening programme. Australasian Radiology. 1995;39(1):18–23.
37 Chung HL, Bevers TB, Legha RS, et al. Nipple discharge imaging evaluation with mammography, ultrasound, galactography, and MRI. Academic Radiology. 2023;30(5):783–97.
38 Makineli S, van Wijnbergen JWM, Vriens MR, et al. Role of duct excision surgery in the treatment of pathological nipple discharge and detection of breast carcinoma: systematic review. BJS Open. 2023;7(4):zrad066.

10

Breast Sepsis

Rasheed Elayyan and Sarah Downey

Mastitis is an inflammatory process involving the breast tissue that may not necessarily be associated with ongoing infection (1). For this reason, mastitis can be classified as either infectious or non-infectious.

The condition most frequently occurs in lactating women when it is referred to as lactational or puerperal mastitis. Non-Lactational mastitis has a broader range of presentations with a spectrum of clinical manifestation caused by a variety of infectious agents. These can often present management challenges and may be recalcitrant to treatment with different antibiotics (2, 3). These non-lactational forms of mastitis include periductal mastitis and idiopathic granulomatous mastitis.

10.1 Lactational Mastitis

The American Academy of Pediatrics and the World Health Organization (WHO) advocate a policy of exclusive breastfeeding for the first six months of a child's life based on the documented nutritional and immunological benefits attributable to breast milk. This guidance encourages continuation of breastfeeding while supplementary foods are being introduced after six months, with a recommendation to continue breastfeeding for a period of 12 months or more, provided both mother and infant are content with this (4). It is important to acknowledge that the well-being of both mother and infant can be adversely affected by the morbidity associated with lactational mastitis.

Breast infection constitutes one of the commonest benign breast conditions with puerperal sepsis occurring with notable frequency during pregnancy and the postpartum period (5). Lactational mastitis is the most prevalent form of breast sepsis and affects lactating women with reported incidence ranging from 2% to 30% (6). A study conducted amongst breastfeeding women in Glasgow found a mastitis rate of 18% (7), which accords with similar studies from Australia. These results therefore suggest that almost one in five lactating women may experience mastitis (8, 9). The condition is most likely to occur in the initial few weeks following delivery, especially during the second and third weeks postpartum. Furthermore, between 75% and 95% of cases occur in infants under the age of three months (10, 11). Nonetheless, it is important to appreciate that mastitis can potentially develop at any stage throughout the lactation period.

From a pathological perspective, lactational mastitis is a cellulitic process that affects the interlobular connective tissue within the breast parenchyma and, as previously stated, can be infectious or non-infectious (12, 13).

Bacteria originating from the infant's mouth have a tendency to enter the nipple surface through small traumatic cracks or fissures. When this initial physical line of defence is broken, the nutrient-rich mother's milk creates an ideal environment for these organisms to multiply rapidly. This bacterial proliferation, combined with overproduction and stasis of milk contents, can lead to stagnation and worsen the condition of mastitis (5, 14).

In 1958, Gunther (15) made the clinical observation that mastitis usually arises as a consequence of milk stasis within the breast. It was emphasised that regular and efficient emptying of milk from the breast as it forms could mitigate the chance of this mastitis developing. Gunther suggested that any subsequent infection was not the primary cause but rather a consequence of the stagnant milk providing an environment conducive to bacterial growth.

Elevated pressure caused by stagnant or excess milk within the alveoli can trigger lactational mastitis despite the absence of overt infection. If the alveolar cells become excessively swollen, milk can leak into the surrounding connective tissues. The presence of milk outside the ductal system of the breast can elicit a localised immune reaction that is followed by inflammation and oedema. If milk escapes from the alveolar cells and enters the bloodstream through the mammary capillary system, the patient may experience an

DOI: 10.1201/9781003394785-10

immune response characterised by fever and general malaise (16).

Skin commensals are usually responsible for lactational mastitis with *Staphylococcus Aureus* being the predominant culprit. There have been rising numbers of mastitis cases attributed to methicillin-resistant *Staphylococcus aureus* (MRSA), which underlines the importance of recognising any associated risk factors. Additional pathogens include *Streptococcus pyogenes, Escherichia coli, Bacteroides* spp., and coagulase-negative staphylococci that are each considered to be potential causative agents (17).

The diagnosis of lactational mastitis is clinical; breast examination and observation of vital signs will usually lead to a correct diagnosis. Patients with lactational mastitis typically present with localised breast discomfort, tenderness, erythema, and engorgement. It may be accompanied by systemic symptoms, such as fever, malaise, rigors, nausea, and vomiting. In order to ascertain the cause of mastitis, a thorough feeding history must be taken for each patient with identification of possible risk factors. If there are serious concerns about breastfeeding technique, a full assessment should be conducted and preferably done in conjunction with an appropriately trained healthcare provider, such as a midwife.

Lactational mastitis that is not complicated by sepsis is considered to be a 'self-limiting' condition that can resolve spontaneously with self-care measures. The three important principles underpinning the successful conservative management of lactational mastitis are:

1. Breast emptying
2. Application of heat
3. Rest

Consistent and effective milk removal is essential for treatment of mastitis and reducing the risk of complications such as abscess formation or recurrent mastitis (18, 19). If breastfeeding is not feasible or does not achieve complete emptying of milk from the breast, the mother should manually express milk from the affected breast using a breast pump; a combined approach using both methods may be optimal for some women. Women may fear transmission of any infection to their infant and should receive adequate information to reassure them that this practice is unlikely to cause any harm. Manoeuvres such as application of hot compressors combined with gentle breast massage will aid the flow and encourage evacuation of milk. Cold compressors can be employed in the intervals between these sessions of feeding or milk expression to reduce swelling and erythema (20, 21). Measures that will help control symptoms and hasten recovery include simple analgesics (such as paracetamol or ibuprofen), local management of sore/cracked nipples, rest, avoidance of bra wearing (especially at night), family support, nutritious feeding, and adequate fluid intake.

Despite adherence to these suggested self-management measures, for some patients there is no improvement and symptoms can remain severe or even worsen. If symptoms worsen within 12–24 hours from the initial onset, and/or microbiological cultures of milk are positive, then oral antibiotics should be promptly prescribed (16, 22).

White cell count, inflammatory markers, and bacterial cultures are valuable parameters in differentiating between infectious and non-infectious mastitis (23). A mid-stream clean-catch culture of milk breast will yield results that guide antibiotic treatment according to sensitivity.

The first-line treatment is flucloxacillin, which is particularly effective against *Staphylococcus aureus*. In cases of penicillin allergy, suitable alternatives include erythromycin and clarithromycin. Second-line antibiotics (amoxycillin with clavulanic acid or clindamycin [for those with penicillin allergy]) may be considered. The prescribed course of antibiotic treatment typically extends for a duration of 10 to 14 days. Patients should be advised to seek medical advice, if the symptoms fail to settle after 48 hours of commencing antibiotics. Alternative diagnoses should be considered in those circumstances when there is no improvement or progression of symptoms after first- and second-line antibiotic treatment. According to NICE guidelines, patients with mastitis should be referred to the emergency department for urgent admission in cases showing:

- Presence of systemic sepsis with signs of fever, chills, and tachycardia
- Rapid progression
- An immunocompromised or haemodynamically unstable patient

10.2 Breast Abscess

If left untreated, mastitis can lead to destruction of parenchymal tissue, potentially resulting in the formation of an abscess which is a localised purulent collection within the breast tissue. An abscess may be the initial presentation of breast infection without any preceding mastitis. These de novo abscesses are mostly lactational in women of childbearing age, but older premenopausal women and men can develop non-puerperal abscesses (Figure 10.1) (24).

Breast abscesses in lactating and non-lactating women are essentially different clinical entities with each type having a distinct aetiology. Despite the observation of a declining incidence in recent years, lactational breast abscesses continue to predominate (25). Between 3 and 11% of mastitis patients will have a breast abscess as an associated complication with an estimated incidence of 0.1–3% in breastfeeding mothers (26–28). Lactational abscesses tend to occur in the peripheral zones of the breast in comparison to non-lactational abscesses that are more often in the sub-areolar region (29). Risk factors that increase the likelihood of developing a lactational breast abscess include a first pregnancy over the age of 30 years, pregnancy lasting beyond 41 weeks, and previous episodes of mastitis (30, 31).

Women tend to develop non-lactational abscesses towards the end of their reproductive years (32). Abscesses in the sub-areolar region represent almost 90% of non-lactational breast abscesses (33). Rarer forms of non-lactational abscesses may be attributable to granulomatous, bacterial, or fungal aetiologies but can also be linked to cutaneous infections, including sebaceous cyst with abscess formation (Figure 10.2). Those patients with a breast abscess that is unrelated to lactation have a higher likelihood of developing recurring infections. This applies particularly to patients who regularly smoke but is also pertinent to diabetic patients with poor monitoring of blood sugar levels. Central periareolar non-lactational abscesses are commonly related to the pathological condition of periductal mastitis (34).

A breast abscess is diagnosed on clinical criteria and should be suspected in patients with a recent history of mastitis or a previous breast abscess. In addition, there should be a high index of suspicion in patients with systemic sepsis characterised by fever and generalised fatigue, as well as the presence of a severely painful, swollen breast mass associated with redness, warmth, and swelling of the overlying skin (Figure 10.3). On examination, it may be possible to elicit fluctuance and the mass will be tender with vivid changes in skin coloration.

The conventional method for definitive treatment of a breast abscess has been surgical incision and drainage. However, this can be associated with several disadvantages, including potential cosmetic detriment, challenges with breastfeeding, requirement for general anaesthesia, prolonged healing, the possibility of milk duct fistula formation, and the need for frequent dressing changes. A diagnostic breast ultrasound can demonstrate the presence or otherwise of a collection of pus and this can be drained percutaneously with needle aspiration (Figure 10.4). The latter serves

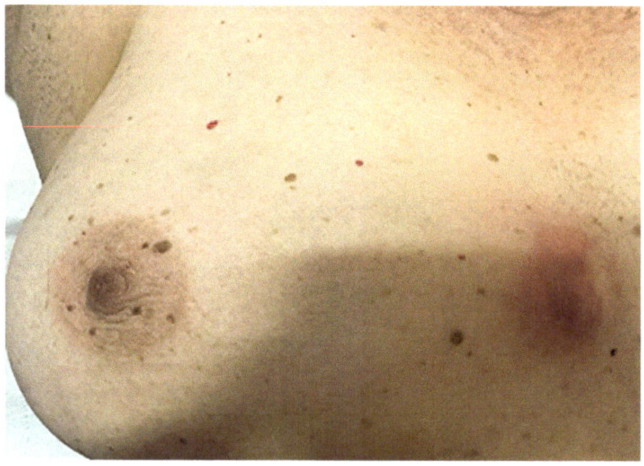

FIGURE 10.2
Infected sebaceous cyst with abscess formation.

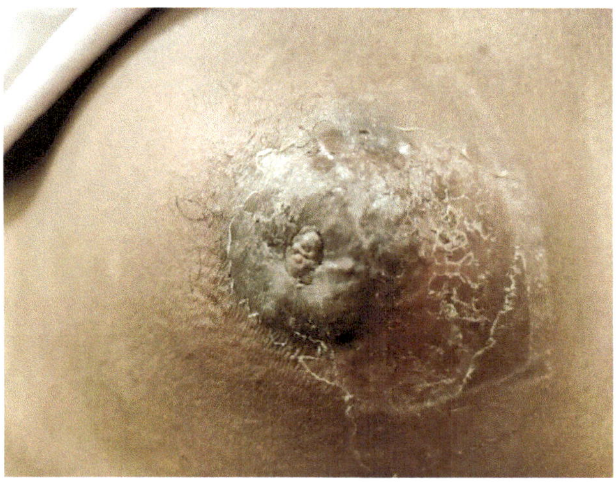

FIGURE 10.1
Male breast abscess.

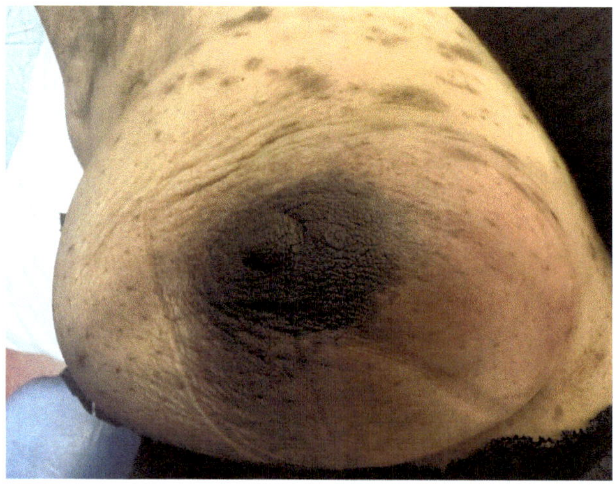

FIGURE 10.3
Breast abscess: hot, red, and tender lump.

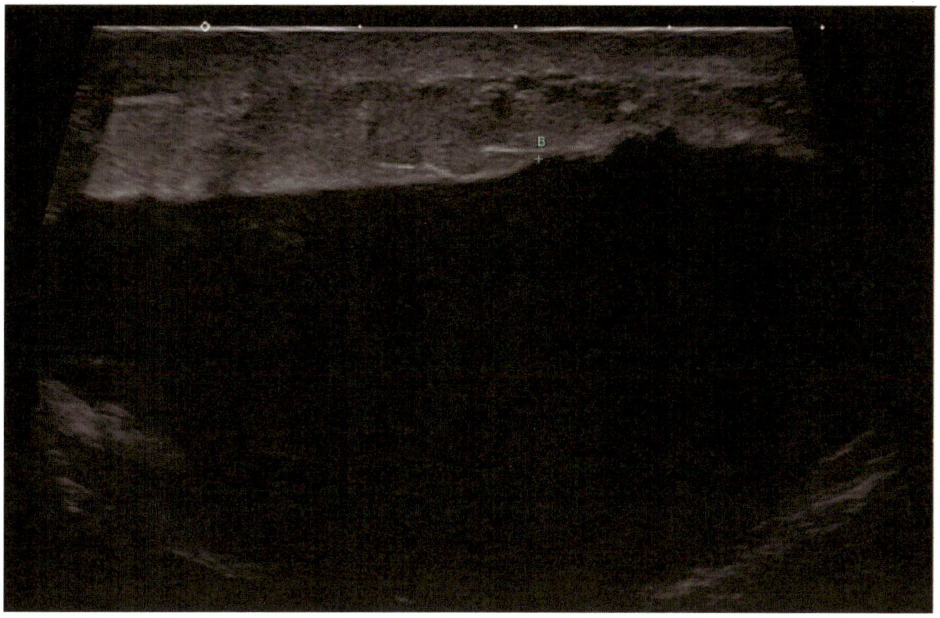

FIGURE 10.4
Breast abscesses generally appear on ultrasound as poorly defined masses with central hypoechoic area. They can also show signs of internal septations, debris, posterior enhancement, and thick surrounding walls that are eccentrically oriented. A 61 mm breast abscess which was drained to dryness under ultrasound guidance.

as both a diagnostic and therapeutic procedure and it may be necessary to repeat needle aspiration (typically 2–3 times) to achieve complete resolution (35–37). Ultrasound-guided aspiration should be performed within 24 hours of presentation and combined with initiation of empirical antibiotic treatment pending culture and sensitivity results. A policy of serial aspiration is associated with reduced loss of breast tissue compared with an open procedure. Nonetheless, surgical intervention should be promptly undertaken when the abscess cannot be adequately managed with percutaneous aspiration and there is potential compromise of skin viability (especially in the young patients).

10.3 Subclinical Mastitis

Subclinical mastitis (SCM) is an asymptomatic inflammatory process that affects the breast parenchyma in lactating mothers (38). Studies involving different ethnic populations have yielded diverse findings in terms of demographics, with some groups having a prevalence as high as 66%. It is noteworthy that the majority of these cases occur during the early months of breastfeeding and the incidence of SCM decreases with the passage of time (38–40).

Human milk contains both pro- and anti-inflammatory cytokines; the newborn infant is assumed to be protected by anti-inflammatory cytokines (41, 42), whilst inflammatory cytokines (including interleukin-8 [IL-8]) may be more crucial for defending the breast from infection. Mastitis generally causes higher levels of IL-8, thereby reflecting the existence of an inflammatory reaction within breast tissue (43, 44). The diagnosis of subclinical mastitis is reliant upon detection of an elevated sodium-potassium ratio and a raised concentration of IL-8 in the in the absence of any clinical symptoms of mastitis. The increased levels of both sodium and IL-8 indicates that an inflammatory process is ongoing.

10.4 Periductal Mastitis

Periductal mastitis was first identified by Birkett in 1850 as a 'morbid condition of lactiferous ducts' (45). In 1921 Bloodgood described the pathological hallmarks of the disease as ductal dilatation and periductal inflammation (46). Zuska and colleagues reported that mammary fistula formation can be associated with the disease in 1951, which temporarily became known as Zuska's disease (29).

Periductal mastitis, which is termed plasma cell mastitis, is a form of chronic non-lactational mastitis. Histopathologically, it is defined as chronic inflammation of the breast associated with dilation of mammary ducts, abscess formation and plasma cell infiltration (47). Squamous metaplasia that results from persistent inflammation is also linked to periductal mastitis. Squamous metaplasia has been proposed to cause partial duct obstruction, which can then dilate and result in further inflammation and infection.

It remains unclear what causes periductal mastitis despite much research into this condition. Smoking, obesity, and diabetes mellitus are among several factors that have been linked to an elevated risk. Nonetheless, none of these factors have been epidemiologically validated; rather, they are all identified based on reports of small case series (48, 49). Although heavy smokers are typically diagnosed with periductal mastitis, and many suggest smoking may contribute to the condition's genesis by directly causing duct damage and subsequent inflammation or it may cause a localised hypoxic effect, a few other studies provide contradictory results to this conclusion (50). The precise contribution of bacterial infection to periductal mastitis has long been a topic of discussion in terms of aetiology. It was believed that bacterial infection can contribute to development of periductal mastitis. However, studies to date are inconclusive because some patients with periductal mastitis have sterile lesions devoid of bacterial infiltration (51). On the other hand, some studies have revealed that between 62% and 85% of patients with periductal mastitis have bacteria isolated in cultures. The most frequent pathogens are *Staphylococcus aureus*, *Pseudomonas aeruginosa*, *Enterococcus*, *Bacteroides*, and *Proteus* spp. (51).

Clinically, patients with periductal mastitis may present with nipple discharge, a subareolar mass that is either painless or painful, nipple retraction, periareolar abscess formation, or in extreme cases, a mammary duct fistula (52). The three most common presentations in descending order of frequency are (1) a subareolar mass, (2) abscess formation, and (3) mammary duct fistula. These clinical manifestations typically lack specificity and their appearance can be mistaken for breast cancer on imaging (53, 54).

A proposed clinical classification of periductal mastitis was suggested by Zhang and colleagues who divided the condition into 4 categories (52). Type I is a breast mass without any evidence of abscess formation or fistula, Type IIa is a breast mass with an abscess measuring ≤3 cm, Type IIb is a breast mass with an abscess >3 cm, Type III denotes a mammary duct fistula with or without a breast mass, whilst Type IV is a breast mass with both abscess and fistula formation.

Cessation of smoking is strongly advocated as an adjunctive measure for patients diagnosed with periductal mastitis. The initial treatment of this condition includes antibiotics and drainage of any abscess that is present. However, the standard treatment for refractory non-self-limiting cases is surgery. Various techniques can be employed, including wide surgical resection, fistulectomy, and extended excisions involving transfer of a random breast dermal graft. In appropriately selected patients, these procedures have each proven to be effective methods for the various types of periductal mastitis and are associated with low recurrence rates together with favourable cosmetic outcomes (52).

Although periductal mastitis is a relatively uncommon condition, there is a finite chance of recurrence following treatment and this can lead to much morbidity and be a cause of severe pain with a protracted course of disease.

10.5 Tuberculous Mastitis

Tuberculosis is a chronic granulomatous disease mostly caused by *Mycobacterium tuberculosis* and is one of the most prevalent infections worldwide. The condition can affect any organ and shows a plethora of manifestations. Breast tuberculosis (otherwise termed tuberculous mastitis) is a rare extra pulmonary manifestation of tuberculosis. It is rare in Western countries with an incidence of <1% in histological specimens from breast lesions (55). The incidence is higher in those countries where tuberculosis is endemic, such as the Indian subcontinent, where rates as high as 4% are reported (56). The first ever published case of breast tuberculosis was described in 1829 by Sir Astley Cooper, who reported it as 'scrofulous swelling of the bosom' (57). Lactating women appear to be at higher risk of contracting tuberculous mastitis and thus is likely a consequence of increased blood supply to the breasts and dilated ducts, rendering them more susceptible to lacerations and infections (58). Breast tuberculosis can be primary or secondary; routes of dissemination include direct extension from the chest wall tissues, lymphatic spread via axillary lymph nodes, haematogenous spread in the bloodstream, or spread through traumatised skin or ducts (59–61).

McKeown and Wilkinson were the first authors to categorise breast tuberculosis into five distinct types: (1) nodular tubercular mastitis, (2) disseminated or confluent tubercular mastitis, (3) sclerosing tubercular mastitis, (4) acute miliary tubercular mastitis, and (5) tuberculous mastitis obliterans. The most common type is nodular caseous tuberculous mastitis (62). More recently, Tewari has proposed a reclassification of breast tuberculosis into three categories: nodular, disseminated, and abscess varieties. This updated classification accounts for the evolving changes observed in the clinical presentation of tuberculosis over the past two decades (63).

There are no clearly defined clinical characteristics that specifically suggest breast tuberculosis. Therefore, making a diagnosis can be challenging due to varied clinical presentations. Tuberculous mastitis can be mistaken for breast carcinoma or a pyogenic abscess (64, 65). Tuberculous mastitis is usually unilateral; rarely affects men, with a male-to-female ratio of 1 to 30 (66); and should always be considered in immunocompromised individuals (66). Although both breasts are susceptible to infection, bilateral involvement occurs in only 3% of patients with breast tuberculosis (67). The most common presentation of breast tuberculosis is in the form of a lump. The most frequent site for these lumps is the central or upper outer quadrant of the breast (68). The lump may resemble breast carcinoma and can be firm with irregular borders. Moreover, the lump may be adherent to skin, muscle, or even to chest wall (61, 69). Fistula formation, nipple retraction, or skin tethering may occur, but nipple discharge is infrequent (58). The lump may become an inflammatory mass followed by abscess formation and diffuse mastitis. Peau d'orange is a common finding in patients with widespread axillary nodal tuberculosis.

Diagnosis of breast tuberculosis demands a high index of suspicion; all suspected lesions should be evaluated pathologically and/or microbiologically. Breast tuberculosis should be considered as a potential diagnosis when evaluating cases of painful breast masses, discharging sinuses, mastitis, or a breast abscess that does not respond to standard treatment. The commonly performed Mantoux test does not provide a conclusive diagnosis but does confirm prior exposure to the tubercle bacillus (65). In 60% of patients, ultrasonography detects a hypoechoic mass, and breast ultrasound has the potential to identify fistulous or sinus tracts which are characteristic of tuberculosis mastitis. Mammography is unhelpful in young women with dense breasts and cannot differentiate tuberculosis from breast carcinoma. The most reliable method to diagnose breast tuberculosis is detection of *Mycobacterium tuberculosis* with Ziehl–Neelsen staining or culture. Unfortunately, histochemical approaches are not feasible; reliance solely on culture for definitive diagnosis of tuberculous mastitis has drawbacks, including delayed results and the possibility of false-negative results that are more likely in samples with a low bacterial count (59). Polymerase chain reaction (PCR) has a high sensitivity for diagnosing breast tuberculosis. Although infrequently utilised, it is recommended in those situations where culture results are negative or there is difficulty distinguishing from other forms of granulomatous mastitis (65). Histopathological examination of the lesion reveals a chronic granulomatous inflammation with characteristic caseous necrosis and Langhans-type giant cells—these latter features play a crucial role in diagnosing the majority of cases of tuberculous mastitis (65).

The primary treatment for breast tuberculosis involves medical therapy, using anti-tuberculous therapy. Guidelines for treatment of breast tuberculosis are not well established, so treatment tends to follow guidelines derived for pulmonary tuberculosis. The success rate for medical therapy is very high and exceeds 90% in most series when a 6-month course of antituberculous therapy is administered (70).

10.6 Mondor's Disease (Superficial Thrombophlebitis)

In 1939 the French surgeon Henri Mondor first described the condition that now bears his name. Mondor's disease is a syndrome of superficial thrombophlebitis with sclerosis that affects the subcutaneous veins of the anterior thoracic wall (71). Mondor's disease can impact various venous drainage systems, but the superior epigastric vein is the most frequently affected and produces a noticeable cord-like structure in the inferior outer quadrant of the breast. Mondor's disease characteristically involves the lower and outer parts and rarely affects the upper inner portion of the breast (71).

The precise pathophysiology of Mondor's disease remains unclear, but the condition is idiopathic in 50–60% of the cases (72). It is believed to be triggered by a variety of factors, including direct local trauma, excessive physical activity, recent breast surgery and some systemic conditions such as breast cancer or hypercoagulable states (73). Clinically, an acute painful cord-like hardening of a superficial vein associated with overlying erythema is the main presentation. Mondor's disease is a self-limiting condition that normally resolves within a few weeks and therefore symptomatic treatment only is recommended. Measures including local application of heat, provision of adequate breast support together with oral or topical non-steroidal anti-inflammatory drugs (NSAIDs) can be used to alleviate symptoms.

10.7 Idiopathic Granulomatous Mastitis

Two principal types of granulomatous mastitis are recognised. The specific form of granulomatous mastitis can be attributed to a known cause whether this be an infectious or non-infectious aetiology. In contrast, the nonspecific or idiopathic form has no identifiable cause and is usually referred to as idiopathic granulomatous mastitis, a condition that was first reported by Kessler and Wooloch in 1972 (74, 75).

Idiopathic granulomatous mastitis is an uncommon chronic inflammatory breast disease that exhibits clinical and radiographic features of both malignant and inflammatory breast conditions including carcinomas and abscesses, respectively.

Three theories for the aetiology of idiopathic granulomatous mastitis have been postulated, and these are autoimmune, infectious, and hormonal based mechanisms of pathogenesis (76). Autoimmunity is currently considered to be the most probable cause (76–78). Thus, a T-lymphocytic predominance has been observed histologically in most cases of idiopathic granulomatous mastitis and the marked response to steroids that has been demonstrated in multiple trials collectively support this condition being an autoimmune disorder (76, 79).

In terms of a potential infectious cause, there is a consensus that infection may be associated with idiopathic granulomatous mastitis but is not a direct causative factor. Taylor and colleagues documented *Corynebacterium* infection in 34 cases of women with granulomatous mastitis (80). This bacterium is gram-positive and part of the normal skin flora. It is the most commonly identified bacterial strain in cases of idiopathic granulomatous mastitis (81).

Although idiopathic granulomatous mastitis is most frequently encountered in women of childbearing age, cases have been reported amongst older women and also men (82). These findings suggest that a hormonal aetiology is much less likely as a main cause for the condition.

The diagnosis of idiopathic granulomatous mastitis is by exclusion, and there should be a high index of suspicion in the absence of any clear consensus pertaining to aetiology. The disease has a very broad range of clinical manifestations and may present as a breast mass, an abscess, nipple retraction, peau d'orange or axillary lymphadenopathy (Figure 10.5) (83, 84). Management of idiopathic granulomatous mastitis is a challenge for both the clinician and the patient who frequently has to suffer a protracted disease course with a considerable negative impact on their quality of life. As this is a diagnosis of exclusion, other causes of mastitis should be ruled out before considering a diagnosis of idiopathic granulomatous mastitis. It is particularly important to exclude malignancy (85). It is also essential to exclude tuberculous mastitis where primary treatment with steroids would otherwise exacerbate mycobacterial infection. For this reason, all tissue samples should undergo Ziehl–Neelsen staining for acid-fast bacilli (86).

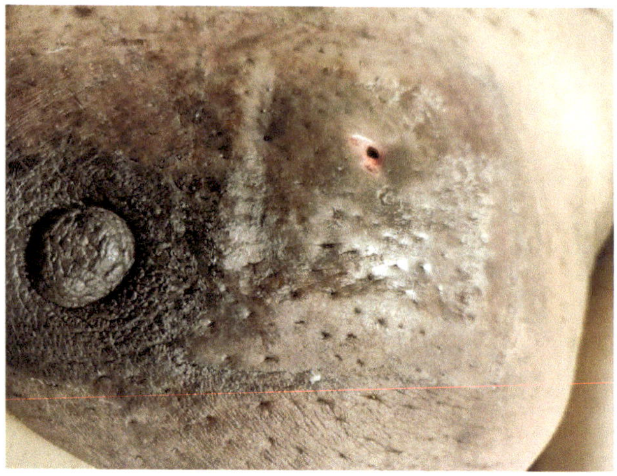

FIGURE 10.5
A case of biopsy proven idiopathic granulomatous mastitis with abscess formation and peau d'orange changes. The sinus at the abscess drainage site is noted. Tuberculosis ruled out. The patient was started on steroids.

No particular radiological features exist that can definitively point towards a diagnosis of idiopathic granulomatous mastitis, and therefore, histological examination is crucial for a definitive diagnosis. Histologically, idiopathic granulomatous mastitis is defined by the existence of non-caseating granulomas located around breast lobules, consisting of histiocytes and Langhans giant cells. Additionally, there is a chronic inflammatory pattern with lymphocytes and plasma cells with micro-abscess formation (86).

There is no consensus statement or guidelines for management of idiopathic granulomatous mastitis. Multiple treatment options have been discussed in the literature, including corticosteroids, antibiotics, surgical excision, immunosuppressive drugs (namely, methotrexate), and watchful waiting. The approach to management of this enigmatic disease depends on its clinical presentation and severity. Currently, corticosteroids are considered as the primary treatment approach for patients with idiopathic granulomatous mastitis. Numerous studies have demonstrated positive outcomes with administration of these agents. In a prospective study conducted by Pandey and colleagues, almost 80% of patients who received steroid treatment experienced complete resolution of their disease (79). The recommended duration of steroid therapy is between three to six months with an initial high dosage (60 mg prednisolone per day) that can be gradually tapered according to disease response (86).

10.8 Inflammatory Breast Cancer

Whatever the cause and nature of a breast problem, the main aim of assessment is to rule out cancer and manage the patient's symptoms (87). The chance of developing breast cancer is not increased by a diagnosis of mastitis. However, inflammatory breast cancer is a rare form of breast malignancy that resembles mastitis and exhibits signs that can occasionally be mistaken for an infection (88).

Inflammatory breast cancer is an uncommon and aggressive subtype of breast cancer. It represents between 1% and 6% of all breast cancer cases (89). The diagnosis of inflammatory breast cancer is based on clinical features of skin erythema and peau d'orange with involvement of at least 30% of the affected breast skin envelope. Additionally, confirmation of invasive breast cancer should be done through either core biopsy of breast parenchyma or punch biopsy of the skin (90). Dermal-lymphatic invasion is observed in approximately 75% of inflammatory breast cancer cases (91).

Inflammatory breast cancer can be a diagnostic challenge with potential delays in diagnosis. A distinctive feature of these cancers is not forming a discrete tumour mass. Instead, the tumour appears as scattered sheets or cords throughout the breast, making mammography less valuable for diagnosis (92). A prompt and accurate diagnosis at the outset is crucial since a delayed diagnosis of inflammatory breast cancer can adversely affect what is already a poor prognosis disease (Figure 10.6).

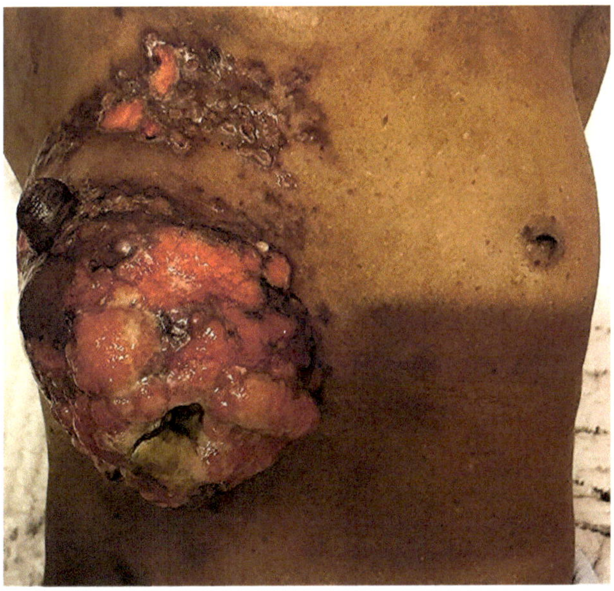

FIGURE 10.6
An extreme case of a neglected inflammatory breast cancer.

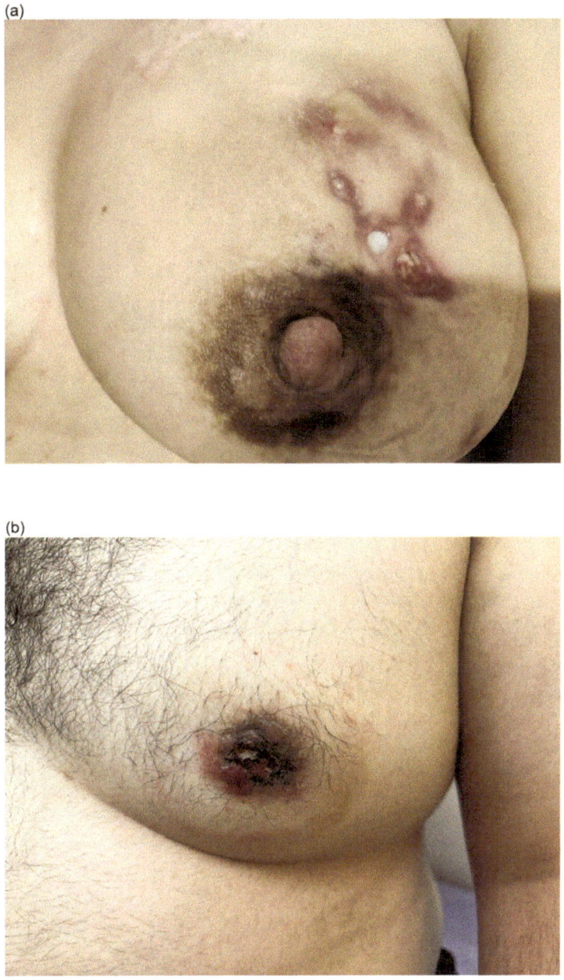

FIGURE 10.7
(a) A 36-year-old female who was 21 weeks pregnant presented with the features of an inflammatory breast lump and was not clinically suspicious for malignancy. She underwent ultrasound examination which was indeterminate and a core biopsy was performed. The inflammatory changes improved after two courses of antibiotics and histology showed benign inflammatory changes only. At 27 weeks the patient had had a pre-term delivery by caesarean section, but within 1 week post-delivery, the inflammatory breast changes recurred. In succeeding weeks, the site of core biopsy can be seen draining milk as a complication of milk duct fistula formation. (b) A 35-year-old male who was treated for nipple changes for a year without improvement. These changes were considered as inflammatory changes and treated accordingly. He was not seen by any breast surgeon during this period and was treated by his GP and dermatologists. Finally one of the dermatologists decided to do a punch biopsy of this ulceration, which surprisingly showed invasive ductal carcinoma of the breast.

10.9 The Threshold for Tissue Biopsy

An important aspect to consider in management of inflammatory breast conditions is the need for tissue diagnosis. The clinical decision whether to take a biopsy or not is often not straightforward. Two cases are discussed to illustrate how the threshold for biopsy needs to be carefully judged for each patient in order to ensure optimal outcomes (Figure 10.7).

> If invasive *breast cancer* is considered a possibility, then tissue biopsy is required to confirm the diagnosis as soon as possible.

References

1. Boakes E, Woods A, Johnson N, Kadoglou N. Breast infection: a review of diagnosis and management practices. Eur J Breast Health. 2018;14(3):136–43.
2. Joseph KA, Luu X, Mor A. Granulomatous mastitis: a New York public hospital experience. Ann Surg Oncol. 2014;21:4159–63.
3. Contreras GA, Rodríguez JM. Mastitis: comparative etiology and epidemiology. J Mammary Gland Biol Neoplasia. 2011;16:339–56.
4. American Academy of Pediatrics Section on Breastfeeding. Breastfeeding and the use of human milk. Pediatrics. 2012; 129:827–41.
5. Scott-Conner CE, Schorr SJ. The diagnosis and management of breast problems during pregnancy and lactation. Am J Surg. 1995;170:401–5.
6. Schoenfeld EM, McKay MP. Mastitis and methicillin-resistant Staphylococcus aureus (MRSA): the calm before the storm? J Emerg Med. 2010;38(4):e31–4.
7. Scott JA, Robertson M, Fitzpatrick J, et al. Occurrence of lactational mastitis and medical management: a prospective cohort study in Glasgow. Int Breastfeed J. 2008;3(21).
8. Amir LH, Forster DA, Lumley J, McLachlan H. A descriptive study of mastitis in Australian breastfeeding women: incidence and determinants. BMC Public Health. 2007;7:62.
9. Kinlay JR, O'Connell DL, Kinlay S. Incidence of mastitis in breastfeeding women during the six months after delivery: a prospective cohort study. Med J Australia. 1998;169(6):310–2.
10. Creasy RK, Resnik R. Maternal and fetal pathophysiology. In: Creasy RK, Resnik R, eds, Maternal-Fetal Medicine: Principles and Practice. Philadelphia, W.B. Saunders, 1984:628.
11. Novy MJ. Disorders of Lactation. Obstetric and Gynecologic Diagnosis and Treatment. Lange Medical Publications, Los Altos, 1984:864–7.
12. Marshall BR, Heppa JK, Zirbel CC. Sporadic puerperal mastitis: an infection that need not interrupt lactation. JAMA. 1975;233:1377–9.
13. Devereux WP. Acute puerperal mastitis: evaluation of its management. Am J Obstet Gynecol. 1970;108:78–81.
14. Marchant DJ. Inflammation of the breast. Obstet Gynecol Clin North Am. 2002;29:89–102.
15. Gunther M. Discussion on the breast in pregnancy and lactation. Proc R Soc Med. 1958;51(Section of General Practice):305–9.
16. Guidelines on the Treatment, Management & Prevention of Mastitis. RQIA. Available at: www.rqia.org.uk/RQIA/files/68/681b5723-6972-4e11-8a09-24cea893d430.pdf (Accessed 3 September 2023).
17. Foxman B, D'Arcy H, Gillespie B, et al. Lactation mastitis: occurrence and medical management among 946 breastfeeding women in the United States. Am J Epidemiol. 2002;155(2):103–14.
18. Betzold CM. An update on the recognition and management of lactational breast inflammation. J Midwif Women's Health. 2007;52(6):595–605.
19. The Academy of Breastfeeding Medicine Protocol Committee. ABM clinical protocol #4: mastitis. Breastfeed Med. 2008;9:177–80.
20. Spencer J. Management of mastitis in breastfeeding women. Am Fam Phys. 2008;78(6):727–31.
21. Wambach KA. Lactation mastitis: a descriptive study of the experience. J Hum Lact. 2003;19(1):24–34.
22. Clinical Knowledge Summaries, NICE, UK. Available at: https://cks.nice.org.uk/topics/mastitis-breast-abscess/management/management-lactating-women/ (Accessed 3 September 2023).
23. Matheson I, Aursnes I, Horgen M, et al. Bacteriological findings and clinical symptoms in relation to clinical outcome in puerperal mastitis. Acta Obstetr Gynecol Scand. 1988;67(8):723–6.
24. Efrat M, Mogilner JG, Iujtman M, et al. Neonatal mastitis: diagnosis and treatment. Isr J Med Sci. 1995;31:558–60.
25. Kataria K, Srivastava A, Dhar A. Management of lactational mastitis and breast abscesses: review of current knowledge and practice. Indian J Surg. 2013;75:430–435.
26. Dixon JM, Khan LR. Treatment of breast infection. BMJ. 2011;342:d396.
27. Amir LH, Forster D, McLachlan H, Lumley J. Incidence of breast abscess in lactating women: report from an Australian cohort. BJOG. 2004;111:1378–81.
28. Dixon JM. Breast infection. BMJ. 2013;347:f3291.
29. Zuska JJ, Crile G, Jr, Ayres WW. Fistulas of lactifierous ducts. Am J Surg. 1951;81:312–7.
30. Bharat A, Gao F, Aft RL. Predictors of primary breast abscesses and Recurrence. World J Surg. 2009;33(12):2582–6.
31. Berens PD. Prenatal, intrapartum, and postpartum support of the lactating mother. Pediatr Clin North Am. 2001;48(2):365–75.
32. AbdelHadi MSA, Bukharie HA. Breast infections in non-lactating women. J Fam Community Med. 2005;12:133–7.
33. Versluijs-Ossewaarde FN, Roumen RM, Goris RJ. Subareolar breast abscesses: characteristics and results of surgical treatment. Breast J. 2005;11:179–82.
34. Rizzo M, Peng L, Frisch A. Breast abscesses in nonlactating women with diabetes: clinical features and outcome. Am J Med Sci. 2009;338(2):123–6.
35. Dixon JM. Repeated aspiration of breast abscesses in lac tating women. BMJ. 1988;297:1517–8.
36. Ulitzsch D, Nyman MKG, Carlson RA. Breast abscess in lactating women: US-guided treatment. Radiology. 2004;232:904–9.
37. Christensen AF, Al-Suliman N, Nielson KR, et al. Ultrasound guided drainage of breast abscesses: results in 151 patients. Br J Radiol. 2005;78:186–8.
38. Aryeetey RNO, Marquis GS, Timms L, et al. Subclinical mastitis is common among ghanaian women lactating 3 to 4 months postpartum. J Hum Lact. 2008;24:263–7.
39. Arsenault JE, Aboud S, Manji KP, et al. E vitamin supplementation increases risk of subclinical mastitis in HIV-infected women. J Nutr. 2010;140:1788–92.
40. Nussenblatt V, Lema V, Kumwenda N, et al. Epidemiology and microbiology of subclinical mastitis among HIV-infected women in Malawi. Int J STD AIDS. 2005;16:227–32.
41. Dinarello CA. Interleukin-1. Rev Infect Dis. 1984;6(1):51–95.
42. Soder O. Isolation of interleukin-1 from human milk. Int Archiv Allergy Appl Immunol. 1987;83(1):19–23.
43. Filteau SM, Lietz G, Mulokozi G, et al. Milk cytokines and subclinical breast inflammation in Tanzanian women: effects of dietary red palm oil or sunflower oil supplementation. Immunology. 1999;97:595–600.
44. Willumsen JF, Filteau SM, Coutsoudis A, Uebel KE, Newell ML, Tomkins AM. Subclinical mastitis as a risk factor for mother-infant HIV transmission. Adv Exp Med Biol. 2000;478:211–23. doi: 10.1007/0-306-46830-1_19. PMID: 11065074.
45. Birkett J. The Diseases of the Breast and Their Treatment, Longmans, London, 1850.

46. Bloodgood JC. The clinical picture of dilated ducts beneath the nipple frequently to be palpated as a doughy wormlike mass: the varicocele tumour of the breast. Surg Gynecol Obstet. 1923;36:486–95.
47. Liu L, Zhou F, Wang P, et al. Periductal mastitis: an inflammatory disease related to bacterial infection and consequent immune responses? Mediators Inflamm. 2017;2017:5309081.
48. Gollapalli V, Liao J, Dudakovic A, et al. Risk factors for development and recurrence of primary breast abscesses, J Am Coll Surg. 2010;211(1):41–8.
49. Risager R, Bentzon N. Smoking and increased risk of mastitis. Ugeskrift Laeger. 2010;172(33):2218–21.
50. Oltean HN, Soliman AS, Omar OS, et al. Risk factors for chronic mastitis in Morocco and Egypt. Int J Inflamm. 2013;Article ID:184921.
51. Bundred NI, Dixon NJ, Lumsden AB, et al. Are the lesions of duct ectasia sterile? Br J Surg. 1985;72(10):844–5.
52. Zhang Y, Zhou Y, Mao F, Guan J, Sun Q. Clinical characteristics, classification and surgical treatment of periductal mastitis. J Thorac Dis. 2018;10(4):2420–7.
53. Lequin MH, van Spengler J, van Pel R, et al. Mammographic and sonographic spectrum of non-puerperal mastitis. Eur J Radiol. 1995;21(2):138–42.
54. Tomczak R, Rieber A, Zeitler H, et al. The value of MR-mammography at 1.5 tesla in the differential diagnosis of non-puerperal mastitis and inflammatory breast carcinoma. RöFo Fortschritte auf dem Gebiete der Röntgenstrahlen und der Nuklearmedizin. 1996;165(2):148–51.
55. Kalac N, Ozkan B, Bayiz H, et al. Breast tuberculosis. Breast. 2002;11:346–9.
56. Tse GM, Poon CS, Ramachandram K, et al. Granulomatous mastitis: a clinicopathological review of 26 cases. Pathology. 2004;36:254–7.
57. Cooper A. Illustrations of the Diseases of the Breast. Longman, Rees, Orme, Brown and Green, London, 1829.
58. Maroulis I, Spyropoulos C, Zolota V, Tzorakoleftherakis E. Mammary tuberculosis mimicking breast cancer: a case report. J Med Case Rep. 2008;2:34.
59. Da Silva BB, Lopes-Costa PV, Pires CG, et al. Tuberculosis of the breast: analysis of 20 cases and a literature review. Trans R Soc Trop Med Hygiene. 2009;103:559–63.
60. Fadaei-Araghi M, Geranpayeh L, Irani S, et al. Breast tuberculosis: report of eight cases. Arch Iran Med. 2008;11:463–5.
61. Jah A, Mulla R, Lawrence FD, et al. Tuberculosis of the breast: experience of a UK breast clinic serving an ethnically diverse population. Ann R Coll Surg Engl. 2004;86:416–9.
62. Mckeown KC, Wilkinson KW. Tuberculous diseases of the breast. Br J Surg. 1952;39:420.
63. Tewari M, Shukla HS. Breast tuberculosis: diagnosis, clinical features, and management. Indian J Med Res. 2005;122:103–10.
64. Baharoon S. Tuberculosis of the breast. Ann Thorac Med. 2008;3:110–4.
65. Marinopoulos S, Lourantou D, Gatzionis T, et al. Breast tuberculosis: diagnosis, management and treatment. Int J Surg Case Rep. 2012;3:548–50.
66. Mirsaeidi S, Masjedi M, Mansouri S, Velayati A. Tuberculosis of the breast: report of 4 clinical cases and literature review. East Mediterr Health J. 2007;13(3):670–6.
67. Hale JA, Peters GN, Cheek JH. Tuberculosis of the breast: rare but still exist. Review of the literature and report of an additional case. Am J Surg. 1985;150:620–4.
68. Morsad F, Ghazli M, Boumzgou K, et al. Mammary tuberculosis: a series of 14 cases. J Gynecol Obstet Biol Reprod. 2001;30:331–7.
69. Teo TH, Ho GH, Chaturverdi A, Khoo BK. Tuberculosis of the chest wall: unusual presentation as a breast lump. Singapore Med J. 2009;50:e97–9.
70. Thimmappa D, Mallikarjuna MN, Vijayakumar A. Breast tuberculosis. Indian J Surg. 2015;77(Suppl 3):1378–84.
71. Amano M, Shimizu T. Mondor's disease: a review of the literature. Intern Med. 2018;57(18):2607–12.
72. Pugh CM, DeWitty RL. Mondor's disease. J Natl Med Assoc. 1996;88(6):359–63.
73. Rountree KM, Barazi H, Aulick NF. Mondor Disease. In: StatPearls [Internet]. StatPearls Publishing, Treasure Island, FL, 2023. Available at: https://www.ncbi.nlm.nih.gov/books/NBK538282/.
74. Altintoprak F, Kivilcim T, Ozkan OV. Aetiology of idiopathic granulomatous mastitis. World J Clin Cases. 2014;2:852–8.
75. Kessler EWY. Granulomatous mastitis: a lesion clinically simulating carcinoma. Am J Clin Pathol. 1972;58:642–6.
76. Sheybani F, Sarvghad M, Naderi H, Gharib M. Treatment for and clinical characteristics of granulomatous mastitis. Obstet Gynecol. 2015;1:125–801.
77. Sheybani F, Naderi H, Gharib M, et al. Idiopathic granulomatous mastitis: long-discussed but yet-to-be-known. Autoimmunity. 2016;18:236–9.
78. Aghajanzadeh M, Hassanzadeh R, Sefat SA, et al. Granulomatous mastitis: presentations, diagnosis, treatment and outcome in 206 patients from the north of Iran. Breast. 2015;1:456–60.
79. Pandey TS, Mackinnon JC, Bressler L, et al. Idiopathic granulomatous mastitis: a prospective study of 49 women and treatment outcomes with steroid therapy. Breast J. 2014;20:258–66.
80. Taylor GB, Paviour SD, Musaad S, et al. A clinicopathological review of 34 cases of inflammatory breast disease showing an association between corynebacteria infection and granulomatous mastitis. Pathology. 2003;1:109–19.
81. Mathelin C, Riegel P, Chenard MP, et al. Granulomatous mastitis and corynebacteria: clinical and pathologic correlations. Breast J. 2005;11:357.
82. Gautier N, Lalonde L, Tran D, et al. Chronic granulomatous mastitis: imaging, pathology and management. Eur J Radiol. 2013;82:165–75.
83. Baslaim MM, Khayat HA, Al-Amoudi SA. Idiopathic granulomatous mastitis: a heterogeneous disease with variable clinical presentation. World J Surg. 2007;31(8):1677–81.
84. Kiyak G, Dumlu EG, Kilinc I, et al. Management of idiopathic granulomatous mastitis: dilemmas in diagnosis and treatment. BMC Surg. 2014;14:66.
85. Lei X, Chen K, Zhu L, et al. Treatments for idiopathic granulomatous mastitis: systematic review and meta-analysis. Breastfeed Med. 2017;12:415–21.
86. Benson JR, Dumitru D. Idiopathic granulomatous mastitis: presentation, investigation and management. Fut Oncol. 2016;12:1381–94.
87. Morrow M. Evaluation of common breast problems. Am Fam Phys. 2000;61:2371–85.
88. Guray MS. Benign breast diseases: classification, diagnosis and management. Oncologist. 2006;11:435–49.
89. Hance KW, Anderson WF, Devesa SS, et al. Trends in inflammatory breast carcinoma incidence and survival: the surveillance, epidemiology, and end results program at the National Cancer Institute. J Natl Cancer Inst. 2005;97(13):966–75.
90. Fouad TM, Barrera AM, Reuben JM, Lucci A, Woodward WA, Stauder MC, Lim B, DeSnyder SM, Arun B, Gildy B, Valero V. Inflammatory breast cancer: a proposed conceptual shift in the UICC-AJCC TNM staging system. Lancet Oncol. 2017;18:e228–32.
91. Bonnier P, Charpin C, Lejeune C, Romain S, Tubiana N, Beedassy B, Martin PM, Serment H, Piana L. Inflammatory carcinomas of the breast: a clinical, pathological, or a clinical and pathological definition? Int J Cancer. 1995;62:382–5.
92. Dawood S, Valero V. Clinical aspects of inflammatory breast cancer: diagnosis, criteria, controversy. In: Ueno NT, Cristofanilli M, eds, Inflammatory Breast Cancer: An Update, Springer, New York, 2012:11–20.

11

Gynaecomastia

An Overview with a Focus on the Surgical Management

Matthew G. Wedlich, Christian M. Asher, and Charles M. Malata

11.1 Introduction

Gynaecomastia is the benign overgrowth of male breast tissue and has been quantified as the presence of more than 2 cm of palpable, firm, subareolar glandular and ductal tissue (1). It is to be distinguished from 'pseudogynaecomastia' or lipomastia, which is fatty enlargement of the breasts without glandular proliferation.

Gynaecomastia is a benign, relatively common condition, affecting an estimated 35% of all men (2), around 10.2 million men in England. Prevalence increases with age, affecting approximately one third of healthy young adult men, half of healthy older men and nearly three quarters of hospitalised elderly men (3).

In both sexes, mammary tissue develops from both ectoderm and mesoderm in utero, forming the parenchyma and stroma, respectively (4). In normal development, females produce higher levels of oestrogen during puberty promoting breast growth. Males produce less oestrogen and higher levels of androgens, including testosterone, directly antagonising breast development (5). The three main types of oestrogens produced in the body are oestradiol, oestriol, and oestrone. Normal adult testes secrete 15% of the oestradiol and 5% of the oestrone in the circulation, with the remainder produced by androgen aromatisation in liver, muscle, and adipose tissue (Figure 11.1).

Dysregulation of the hormonal axis, with an increase in the oestrogen: testosterone ratio, underpins the aetiology of gynaecomastia. Excess oestrogen stimulates male breast tissue growth directly, and indirectly through suppressing the release of luteinising hormone from the pituitary (thus decreasing testicular testosterone production) and increasing levels of sex hormone-binding globulin (SHBG) (6). SHBG is a circulating transport protein that binds testosterone with a higher affinity than it binds oestrogens. This results in a relative decrease in the free androgen concentration (7).

Additional risk for gynaecomastia development is posed by extra-glandular aromatisation of testosterone and androstenedione into oestradiol and estrone, respectively. This includes skin fibroblasts, adipose tissue, and a by-product of common enzymatic pathways (Figure 11.1). As a result, obesity itself leads to increased oestrogen activity and predisposes to gynaecomastia.

11.2 Aetiology of Gynaecomastia

Causes of gynaecomastia can be broadly classified into physiological and non-physiological.

11.2.1 Physiological

Physiological causes account for 25% of cases. These are periods where natural changes in male hormone levels cause an imbalance of oestrogen and testosterone, favouring oestrogen. There are three main peaks: neonatal, adolescent, and senile. *In utero*, androgenic precursors such as dehydroepiandrosterone (DHEA) are broken down into oestrone and oestradiol by the placenta. A transient excess crossing the placenta results in transient neonatal gynaecomastia.

In childhood, breast development in males is usually quiescent, with some proliferation of ductal tissue and surrounding breast mesenchyme followed by ductal involution and atrophy. During early puberty, increasing androgen production, however, leads to an increased proportion of androgens converted to oestrogen. Clinically this can present as gynaecomastia. Ninety per cent of cases resolve by the end of puberty, but until this time, it can be an emotionally challenging period (9).

DOI: 10.1201/9781003394785-11

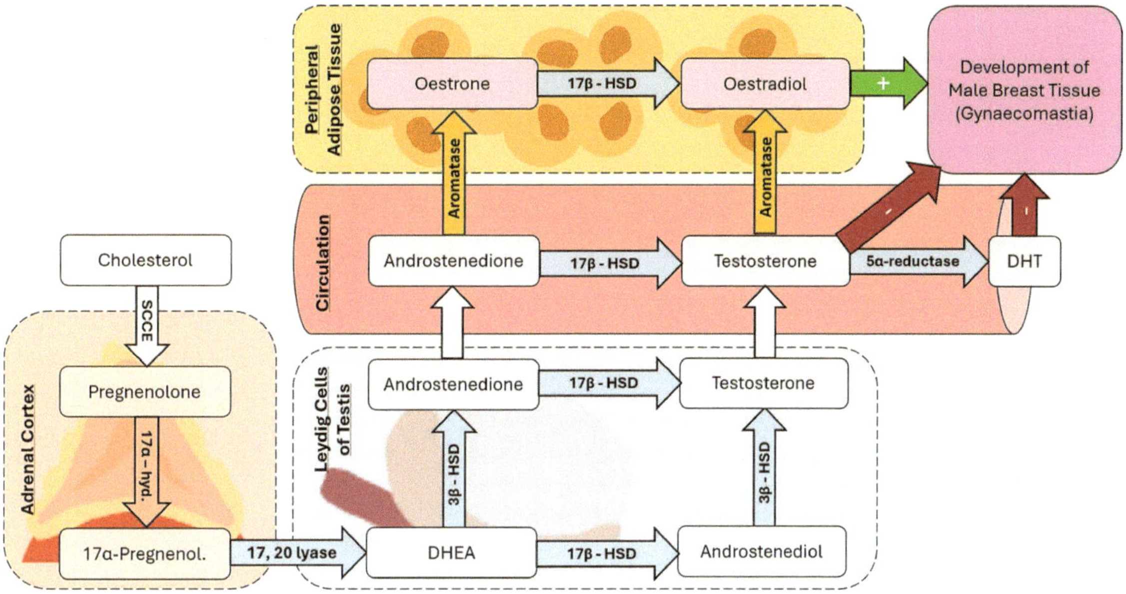

FIGURE 11.1

Steroid hormone synthesis. Androgen precursors are produced from cholesterol in the adrenal cortex, before being converted to DHEA its derivatives, androstenedione and testosterone. These are converted to oestrone and oestradiol through aromatase in peripheral adipose tissue. Testosterone and its derivative DHT antagonise breast tissue growth, whilst oestrogens promote it. (Key: SCCE—side chain cleaving enzyme, DHEA—dehydroepiandrosterone, HSD—hydroxysteroid dehydrogenase, DHT—dihydroxytestosterone.)

Source: **Adapted from (8) under CCO licence.**

Senile gynaecomastia affects up to 65% of men over the age of 70 due to several factors. Testosterone production declines with age. Elderly patients proportionally carry more subcutaneous fat, leading to a greater incidence of peripheral aromatisation (of male sex hormones to female sex hormones), promoting breast tissue growth. The higher proportion of subcutaneous fat with age compounds the clinical appearance of gynaecomastia.

11.2.2 Pathological

Pathological causes of gynaecomastia are largely iatrogenic, accounting for 10–25% of cases. Mechanisms include increased oestrogen activity, decreased testosterone synthesis and androgen receptor blockade (Table 11.1).

Testosterone levels can be decreased due to direct traumatic injury to the testes, infection, iatrogenic (orchidectomy), congenital absence (congenital anorchia), or secondary to an invasive tumour physically destroying testosterone-producing Leydig cells (Table 11.1).

Gynaecomastia can also be indicative of disorders of sexual differentiation (Table 11.1). Klinefelter's syndrome (XXY) and its characteristic hypogonadism are often accompanied by lower testosterone production—with one study finding 70.4% of Klinefelter patients to have low testosterone levels (10). Gynaecomastia may therefore be a clinical feature. In these cases, however, the breast tissue carries a 20-fold increased risk of malignant transformation, requiring careful evaluation (11). Treatment for gynaecomastia in Klinefelter's patients should not include liposuction due to the risk of seeding and the inability to histologically examine this tissue.

In testicular feminisation or androgen insensitivity syndrome, the cells do not respond to the androgens, leading to varying effects on secondary sexual characteristics, from mild, partial, and complete (Table 11.1).

Medication and recreational drugs account for approximately 20% of cases; however, not all mechanisms have been fully identified (12) (Table 11.2).

The phenothiazine antipsychotic drugs stimulate prolactin, directly affecting oestrogen and testosterone levels (24). Use of cimetidine, in comparison to other common antacids (ranitidine, misoprostol, omeprazole), is associated with a substantially greater risk of gynaecomastia (22). This is mediated by a reversible defect in 17-β-hydroxysteroid dehydrogenase (17-β HSD). The relative risk of gynaecomastia for current users of cimetidine compared with non-users was 7.2 (95% confidence interval 4.5 to 11.3).

TABLE 11.1

Pathological Causes of Gynaecomastia Classified According to Effect on Hormonal Axis

Category	Increased Oestrogen	Decreased Testosterone
Liver	Cirrhosis: ↑ oestrogen through decreased metabolism ↑ SHBG leading to ↓ free testosterone. Alcoholic liver disease (ALD): ethanol directly disrupts testosterone synthesis	
Adipose tissue	Obesity: peripheral aromatisation leads to ↓ testosterone and ↑ oestrogen	
Gonadal	No effect	Testicular absence/damage: • Orchidectomy • Viral or bacterial orchitis • Congenital anorchia
Renal/adrenal	Adrenal tumours: release of feminising hormones [feminising adrenal tumours (FAT)]	Renal failure: uraemia is gonadotoxic
Tumours	Prolactinomas: can alter both oestrogen and testosterone levels Paraneoplastic release of hCG ↑ oestrogen	Testicular tumours: direct destruction of Leydig cells
Congenital	No effect	Klinefelter's syndrome (XXY): hypogonadism Androgen insensitivity syndrome: effective absence of testosterone

TABLE 11.2

Drugs/Chemical Substances Linked to Development of Gynaecomastia

Drug	Theorised Mechanism of Action
Topical oestrogen creams (direct or indirect exposure) (13)	Oestrogenic activity
Digoxin (14)	Structural similarity to oestrogen—hence agonist activity
hCG (15) Clomiphene (withdrawal) (16)	Increased oestrogen formation
Ketoconazole (17) Metronidazole (18) Spironolactone (19) Cytotoxic chemotherapy (20)	Inhibition of testosterone synthesis
Finasteride/dutasteride (21) Cimetidine (22) Bicalutamide (23)	Inhibition of testosterone/DHT action
Phenothiazines (24)	Stimulation of prolactin—directly affecting oestrogen and testosterone levels
Amiodarone, verapamil, isoniazid, proton pump inhibitors, marijuana (25)	Unknown

A strong dose-response relation was observed, with a daily dose of over 1 gram resulting in 40 times the risk of developing gynaecomastia. The risk was highest 7 to 12 months after starting cimetidine (26). Digoxin, an oestrogen receptor agonist, and spironolactone, an androgen receptor antagonist, possess molecular moiety to steroid hormones allowing occupation of oestrogen and/or androgen receptors. Finasteride induces gynaecomastia through its anti-androgen activity, via 5-alpha-reductase blockade (27). Ketoconazole dysregulates the oestrogen-to-testosterone ratio through testosterone synthesis inhibition (28). Another interesting drug cause of gynaecomastia is exposure to antiretroviral therapy (ART), particularly efavirenz. Njunguna et al., in a series of 51 cases (mean age 34 years) of gynaecomastia, reported over a year found that all patients were on efavirenz-based ART with a median onset of 15 months after efavirenz initiation (29). The mechanism is unclear but may be related to low serum testosterone (documented in only 8%). On replacement of efavirenz with an alternative antiretroviral gynaecomastia improved in most patients (69%, 20/29).

Substances of misuse and abuse associated with gynaecomastia include amphetamines, heroin, and methadone. Their mechanisms of action remain poorly understood. Alcohol both inhibits testosterone synthesis and contains phytoestrogens, raising the oestrogen–testosterone ratio. Cannabis is an anti-androgen.

Rarer causes of gynaecomastia include liver cirrhosis (8%), primary hypogonadism (8%), sex cord-gonadal stromal tumours (3%), hyperthyroidism (2%), and chronic renal insufficiency (1%) (30).

11.3 Assessment

Patients presenting with gynaecomastia should be assessed with a thorough clinical history including medications, both prescribed and over the counter, comprehensive physical examination and, if indicated, biochemistry, hormonal assays, and relevant imaging.

11.3.1 Clinical History

A focused history should determine the precise onset of symptoms and their progression over time. Clinicians should explore the effect of gynaecomastia on the patient's day-to-day life, physically, socially, and psychologically, as this can be a distressing (and occasionally 'debilitating') condition for many. The medical history should elicit relevant comorbidities including chronic liver disease, thyroid disease, and obesity (currently or a history of significant or massive weight loss). A systems review should enquire about a reduction in libido or impotence as these may signal hypogonadism or increased prolactin production.

Red-flag features suggestive of malignancy include sudden onset, rapidly growing breast tissue, persistent pain, or persistent/massive gynaecomastia in adolescent patients (unilaterally). Pathognomonic skin changes include *peau d'orange*, skin tethering, large or eccentric breast masses and indurated or craggy breast tissue on clinical examination (31). These clinical findings warrant urgent referral to an oncological breast clinic for triple assessment and expedient management.

A comprehensive list of the patient's prescribed and over-the-counter medications should be acquired. Common offending drugs and their mechanisms of action are listed in Table 11.2. Smoking status, alcohol consumption, and recreational drug use should be explored. The latter two can directly influence the development of gynaecomastia or potentiate the effects of other medications.

11.3.2 Examination

The patient is assessed with a general inspection, followed by a detailed oncological and aesthetic examination.

11.3.2.1 General

Baseline measurements include height, weight, and BMI (normal habitus, overweight, or obese). On general inspection, look for loss of secondary sexual characteristics, as well as hair loss and shiny skin (which can result from a reduction in testosterone levels). Remain astute for findings associated with causative conditions such as orbital proptosis, goitre, evidence of disturbed metabolism, as with thyroid disease.

The overall size and symmetry of the breasts should be noted. Gynaecomastia may be unilateral or bilateral and is often asymmetrical. One should comment on the severity (size—small, moderate, large, or severe), the extent, and distribution (diffuse or discrete). Assess the skin quality (excellent, good, or poor), its elasticity, the presence and degree of skin excess, ptosis, or pseudoptosis. The definition of the inframammary fold (IMF) is worth noting as a well-defined IMF will require disruption in addition to addressing excess breast tissue and skin.

11.3.2.2 Oncological

An oncological breast examination is performed in the standard fashion, both sitting and supine, with all quadrants of the breast assessed. Inspection is repeated with the pectoralis muscle contracted by the patient applying pressure with their hands on their hips. Skin changes, contour irregularities, tethering, abnormalities of the NAC, and any discharge should be noted.

Palpation should encompass all four quadrants of each breast to detect any evidence of breast malignancy. The patient is first positioned with the arms by their sides. Each breast should be palpated in turn, systematically, determining its consistency (soft, firm, hard, rubbery), and the presence of any masses, lumps, or discs. It is useful to assess the skin thickness, elasticity by pinching the affected tissue, and mobility of any masses when the pectoralis muscle contracts (Figure 11.2). This examination is repeated with the patient supine, and the ipsilateral arm positioned behind their head in turn.

Breast cancer is typically hard, craggy to palpation, often not immediately underneath the NAC and eccentric. It can be fixed to the underlying tissues meaning the mass will move with contraction of pectoralis major and not freely mobile. Other features can include skin change and enlarged axillary nodes.

A high index of suspicion for testicular cancer in 20–40-year-olds presenting with sudden onset gynaecomastia is needed, as this is the peak age of onset (32). On examination, this is typically a unilateral painless mass in the scrotum, however, in a minority of cases,

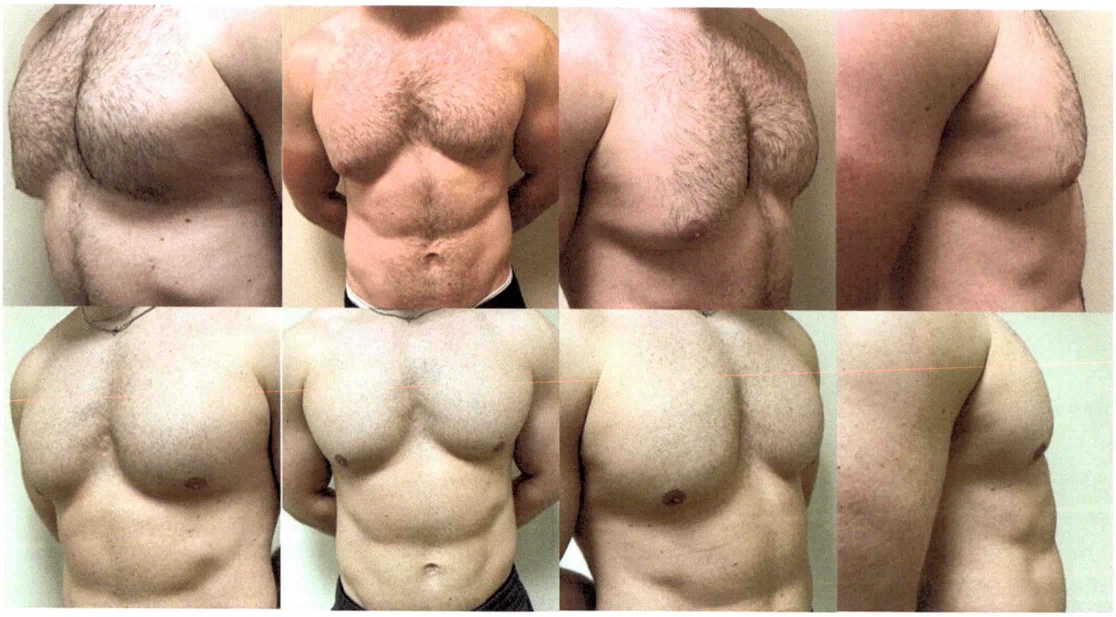

FIGURE 11.2
Right unilateral gynaecomastia treated by open excision in a bodybuilder.

the clinical presentation mimics epididymo-orchitis. Comparison with the contralateral testicle is essential. Concerning clinical findings or identification of a diffuse asymmetrical enlargement warrants further investigation with hormone assays and clinical imaging with ultrasound scan in the first instance.

Further examination should assess for distant lymphadenopathy, abdominal masses, signs of chronic liver disease (jaundice, clubbing, palmar erythema, spider naevi, ascites, ecchymoses) indicating coagulopathy and impaired synthetic function of the liver amongst other peripheral stigmata.

11.3.2.3 Aesthetic

Aesthetic examination is performed from both an anterior and lateral point of view. Establish if there is any chest wall deformity, including the bony chest wall contour and the presence (or absence) of pectoralis major, in reference to Poland's syndrome (33). Determine the laterality of the gynaecomastia (Figure 11.2), symmetry, the extent of surplus tissues (gland and skin), and the degree of ptosis, if present. The male NAC should ideally sit at the mid-humeral line at the level of the fourth intercostal space along the midclavicular line. The composition of the tissue excess (skin, fat, or glandular), evidence of striae, and an overall appreciation for the patient's skin quality should be noted.

Distinguishing true gynaecomastia from pseudogynaecomastia can be challenging as the conditions are often concurrent (34). Pseudogynaecomastia arises due to excess adiposity rather than true breast tissue (glandular) hypertrophy. True gynaecomastia demonstrates a distinct disc of firm or rubbery mobile tissue concentrically located beneath the NAC, whilst pseudogynaecomastia demonstrates more uniform, softer enlargement. This is best assessed by pinching the affected tissue between the thumb and index finger, palpating for firm or rubbery breast tissue growth (Figure 11.3). Pseudogynaecomastia is much more common in obese and elderly patients. Even if this is the case, there may still be a discrete sub-areolar disc projecting the NAC forward. In cases of more severe gynaecomastia, the breast tissue and well-defined IMF may cause a clinical ptosis as in female patients.

Clinical photographs should be taken—with patient consent—to aid with pre-operative planning and to demonstrate the efficacy of later treatment. Gynaecomastia surgery constitutes a significant proportion of complaints made by male patients against breast and plastic surgeons. As such, clinical photographs are a useful adjunct medico-legally. Photographs should encompass both anteroposterior (AP), lateral and oblique views with the patient's arms by the side as well as AP hand on waist with pectoralis major contracted.

11.3.3 Investigations

Investigations (both biochemical and imaging) in gynaecomastia are guided by the history and examination findings (Table 11.2). Biochemical investigations include peripheral blood sampling for hormonal

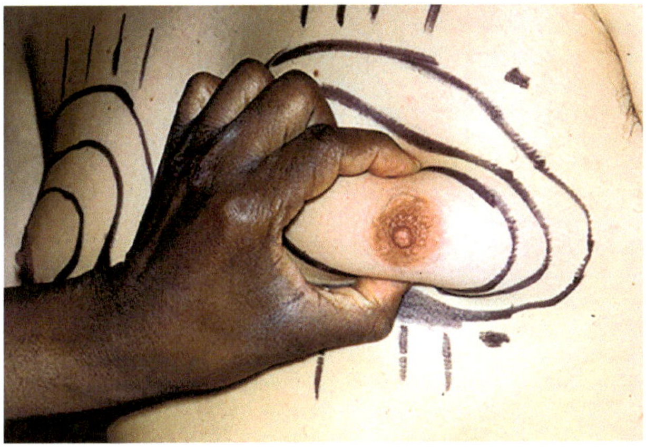

FIGURE 11.3
Pinch test performed to determine extent of breast tissue growth.

profiling, a 9:00 a.m. testosterone level, thyroid function tests, liver function tests, alpha-fetoprotein, and b-HCG in attempts to identify hormonal imbalance or secondary causes (Table 11.3).

Imaging may be of use in distinguishing true gynaecomastia from pseudogynaecomastia, differentiating fibrous tissue from adiposity, in addition to characterising possible underlying malignancy. Modalities include ultrasound, mammogram or CT depending on the clinical context. Core- or fine-needle biopsy is warranted if there is suspicion of breast cancer and should be actively considered in Klinefelter patients presenting with progressive gynaecomastia (11).

TABLE 11.3

Recommended Laboratory Tests in Gynaecomastia including Rationale

Laboratory Tests	Rationale
Testosterone	Low levels Inhibition of gynaecomastia
Oestrogen and bHCG	↑ breast tissue growth
Gonadotrophins—FSH, LH	Hypogonadism ↓ Testosterone levels
Prolactin	Hypogonadism ↓ Testosterone levels ↓ Androgen receptors ↑ Oestrogen and progesterone receptors
Urea and electrolytes	Uraemia causes gonadotoxicity
Liver function tests	Cirrhosis ↓ Oestrogen breakdown and ↑ SHBG causing ↓ free testosterone
Thyroid function tests	Hyperthyroidism ↑ Androgen aromatisation to oestrogen ↑ SHBG ↓ Free testosterone

11.3.4 Classification

Gynaecomastia is most often graded according to the Simon classification (35), which categorises the severity of breast tissue growth and can inform operative management (Figure 11.4). Rohrich and colleagues provided an alternative classification factoring the consistency of the breast tissue (i.e. glandular or fibrous) and the presence or otherwise of ptosis (36) (Table 11.4).

Clinically establishing the grade of severity establishes a platform for management and helps determine the extent of any surgical intervention required (37).

11.4 Management

Treatment options for gynaecomastia are guided by the underlying aetiology and the clinical severity, encompassing conservative, medical, radiological, and surgical options.

11.4.1 Conservative

A conservative approach is appropriate, as determined by aetiology and patient demographic. Neonatal gynaecomastia is self-limiting and similarly adolescent gynaecomastia will often self-resolve within 18

TABLE 11.4

Classifications of Gynaecomastia (Simon et al. vs Rohrich et al.)

Simon Classification of Gynaecomastia (35)	
Grade	**Features**
Grade 1	Small enlargement, no skin excess
Grade 2a	Moderate enlargement, no skin excess
Grade 2b	Moderate enlargement, with skin excess
Grade 3	Marked enlargement, with skin excess
Rohrich Classification of Gynaecomastia (36)*	
Grade	**Features**
Grade I	Minimal hypertrophy (<250 g) without ptosis
IA	Primarily glandular
IB	Primarily fibrous
Grade II	Moderate hypertrophy (250–500 g) without ptosis
IIA	Primarily glandular
IIB	Primarily fibrous
Grade III	Severe hypertrophy (>500 g) with grade 1 ptosis (glandular or fibrous)
Grade IV	Severe hypertrophy with grade 2 or 3 ptosis (glandular or fibrous)

Note: *This classification does not acknowledge fatty-glandular tissue with predominantly fatty tissue, a common occurrence.

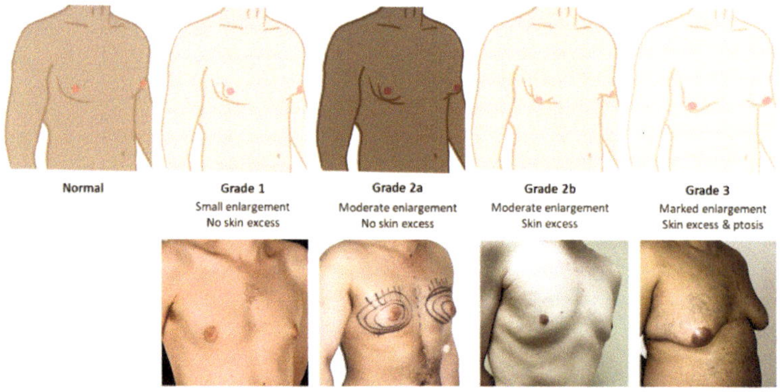

FIGURE 11.4
Simon classification of gynaecomastia (35; image adapted from ref. 2, including representative cases from the senior author's clinical practice).

months once hormonal imbalances equilibrate (1). Some patients are less affected by the presence of small volume gynaecomastia, making invasive treatment inappropriate. Others may not be surgical candidates due to medical comorbidity.

As gynaecomastia is often concurrent with pseudogynaecomastia, the adipose component can be managed through lifestyle modifications. Improved diet, increased activity levels, and optimal medical management of comorbidities such as diabetes and hypothyroidism, which often cause weight gain when poorly controlled. Prescribed drugs can be discontinued if clinically appropriate or alternatives given. Iatrogenic gynaecomastia is often reversed on cessation of the offending drug within months.

11.4.2 Medical or Hormonal Treatment

The focus of medication-based intervention is to correct the imbalance between the androgen–oestrogen axis and diminish further breast tissue growth (Table 11.5). This is indicated in cases of gynaecomastia where the patient is experiencing significant discomfort or negatively socially impacted. It is most effective when administered during the proliferative phase. It is good practice to refer such cases to a specialist endocrine multidisciplinary team (MDT), adult or paediatric. Where gynaecomastia is well established and is fibrotic (and therefore histologically hyalinised), surgery is the most suitable intervention.

The foremost options are tamoxifen (a selective oestrogen receptor modulator) and anastrozole (aromatase inhibitor) (44). These diminish the action and production of oestrogens, respectively. As of 2024, anastrozole is not licenced in the United Kingdom for the treatment of gynaecomastia, and tamoxifen is recommended only for the treatment of gynaecomastia in men with prostate cancer undergoing long-term bicalutamide treatment (45).

11.4.3 Radiotherapy

Radiotherapy is used prophylactically in older men prior to prostate cancer treatment with antiandrogens including bicalutamide–a well-established iatrogenic

TABLE 11.5
Medications Proposed for Treatment of Gynaecomastia

Drug	Mechanism	Patient Population and Evidence
Anastrozole	Aromatase inhibitor	Pubertal gynaecomastia (44 patients): reduction in breast area (–63%) and volume (–57%) (38)
Clomiphene	Selective oestrogen receptor modulator (SERM)	Hypogonadal men (review): overall reduction of symptoms including breast size (39)
Danazol	Androgen and anti-gonadotropin	Idiopathic gynaecomastia (52 patients): significantly improved breast tenderness and degree of breast tissue (40)
Dihydrotestosterone (DHT)	Non-aromatisable androgen	Idiopathic gynaecomastia (40 patients): 25% complete remission, 48% partial remission (41)
Tamoxifen	Selective oestrogen receptor modulator	Prostate cancer patients treated with bicalutamide (anti-androgen) (50 patients): significant reduction in development of gynaecomastia and mastalgia (42)
Testolactone	Aromatase inhibitor	Pubertal gynaecomastia (22 patients): 25% reduction in breast gland diameter (43)

cause of gynaecomastia (46, 47). The doses administered are comparatively lower than those used in adjuvant or neoadjuvant cancer treatment, ranging from 8–16 Gy in divided doses, compared to the 40–50 Gy delivered in breast cancer patients (48). Younger patients, however, should not be exposed to higher doses of ionising radiation due to its established long-term cumulative adverse effects, including the development of radiation-induced malignancy.

11.4.4 Surgery

The most effective treatment modality for gynaecomastia is surgical removal. It is, however, essentially an aesthetic procedure and indications should be considered carefully (Table 11.6), with an appropriate approach selected based on both the patient and clinical severity. Timing of any intervention is tailored to when expectations can align with predictable outcomes. As with all aesthetic procedures, pre-operative counselling over at least two separate consultations is indicated. The first, to assess and establish the options available, discuss risks, benefits, and likely outcomes. The patient is then directed to further information and given time to consider this and alternative options. A second consultation allows considered questions and finalisation of mutually agreed interventions.

Medical optimisation before surgery is essential to reduce anaesthetic and surgical risks in the perioperative period and improve operative outcomes. The patient should be post-pubertal with a stable BMI, ideally, within acceptable limits for cosmetic surgery to ensure predictable surgical outcomes (49).

11.4.4.1 Surgical Approach

Intervening surgeons should be familiar with the range of approaches available and tailor it to the clinical picture and patient preferences, considering post-operative down time, potential scarring and what the patient would deem to be an acceptable outcome. This is not always straightforward but can be facilitated using established algorithms and, where indicated, a combination of techniques, in a single or staged manner (36, 37, 50, 51).

TABLE 11.6

Indications for Surgical Management of Gynaecomastia

- Persistence after puberty (>2 years) without underlying medical cause
- Inadequate response to medical therapy
- Drug induced: prostate cancer treatment, i.e. bicalutamide
- Drug induced: anabolic steroid/cannabis induced
- Marked asymmetry
- Post massive weight loss
- Significant psycho-social morbidity
- Clinically apparent and significant

11.4.4.1.1 Liposuction: Conventional, Ultrasonic, Vaser, and Laser

There are various types of liposuction employable for the treatment of gynaecomastia, in isolation or in a combined approach with minimally invasive techniques, open glandular excision or skin-reducing techniques (52–54) (Table 11.7). Liposuction is most suitable where there is a predominantly fatty breast composition (Figure 11.5).

Incisions for liposuction fluid infiltration and liposuction aspiration are made at aesthetically discrete landmarks including infero-laterally in the inframammary crease, at the superior anterior axillary line or on the NAC, within the pigmented portion or at the junction with the normal breast skin (Figure 11.5 and 30m). The breast and surrounding subcutaneous fat are then infiltrated with standard liposuction fluid. In the senior author's practice this comprises 1 ml of 1 in 1000 adrenaline (1 mg) l s 1% lignocaine added to each litre of Hartmann's solution providing haemostatic control and the delivery of local anaesthetic within the operative field (54). Liposuction is performed with both the palm down and pinch techniques with tapering around the edges to achieve a male chest contour. It also engenders a variable degree of skin retraction and can be used to assist disruption of a well-defined IMF in a clinically significant gynaecomastia, which contributes to the female-shaped breasts.

The use of power and ultrasound during liposuction increases the volume of fat that can be removed, making the process quicker and more efficient than conventional liposuction (traditional liposuction which is also (historically) referred to as suction assisted lipectomy (SAL).

Ultrasound-assisted liposuction (or ultrasonic liposuction) (UAL) emulsifies the fat, facilitating aspiration with less tissue trauma in comparison to traditional liposuction modalities (Figures 11.6 and 11.7). Third-generation UAL, VASER (Solta Medical, Bothell, Washington), delivers power in a pulsed manner through cavitated, loosened fat through the delivery of small gas bubbles (5–10 μm), combining subcutaneous infiltration, emulsification, and suction at lower energy levels (36 Hz) (55). This causes less tissue trauma, provides more targeted fat disruption and, in experienced hands, reduces risk of liposuction-associated complications. It is important, however, to protect the skin from thermal damage of the ultrasonic cannula.

Access incisions are closed with 5/0 Vicryl deep dermal sutures or 5/0 Ethilon and covered with Steri-Strips. Nonabsorbable sutures should remain no

TABLE 11.7

Surgical Approaches to Gynaecomastia

Liposuction—Various Types	Minimally Invasive Options	Open Glandular Excision Techniques	Skin Reduction Techniques
Suction-assisted lipectomy (SAL)	Pull-through technique	Periareolar (Webster)	Concentric mastopexy reduction
Ultrasound-assisted (UAL)	Arthroscopic shaver	Circumareolar	LeJour (vertical scar)
Power-assisted (PAL)	Vacuum-assisted biopsy (VAB)	Transareolar	Wise pattern (inverted T-scar)
Laser-assisted (LAL)	Endoscopic	Circumthelial	Elliptical
Radiofrequency-assisted	Microdebrider	Subcutaneous mastectomy	Lateral wedge ± medial wedge
Vibration Amplification of Sound Energy Resonance (VASER)			Lalonde type (no-vertical-scar with nipple transposition)
			Breast amputation and free nipple-grafting

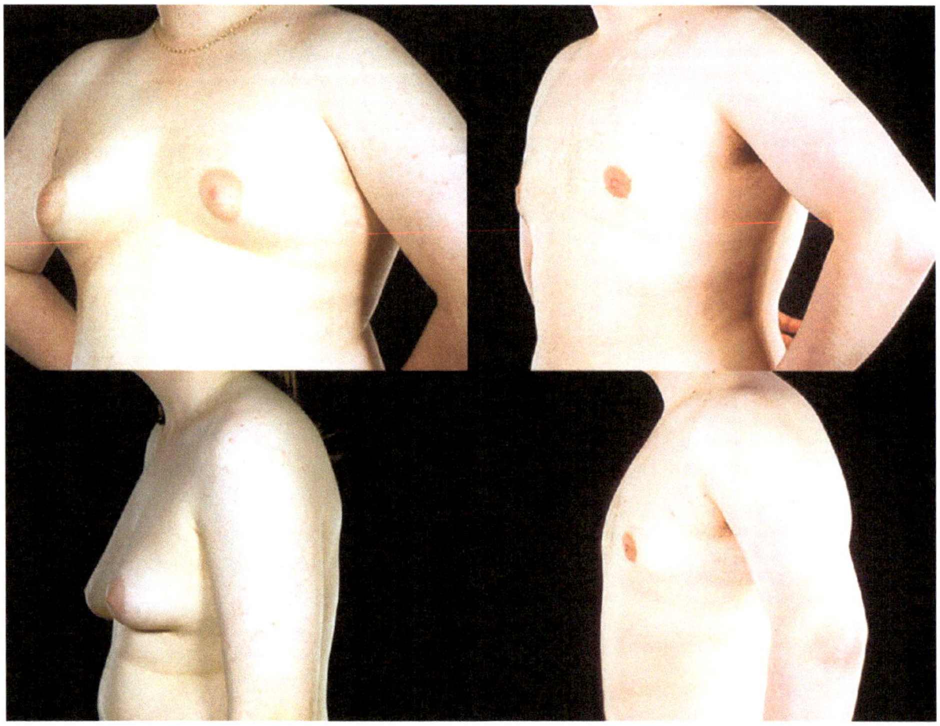

FIGURE 11.5
A 16-year-old patient with Simon Grade 2a fatty gynaecomastia treated with conventional liposuction. Note the hardly noticeable access incisions in the lateral IMF and the anterior axillary line superiorly.

Source: **Ref. 37, with permission.**

longer than 7 days to minimise risk of track marks or railroading. Intra-operative antibiotics are administered routinely but one can consider antibiotic prophylaxis post-operatively (although this is more commonly reserved for cases involving skin resection or open glandular excision). A compression garment is worn for 6 weeks, day and night. In the long term, it is imperative that the patient maintains a stable weight to prevent 'recurrence' and contour deformity because of irregular fat deposition following liposuction. As a single treatment modality, liposuction is not suitable for dense, fibrotic breast tissue and does not address surplus skin, ptosis of the NAC, or pseudoptosis of the breast. For these, direct excision of tissue using minimally invasive or open excision techniques are required with or without skin reduction.

11.4.4.1.2 Minimally Invasive Techniques: Pull Through, VAB, Arthroscopic, and Endoscopic

Minimally invasive techniques in gynaecomastia extend back to the 1990s. They include pull-through techniques, traditionally described in combination with liposuction for small to moderate volume fibro-fatty gynaecomastia without need to address

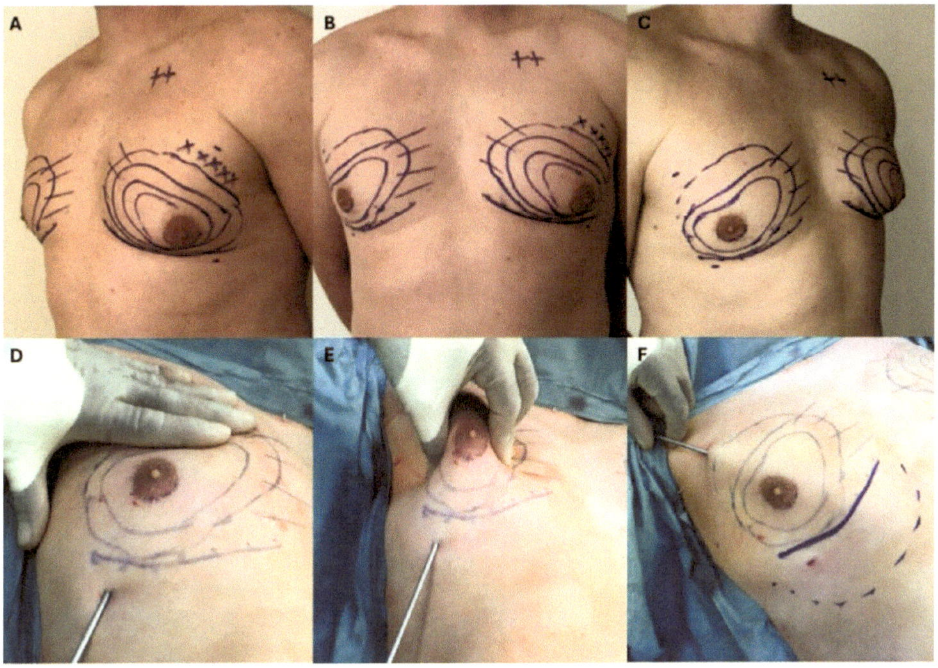

FIGURE 11.6
Pre-operative markings and intra-operative sequence of liposuction. A–C: Pre-operative markings made in the upright position indicating IMF, contour of breast tissue and cannula insertion sites. D–E: Infiltration of LA, conventional liposuction with a 4 mm cannula via an IMF stab incision using palm-down technique (D) and pinch technique (E). F: Liposuction from the AAF incision and disrupting the IMF (straight line just above the inferior stab incision). Note the position of the cannula and the extent of liposuction on the chest wall (dotted line) well below the IMF (solid line) to allow re-draping of the skin and precise inferior periareolar incision after liposuction (see *Figure 11.9*).

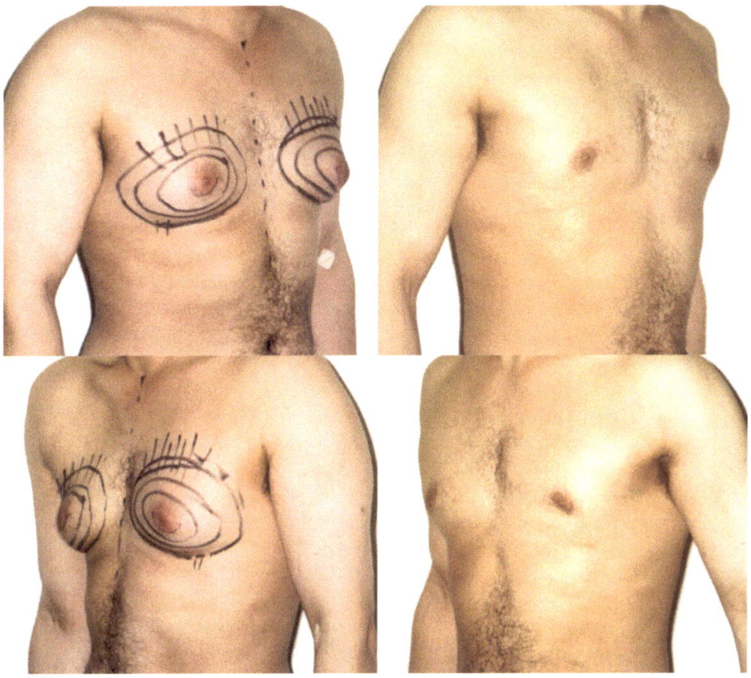

FIGURE 11.7
Bodybuilder presenting with Simon Grade 2a gynaecomastia treated with ultrasound-assisted liposuction (UAL) without recourse to open excision.

Source: **Ref. 54, with permission.**

a significant skin excess. Liposuction via two lateral incisions superiorly and inferiorly is used to mobilise the central fibrous component. This is then extruded through the liposuction ports (56). Endoscopic approaches and arthroscopic shavers are readily available due to their use by other specialties and offer potential for significant reductions in volume without the visible scarring associated with open approaches. Their uptake is yet to be widely published (57).

Several breast surgeons and radiologists have reported the use of vacuum-assisted breast excision techniques (VAB) for treatment of gynaecomastia (58), but these can be complicated by severe internal bleeding/haematoma, which can prove difficult to control or lead to emergency open exploration of the breast. It is better to plan open excision if it is anticipated that the tissue will be too fibrous to deal with by liposuction.

11.4.4.1.3 Open Excision (Webster's Technique) (59)

The time-honoured inferior periareolar access (59), a relatively well concealed approach, is indicated where there is mild to moderate breast tissue which is palpably fibrous without the need to address a skin excess or the size of the NAC. The incision is placed at the lower half of the areola, typically between 3 o'clock and 9 o'clock and should not extend beyond halfway along the circumference of the areola (Figure 11.8 A–B). The NAC is raised on a superiorly based adipodermal pedicle, at least 1 cm thick to prevent central NAC depression (Figure 11.8C, Figure 11.9). Large-calibre serrated dissection scissors such as Bostwick scissors are used to isolate to the lower border of the breast inferiorly, followed by dissection in an ascending trajectory in a plane above the pectoralis major muscle until the cranial edge of the breast tissue is released (Figures 11.8D–G). This gives excellent results and is combined with liposuction of the edges to prevent saucerisation deformity (Figure 11.8H, Figure 11.10). The main drawback is that it does not correct skin excess and ptosis. These can be addressed with skin reducing techniques.

11.4.4.1.4 Skin Reduction Techniques

There are several techniques used to address excess skin in large and/or ptotic breasts as seen in severe gynaecomastia (Grades III and IV). We summarise common approaches illustratively, (for more extensive description of these techniques the reader is referred to previous publications) (60–62).

11.4.4.1.4.1 Concentric Reduction

A circumareolar approach is beneficial where NAC reduction is indicated, access is needed to perform glandular excision and a mild to moderate skin excess needs to be addressed (Figure 11.11). Although the scars are confined to the periphery of the nipple-areolar complex, these are at risk of scar hypertrophy, scar migration, and possible keloid formation. Skin reductions on the larger end of the scale also have a propensity to pucker and the purse string sutures are commonly palpable. There is also the potential for exposure of these nonabsorbable, often braided sutures which poses added risk of infection and a need to be removed.

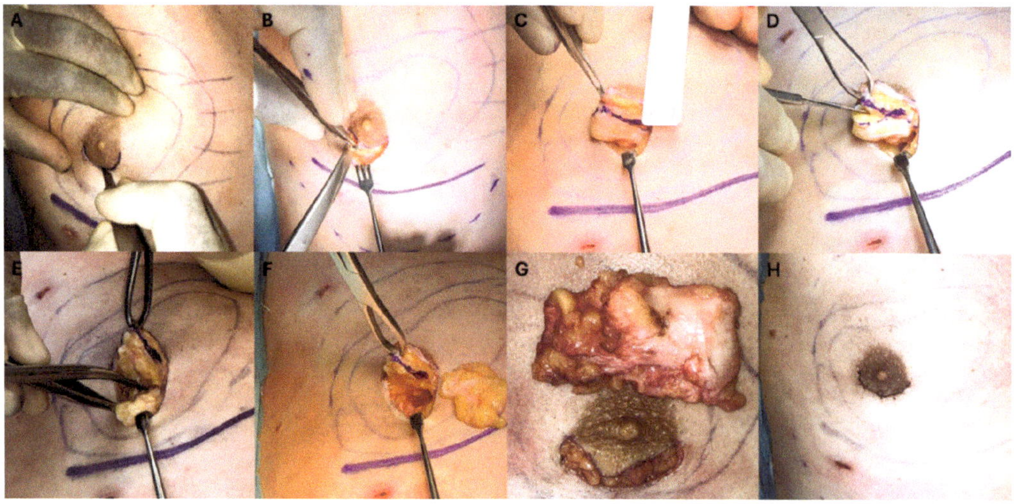

FIGURE 11.8
Intra-operative sequence of open excision of gynaecomastia. A–B: IMF re-marked, peri-areolar incision from 9 o'clock to 3 o'clock. C: Superior adipodermal pedicle measured to ensure 1 cm thickness in the subareolar area. D: Resection of breast tissue from superior adipodermal pedicle. E: Bostwick scissors used to complete dissection superiorly. F: Completion of resection. G: Resected specimen. H: Skin closure using 4–0 Monocryl subcuticular.

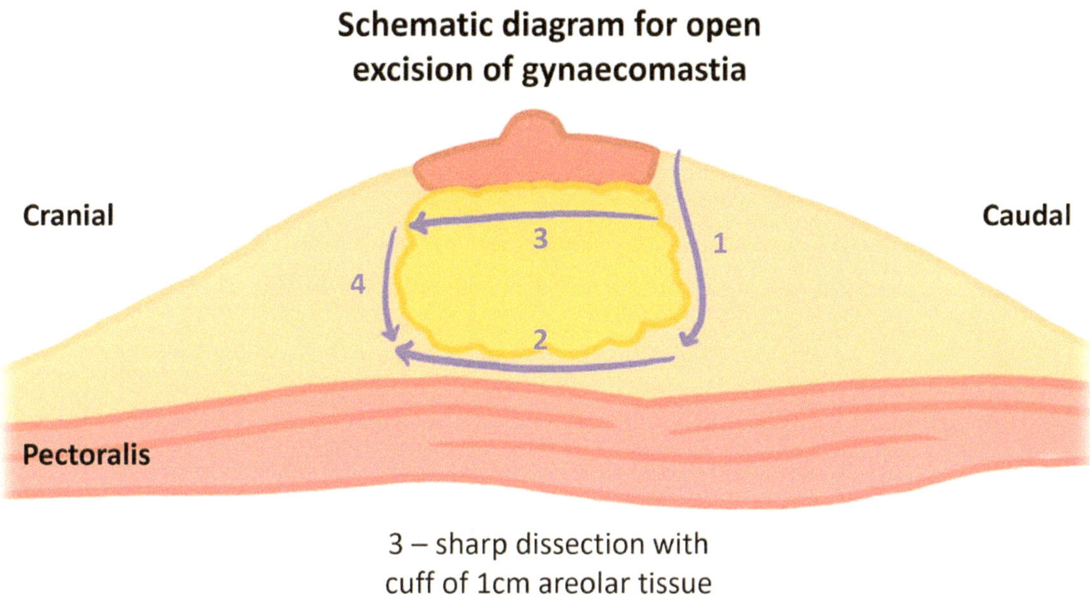

FIGURE 11.9
Open excision of gynaecomastia.

Source: Ref. 37, with permission.

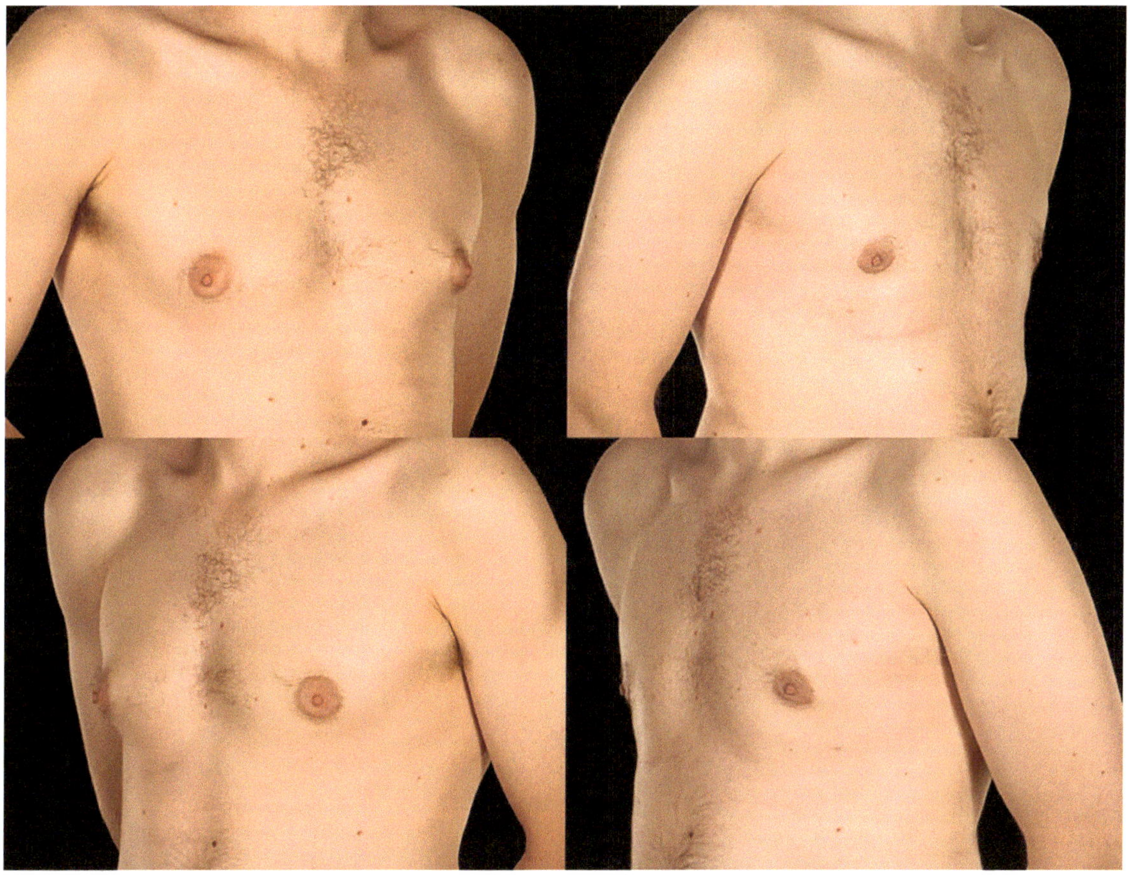

FIGURE 11.10
Simon Grade 1 gynaecomastia treated with open excision (pre- and post-operative images).

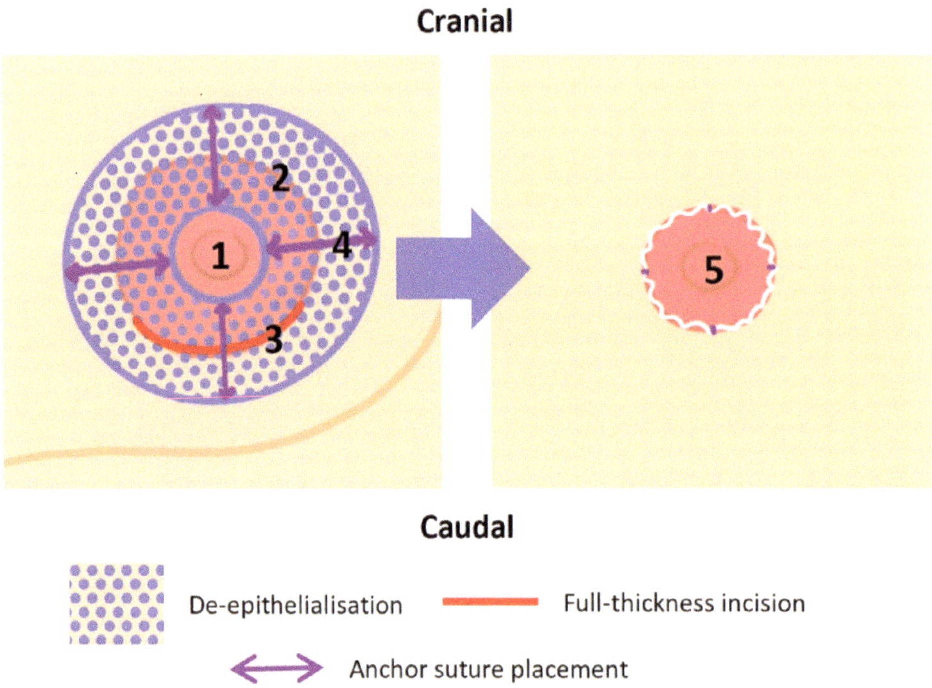

FIGURE 11.11
Concentric reduction. The NAC is reduced to an appropriate diameter. A superior adipodermal pedicle is designed and de-epithelialised, whilst surrounding skin and soft tissue is excised. Anchoring sutures secure the new NAC to surrounding skin whilst purse string and subcuticular sutures secure the skin and prevent stretching of the neo-areola.

Both the pre-existing and new NAC are marked. The average male NAC is 2.6 cm (63). Epidermis is incised along both markings, the skin marked adjacent to the new smaller NAC undermined, outwardly, prior to de-epithelialisation to prevent NAC avulsion. A superiorly based adipo-dermal pedicle is designed and elevated and carefully retracted facilitating access to the glandular tissue requiring excision. Circumferential glandular dissection allows excision but avoiding the pectoralis fascia.

Achieving circular NAC closure commences with anchoring sutures, placed at 12 o'clock, 6 o'clock, 3 o'clock, and 9 o'clock (Figure 11.11). A purse string suture of Ethibond or Gore-Tex is used to prevent stretching of the neo-areola. Further sutures can be distributed equally in between as needed. A subcuticular suture follows, ensuring not to concertina the suture, constricting the NAC irregularly. To avoid puckering sometimes it may be necessary to excise lateral or medial skin wedges.

11.4.4.1.4.2 Lateral +/− Medial Skin Excision

Occasionally de-epithelialised lateral limbs can be added to enable additional elimination of skin excess (Figure 11.12). Orientation of the NAC incision and lateral limbs is based on the trajectory of the skin laxity (obliquely or horizontally) (Figure 11.12). However, sometimes these excisions are not enough, and one may have to resort to traditional female breast reduction techniques is necessary (Figure 11.13).

11.4.4.1.4.3 Traditional Female Breast Reduction Techniques

Both the LeJour and T-scar techniques as employed in female patients have been described for male breasts as well (37, 56). They come into their own when a large-volume skin and tissue excision is required (see the following). Their main drawback is the female pattern scars, and they typically lead to superior fullness which is exactly what is not required in male breast reduction. To avoid this, the senior author recommends combined modality techniques.

11.4.5 Combined Modality Treatment

Often a hybrid approach with liposuction, usually prior to (and often also after) glandular excision and skin reduction, can be applied where clinical examination elicits evidence of adiposity within and around the chest wall, facilitating high-definition contouring. Even in the context of a more fibrous component, liposuction can facilitate disruption of the glandular tissue attachments, and the senior author always performs minor liposuction or uses a liposuction cannula

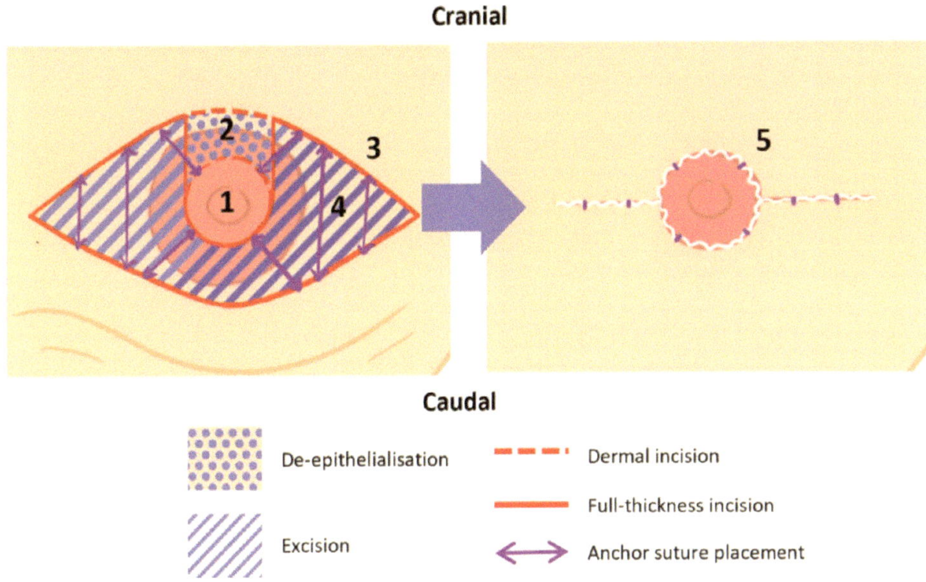

FIGURE 11.12
Reduction with lateral and medial skin excision schematic diagram. The NAC is reduced to an appropriate diameter. As in concentric reduction technique a superior adipodermal pedicle is designed and de-epithelialised, whilst surrounding skin and soft tissue is excised. The area of skin and tissue excision is extended in an ellipse to remove residual skin causing ptosis. Anchoring sutures secure the new NAC to surrounding skin whilst purse string and subcuticular sutures secure the skin and prevent stretching of the neoareola.

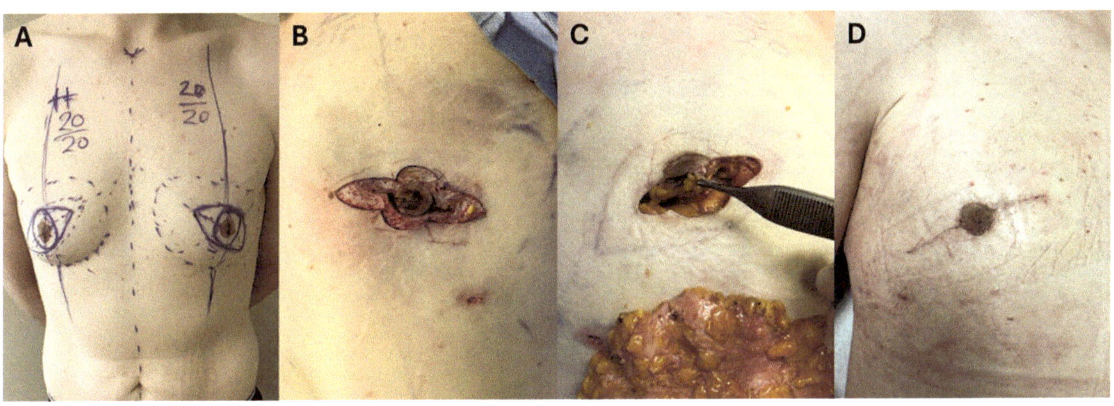

FIGURE 11.13
Reduction with lateral and medial skin excision—intra-operative sequence: after massive weight loss. A) Preoperative marking indicating areas of excess skin to be reduced (dark ellipses) B) De-epithelialised ellipse of skin surrounding nipple-areola complex C) Excess glandular tissue removed via deepening incision inferior to nipple-areola complex D) Healed incisions following surgery.

for pre-tunnelling. The pre-tunnelling also reduces bleeding in addition to facilitating the dissection/resection of the glandular tissue.

11.4.6 Large-Volume Skin and Tissue Excision

To address significant breast tissue excess, correct NAC ptosis and eliminate skin surplus a more radical approach is required. The patient should be counselled on the aesthetic risks in a similar way to a female patient undergoing a reduction mammaplasty or mastopexy. Emphasis should be placed on long and visible scars which may become hypertrophic, stretched or keloid, risk of wound breakdown, impaired nipple sensation, nipple necrosis, asymmetry, and potential for revision surgery. These approaches are always hybrid with liposuction, targeting global fatty excess across the chest in addition to any fat lateral to the breast, providing more definition to the lateral margin of pectoralis major. In all cases of a well-defined IMF, a hybrid approach can be used, as previously detailed, pre-tunnelling with a liposuction cannula, bluntly dissecting and releasing the dermal attachments that are over defining the infra-mammary fold, which reinforce the appearance of a ptotic female breast.

Traditional methods, such as LeJour and Wise pattern skin reduction, are well illustrated elsewhere (56, 58). These produce visible scars that are pathognomonic of female mammaplasty or mastopexy. In a male patient, this is not often perceived as an acceptable outcome. There are a range of alternatives available; the senior author initially used these in dark-skinned patients to reduce the risk of hypertrophic/keloid scar formation or poorly placed scars on the male chest (59) (Figure 11.14), but now applies them to all appropriate patients, with large ptotic breasts. These approaches offer a superior aesthetic outcome without limiting surgical access (Figure 11.14).

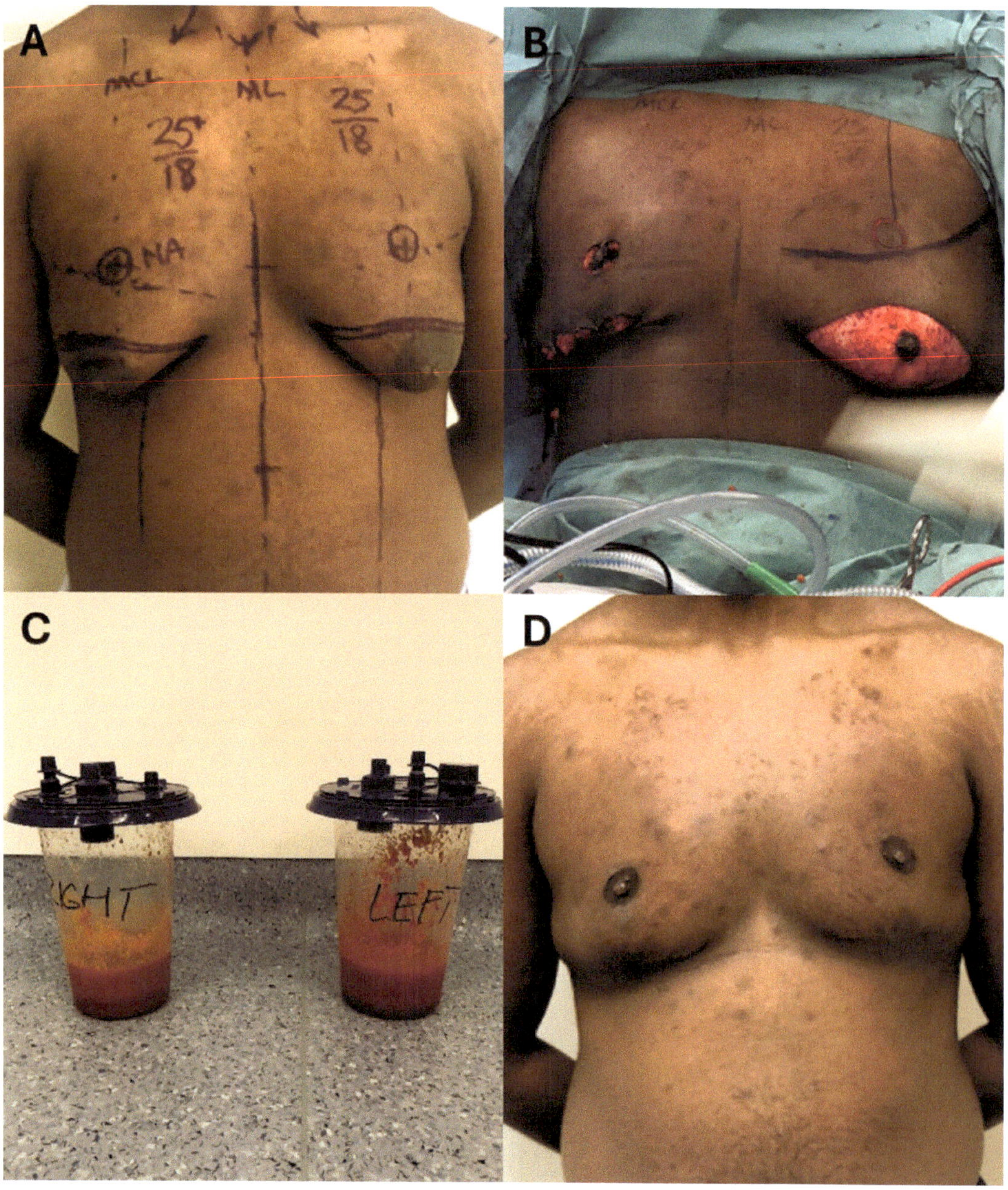

FIGURE 11.14
Lalonde technique employed in a 25-year-old dark-skinned patient. A: Pre-operative markings indicating position of new NAC above the inferior margin of pec major (dashed line) B: Left breast inferior 'melon slice' de-epithelialised and new NAC position incised. Right breast has been reduced with excision of breast tissue and anchoring of adipodermal flap beneath superior flap. C: Fat harvested through liposuction to aid in reduction process. D: Two weeks following surgery.

11.4.6.1 Mastectomy and Free Nipple Graft vs Lalonde Breast Reduction

Large-volume, pendulous breasts, with significant ptosis of the NAC are amenable to an elliptical mastectomy of the ptotic melon slice and free nipple graft, positioned superiorly at the ideal location. This effectively addresses all aspects of true gynaecomastia as first described by Wray et al. in 1974 (64), highlighting its acceptable use for the most severe cases only. NAC grafting risks sequelae, including poor graft take (either partial or total), loss of sensation and depigmentation. In the senior author's experience, it is rarely necessary given the alternatives available but may be better indicated for gender affirmation surgery.

The senior author prefers the Lalonde type no-vertical scar technique (Figures 11.14–11.17) for this cohort of patients with large and severely ptotic breasts (59). Patients are marked as photographed in Figure 11.15. The current NAC is marked accounting for the required concentric reduction. A 2 cm diameter circle is marked to indicate the new NAC position along the breast meridian at the mid-humeral level (Figure 11.15A). The 'melon slice' of ptotic breast is outlined, which can be conceptualised as a plane extending anteriorly from the IMF transecting the excess skin and breast tissue (Figure 11.15B).

Prior to skin incisions or de-epithelialisation liposuction fluid including adrenaline is infiltrated as outlined previously. Care should be taken to ensure no overly superficial liposuction is conducted to thin the future adipodermal flap. The marked skin of the NAC, the new NAC position, and the borders of the inferior melon are incised partially, to dermis (Figure 11.17A). The skin constituting the 'melon slice' surrounding the reduced NAC is then de-epithelialised (Figures 11.17B, 11.17C). The incision is deepened at the superior aspect of the 'melon slice' allowing the NAC to be raised on an inferior adipodermal pedicle at least 1 cm thick composing of the entire de-epithelialised portion (Figures 11.17D, 11.17E). The breast tissue and fat underlying the NAC can then be accessed and excised. A superior skin flap is raised evenly, permitting access to the superior breast tissue requiring excision (Figure 11.17F). The inferior adipodermal flap can then be inset underneath the superior skin flap, with the smaller NAC tunnelled through and fixed in its new position (Figure 11.17G). Skin is closed in a layered approach, leaving a periareolar scar as well as an inferior scar near the IMF (Figure 11.17H).

The Lalonde approach permits correction of Simon Grade 3 gynaecomastia; large breast tissue growth, excess skin, and significant clinical ptosis, whilst avoiding the vertical scars and upper pole fullness generated in traditional female breast reduction patterns. The inferior scar is hidden in the residual skin folds of the corrected IMF (Figure 11.18).

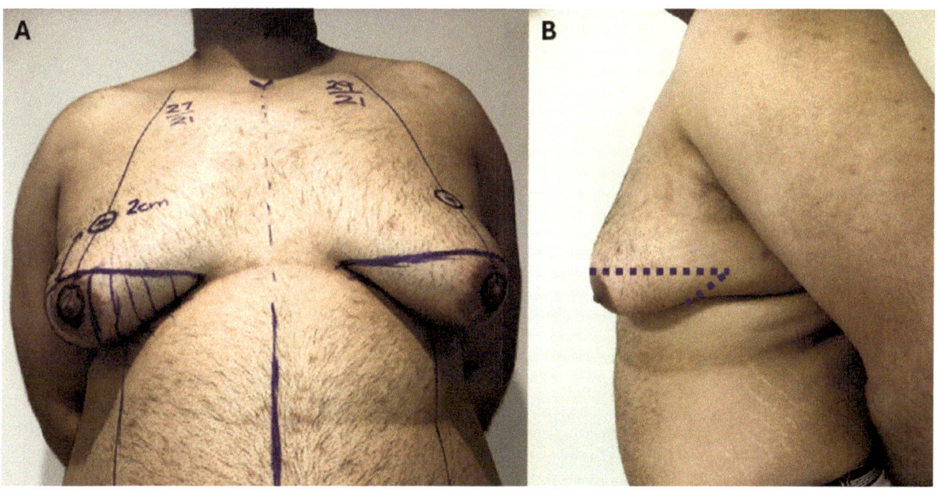

FIGURE 11.15
Lalonde-type male breast reduction skin markings. A: AP view of skin markings. The NAC is marked at a reduced diameter of 2–2.6 cm. The new NAC position is marked at 2 cm diameter along the breast meridian at the mid-humeral level. B: Lateral view of inferior 'melon slice' showing extension of IMF crease and imagined plane transecting ptotic breast tissue and excess skin.

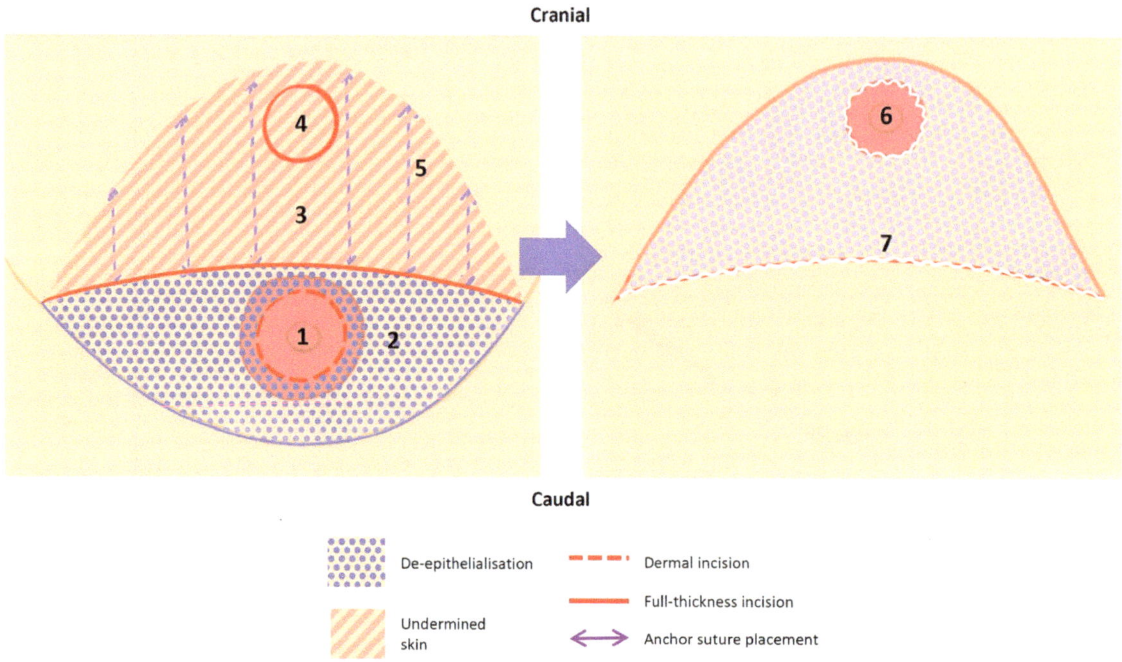

FIGURE 11.16
Lalonde-type male breast reduction. 1: The NAC is reduced to an appropriate diameter of 2–2.6 cm. 2: Inferior 'melon slice' is de-epithelialised. 3: Full-thickness incision made in superior aspect of 'melon slice' allowing excision of underlying breast tissue and undermining of superior skin. 4: Neo-areolar location incised at reduced NAC diameter. 5: Inferior 'melon slice' is hitched to chest wall underneath superior adipodermal flap. 6: Reduced NAC is secured to new location. 7: Inferior wound is closed in layered manner.

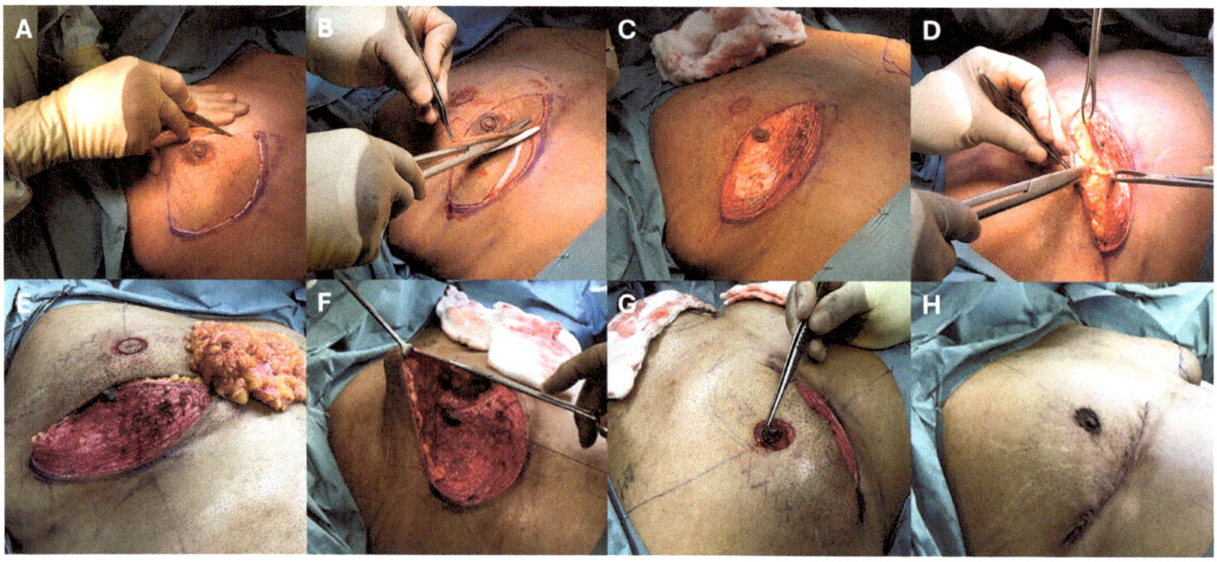

FIGURE 11.17
Lalonde-type male breast reduction: intra-operative sequence. A: Periareolar and 'melon slice' skin incisions are made. B–C: De-epithelialisation of melon portion of skin. D: Developing of inferior adipodermal flap from superior aspect by resection of underlying breast tissue. E: Completed resection of breast tissue with large volume of fat and breast tissue excised. The future position of the smaller neo-areola has been incised superiorly as previously marked. F: The inferior adipodermal flap is fixed (from dermis to pectoral fascia) beneath the superior skin flap. G: The NAC is tunnelled through the neo-areola incision and sutured in place. H: Completed skin closure.

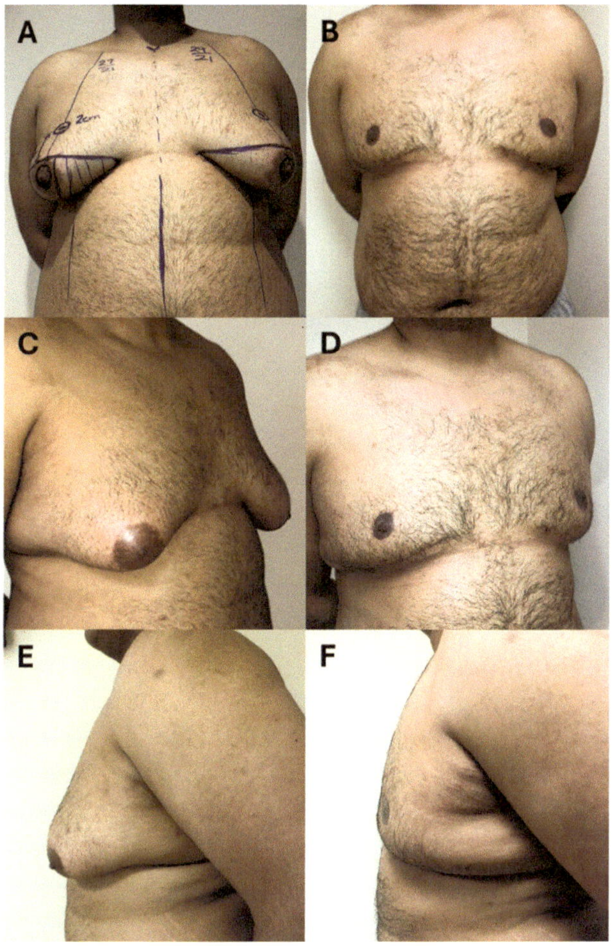

FIGURE 11.18
Pre- and post-operative photos of Lalonde-type male breast reduction. A, C, E: Pre-operative photos prior to Lalonde type breast reduction. This patient presented with Simon Grade 3 gynaecomastia with significant breast tissue growth, clinical ptosis, and skin excess.B, D, F: Post-operative photos following Lalonde type breast reduction, showing removal of breast tissue, reduction in areola size, correction of clinical ptosis and removal of excess skin, and superior transposition of the existing but reduced nipple-areola.

11.5 Conclusion

Approaching gynaecomastia management requires a comprehensive assessment including thorough clinical history and physical examination to determine any underlying aetiology, with relevant investigations and onward referral if indicated.

Surgical management of gynaecomastia is largely an aesthetic procedure and patients should be counselled effectively pre-operatively, gaining an appreciation for their chief concerns, to determine what they would deem an acceptable outcome and to ensure they are aware of the likely outcomes—especially scarring and potential contour deformities. Although severe cases of gynaecomastia mimic the female breast, they should be treated operatively, as a distinct and separate entity. Acceptable outcomes for contouring the female breast are often viewed very differently by male patients.

Based on our experience, we propose a unifying approach seeking to maximise the strengths of each treatment modality whilst minimising the drawbacks of each individual technique. We propose the following algorithmic approach to the management of gynaecomastia, which aims to achieving the best possible outcome in this highly demanding group of patients.

We promote liposuction as a starting point for all cases of gynaecomastia (Figure 11.19)—not only due to its ability to remove adipose tissue but also to facilitate subsequent open excision if required. It is technically easier to undertake prior to open excision. Ultrasound-assisted liposuction (UAL) is used in preference to conventional liposuction when available due to, improved clinical efficacy and superior post-operative skin contraction.

All patients undergoing liposuction for gynaecomastia should be routinely consented for open, peri-areolar excision in the event that liposuction leaves significant residual stromal tissue (Figure 11.19). This would be felt as a palpable lump beneath the areola on reassessment of breast consistency following liposuction, allowing a single-stage approach.

If skin excess or ptosis is apparent, it is preferentially addressed during the original operation. Choice of skin reduction technique is largely surgeon dependent; however, we favour a periareolar concentric reduction where possible (Figure 11.19). Larger volumes of skin excess may warrant more extensive approaches including LeJour or Lalonde pattern reductions.

Gynaecomastia presents a unique challenge in diagnosis and treatment, with detailed and thorough assessment to assist approach and operative planning. The patient's wishes must be upheld foremost when weighing up treatment options. We propose the follow algorithm an algorith for how this condition can be optimally managed to achieve robust outcomes and maximise patient satisfaction.

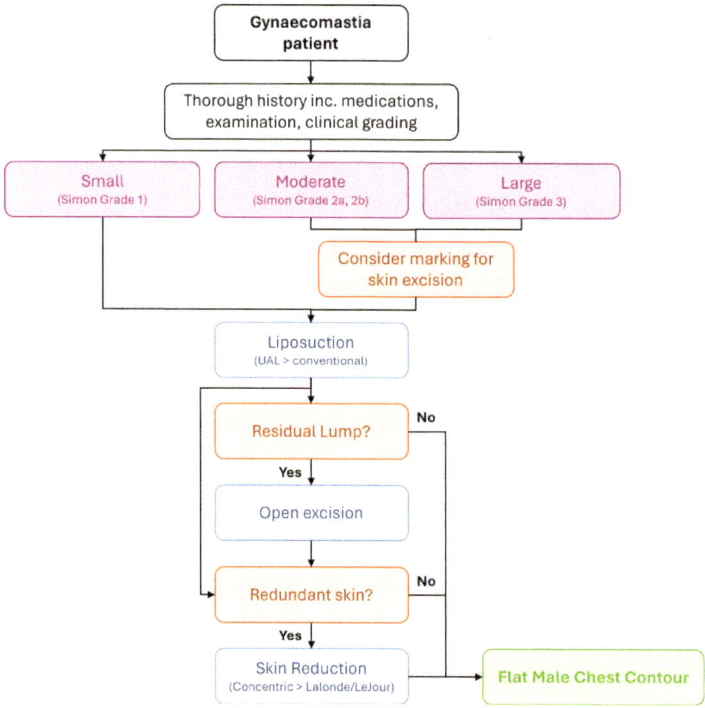

FIGURE 11.19
Proposed algorithmic approach to gynaecomastia.

Source: **Adapted from ref. 37.**

References

1. Niewoehner CB, Schorer AE. Gynaecomastia and breast cancer in men. BMJ. 2008;336(7646):709–13.
2. Thiruchelvam P, Walker JN, Rose K, Lewis J, Al-Mufti R. Gynaecomastia. BMJ. 2016;354:i4833.
3. Nuttall FQ. Gynecomastia as a physical finding in normal men. J Clin Endocrinol Metable. 1979;48(2):338–40.
4. Macias H, Hinck L. Mammary gland development. Wiley Interdiscip Rev Dev Biol. 2012;1(4):533–57.
5. Watson CJ, Khaled WT. Mammary development in the embryo and adult: new insights into the journey of morphogenesis and commitment. Development. 2020;147(22):dev169862.
6. Narula HS, Carlson HE. Gynaecomastia: pathophysiology, diagnosis and treatment. Nat Rev Endocrinol. 2014;10(11):684–98.
7. Thaler MA, Seifert-Klauss V, Luppa PB. The biomarker sex hormone-binding globulin: from established applications to emerging trends in clinical medicine. Best Pract Res Clin Endocrinol Metable. 2015;29(5):749–60.
8. Häggström M, Richfield D. Diagram of the pathways of human steroidogenesis. Wikiversity J Med. 2014;1(1).
9. Daniels J, Brickstock A, Charlton R. Gynaecomastia. BMJ. 2022;379:e069771.
10. Carto C, Loloi J, Campbell K, Ramasamy R. Testosterone therapy in men with Klinefelter syndrome: analysis of a global federated research network. Androg Clin Res Ther. 2022;3(1):208–12.
11. Brown PW, Terz JJ. Breast carcinoma associated with Klinefelter syndrome: a case report. J Surg Oncol. 1978;10(5):413–5.
12. Gikas P, Mokbel K. Management of gynaecomastia: an update. Int J Clin Pract. 2007;61(7):1209–15.
13. Felner EI, White PC. Prepubertal gynecomastia: indirect exposure to estrogen cream. Pediatrics. 2000;105(4):E55.
14. Biggar RJ. Molecular pathways: digoxin use and estrogen-sensitive cancers—risks and possible therapeutic implications. Clin Cancer Res. 2012;18(8):2133–7.
15. Forst T, Beyer J, Cordes U, et al. Gynaecomastia in a patient with a hCG producing giant cell carcinoma of the lung. Case report. Exp Clin Endocrinol Diabetes. 1995;103(1):28–32.
16. Lee PA. The occurrence of gynecomastia upon withdrawal of clomiphene citrate treatment for idiopathic oligospermia. Fertil Steril. 1980;34(3):285–6.
17. Pont A, Williams PL, Loose DS, et al. Ketoconazole blocks adrenal steroid synthesis. Ann Intern Med. 1982;97(3):370–2.
18. Fagan TC, Johnson DG, Grosso DS. Metronidazole-induced gynecomastia. JAMA. 1985;254(22):3217.
19. Overdiek JW, Merkus FW. Spironolactone metabolism and gynaecomastia. Lancet. 1986;1(8489):1103.
20. Saeter G, Fosså SD, Norman N. Gynaecomastia following cytotoxic therapy for testicular cancer. Br J Urol. 1987;59(4):348–52.
21. Carlin BI, Seftel AD, Resnick MI, Findlay J. Finasteride induced gynecomastia. J Urol. 1997;158(2):547.
22. Delle Fave GF, Tamburrano G, De Magistris L, et al. Gynaecomastia with cimetidine. Lancet. 1977;1(8025):1319.
23. Mahler C, Denis L. Clinical profile of a new non-steroidal antiandrogen. J Steroid Biochem Mol Biol. 1990;37(6):921–4.
24. Rivera JL, Lal S, Ettigi P, et al. Effect of acute and chronic neuroleptic therapy on serum prolactin levels in men and women of different age groups. Clin Endocrinol (Oxf). 1976;5(3):273–82.
25. Deepinder F, Braunstein GD. Drug-induced gynecomastia: an evidence-based review. Expert Opin Drug Saf. 2012;11(5):779–95.
26. García Rodríguez LA, Jick H. Risk of gynaecomastia associated with cimetidine, omeprazole, and other antiulcer drugs. BMJ. 1994;308(6927):503–6.

27. Trost L, Saitz TR, Hellstrom WJ. Side effects of 5-alpha reductase inhibitors: a comprehensive review. Sex Med Rev. 2013;1:24–41.
28. Eckman A, Dobs A. Drug-induced gynecomastia. Expert Opin Drug Saf. 2008;6:691–702.
29. Njuguna C, Swart A, Blockman M, et al. Cases of antiretroviral-associated gynaecomastia reported to the National HIV & Tuberculosis Health Care Worker Hotline in South Africa. AIDS Res Ther. 2016;13:40.
30. Derkacz M, Chmiel-Perzyńska I, Nowakowski A. Gynecomastia: a difficult diagnostic problem. Endokrynol Pol. 2011;62(2):190–202.
31. Association of Breast Surgery Summary Statement. Investigation and Management of Gynaecomastia in Primary & Secondary Care. [Internet] 2019. https://associationofbreastsurgery.org.uk/media/65097/abs-summary-statement-gynaecomastia-2019.pdf.
32. Cheng L, Albers P, Berney DM, et al. Testicular cancer. Nat Rev Dis Primers. 2018;4(1):29.
33. Moir CR, Johnson CH. Poland's syndrome. Semin Pediatr Surg. 2008;17(3):161–6.
34. Baumann K. Gynecomastia: conservative and surgical management. Breast Care (Basel). 2018;13(6):419–24.
35. Simon BE, Hoffman S, Kahn S. Classification and surgical correction of gynecomastia. Plast Reconstr Surg. 1973;51(1):48–52.
36. Rohrich RJ, Ha RY, Kenkel JM, Adams WP Jr. Classification and management of gynecomastia: defining the role of ultrasound-assisted liposuction. Plast Reconstr Surg. 2003;111(2):909–23; discussion 924–5.
37. Fruhstorfer BH, Malata CM. A systematic approach to the surgical treatment of gynaecomastia. Br J Plast Surg. 2003;56(3):237–46.
38. Mauras N, Bishop K, Merinbaum D, et al. Pharmacokinetics and pharmacodynamics of anastrozole in pubertal boys with recent-onset gynecomastia. J Clin Endocrinol Me table. 2009;94(8):2975–8.
39. Wheeler KM, Sharma D, Kavoussi PK, et al. Clomiphene citrate for the treatment of hypogonadism. Sex Med Rev. 2019;7(2):272–6.
40. Jones DJ, Holt SD, Surtees P, et al. A comparison of danazol and placebo in the treatment of adult idiopathic gynaecomastia: results of a prospective study in 55 patients. Ann R Coll Surg Engl. 1990;72(5):296–8.
41. Kuhn JM, Roca R, Laudat MH, et al. Studies on the treatment of idiopathic gynaecomastia with percutaneous dihydrotestosterone. Clin Endocrinol (Oxf). 1983;19(4):513–20.
42. Perdonà S, Autorino R, De Placido S, et al. Efficacy of tamoxifen and radiotherapy for prevention and treatment of gynaecomastia and breast pain caused by bicalutamide in prostate cancer: a randomised controlled trial. Lancet Oncol. 2005;6(5):295–300.
43. Zachmann M, Eiholzer U, Muritano M, et al. Treatment of pubertal gynaecomastia with testolactone. Acta Endocrinol Suppl (Copenh). 1986;279:218–26.
44. Berger O, Landau Z, Talisman R. Gynecomastia: a systematic review of pharmacological treatments. Front Pediatr. 2022;10:978311.
45. British National Formulary. Tamoxifen. 2024. Accessed February 2024. Available at: https://bnf.nice.org.uk/drugs/tamoxifen/#:~:text=Initially%2020%20mg%20daily%20on,of%20cycle%20if%20menstruation%20occurs.
46. Tunio MA, Al-Asiri M, Al-Amro A, et al. Optimal prophylactic and definitive therapy for bicalutamide-induced gynecomastia: results of a meta-analysis. Curr Oncol. 2012;19(4):e 280–8.
47. Safran T, Abi-Rafeh J, Alabdulkarim A, et al. Radiotherapy for prevention or management of gynecomastia recurrence: future role for general gynecomastia patients in plastic surgery given current role in management of high-risk prostate cancer patients on anti-androgenic therapy. J Plast Reconstr Aesthet Surg. 2021;74(11):3128–40.
48. Kim CS, Algan O. Radiation Therapy for Early-Stage Breast Cancer. In: StatPearls [Internet]. StatPearls Publishing, Treasure Island, FL, 2023. Available at: https://www.ncbi.nlm.nih.gov/books/NBK459174/.
49. King C, Moir G, Laing H, et al. Information for commissioners of plasticsurgeryservices.[Internet]2006.Availableat:https://www.bapras.org.uk/docs/default-source/commissioning-and-policy/information-for-commissioners-of-plastic-surgery-services.pdf?sfvrsn=ba572cc3_2.
50. Petty PM, Solomon M, Buchel EW, Tran NV. Gynecomastia: evolving paradigm of management and comparison of techniques. Plast Reconstr Surg. 2010;125(5):1301–8.
51. Adekunle A, Malata CM. Gynecomastia: evolving paradigm of management and comparison of techniques. Plast Reconstr Surg. 2012;129(2):366e–7e.
52. Teimourian B, Perlman R. Surgery for gynecomastia. Aesthetic Plast Surg. 1983;7(3):155–7.
53. Rohrich RJ, Beran SJ, Kenkel JM, et al. Extending the role of liposuction in body contouring with ultrasound-assisted liposuction. Plast Reconstr Surg. 1998;101(4):1090–102; discussion 1117–9.
54. Hodgson EL, Fruhstorfer BH, Malata CM. Ultrasonic liposuction in the treatment of gynecomastia. Plast Reconstr Surg. 2005;116(2):646–53; discussion 654–5.
55. Ruff PG 4th, Garcia O Jr, Nykiel MJ, Galanis CJ. Consensus-based recommendations for vibration amplification of sound energy at resonance ultrasound-assisted liposuction. Plast Reconstr Surg Glob Open. 2023;11(7):e5110.
56. Morselli PG. "Pull-through": a new technique for breast reduction in gynecomastia. Plast Reconstr Surg. 1996;97(2):450–4.
57. Belza CC, Blum JD, Neubauer D, et al. A retrospective review of arthroscopic shaver utilization in adolescent gynecomastia. Plast Reconstr Surg Glob Open. 2023;11(10):e5336.
58. Iwuagwu O, Drew P. Vacuum-assisted biopsy device-diagnostic and therapeutic applications in breast surgery. Breast. 2004;13(6):483–7.
59. Webster, JP. Mastectomy for gynecomastia through a semicircular intra-areolar incision. Ann Surg. 1946;124:557–75.
60. Malata CM, Wong KY. Gynaecomastia surgery. In: Nahabedian MY, Neligan P, eds, Neligan's Plastic Surgery, 4th edition. Volume 5m Breast. Elsevier, London, 2018:174–95.
61. Malata CM, Coulson SG. Male breast reduction: liposuction versus excision. In: Gabriel N, Storm-Dickerson, eds, Spear's Surgery of the Breast: Principles and Art, 4th edition. Lippincott Williams & Wilkins, Philadelphia, 2020. 43:416–40.
62. Kazzazi F, Malata CM. Application of the Lalonde (horizontal-only scar) breast reduction technique for correction of gynaecomastia in dark skinned patients. Gland Surg. 2019;8(3):287–93.
63. Maas M, Howell AC, Gould DJ, Ray EC. The ideal male nipple-areola complex: a critical review of the literature and discussion of surgical techniques for female-to-male gender-confirming surgery. Ann Plast Surg. 2020;84(3):334–40.
64. Wray RC Jr, Hoopes JE, Davis GM. Correction of extreme gynaecomastia. Br J Plast Surg. 1974;27(1):39–41.

12

Advising the Breast Cancer Patient

Environmental Risk, Familial and Genetic Risk, Risk-Reducing Strategies, Risk Assessment Tools, Pregnancy, and Fertility

Victoria Harmer and Susanne Cruickshank

Breast cancer evokes a wide range of reactions and is not just a physical disease but also one which impacts on the psychological, emotional, and social needs of an individual.[1,2] Both a cancer diagnosis and the treatment process can change self-esteem, perception of the body, quality of life, daily life activities, sexual life, personal and social roles, family members, and the environment of the patient.

Maguire and colleagues[3] were the first to identify the specific emotional and psychological needs of women after a breast cancer diagnosis, and the importance of providing both psychological as well as physical care to aid recovery. This work laid the foundation for the unique role of the breast care nurse. Today, breast care nurses or clinical breast cancer nurse specialists are integral members of the multidisciplinary team supporting patients navigating through the different modalities of their treatment trajectory.[1]

Some understanding of the wider impact of a breast cancer diagnosis is necessary to have meaningful conversations about risk reducing strategies. Although survival remains a key metric of overall cancer control, increasingly clinicians are balancing the risk of breast cancer recurring and risk of persistent and debilitating toxicities. Risks associated with a cancer recurring are often difficult to quantify or indeed explain as 'a risk is something that might happen in the future' and the prediction of risk in breast cancer is not an exact science. Add in human factors, external and internal influences (Figure 12.1), and this becomes a complex interaction that requires skills from a range of professionals including doctors, nurses, allied health professionals, psychologists, and counsellors.

Despite significant reductions in breast cancer mortality, more than half of women treated for breast cancer live with an ongoing fear that their disease will recur[4,5] and for which many seek help from health professionals, family and friends, and the third sector. It is described internationally as 'Fear, worry, concern that the cancer may recur or progress'.[6] Internal influences, for example, previous mental health issues, chronic illness, health literacy, relationships, and external influences, such as media and charity communications, may impact a person's ability to absorb information.

What this means clinically is that telling someone their outcome is good and sharing up to date evidence to support your argument may not necessarily reassure them, reduce anxiety, or indeed change their perception of their personal risk. In an era of personalised medicine[7] we should not lose sight of the emotional toll that cancer can have on an individual and how this may impact on their reactions and behaviour.[8] Careful use of language at every patient/health professional interaction is vital (see Box 12. 1).

DOI: 10.1201/9781003394785-12

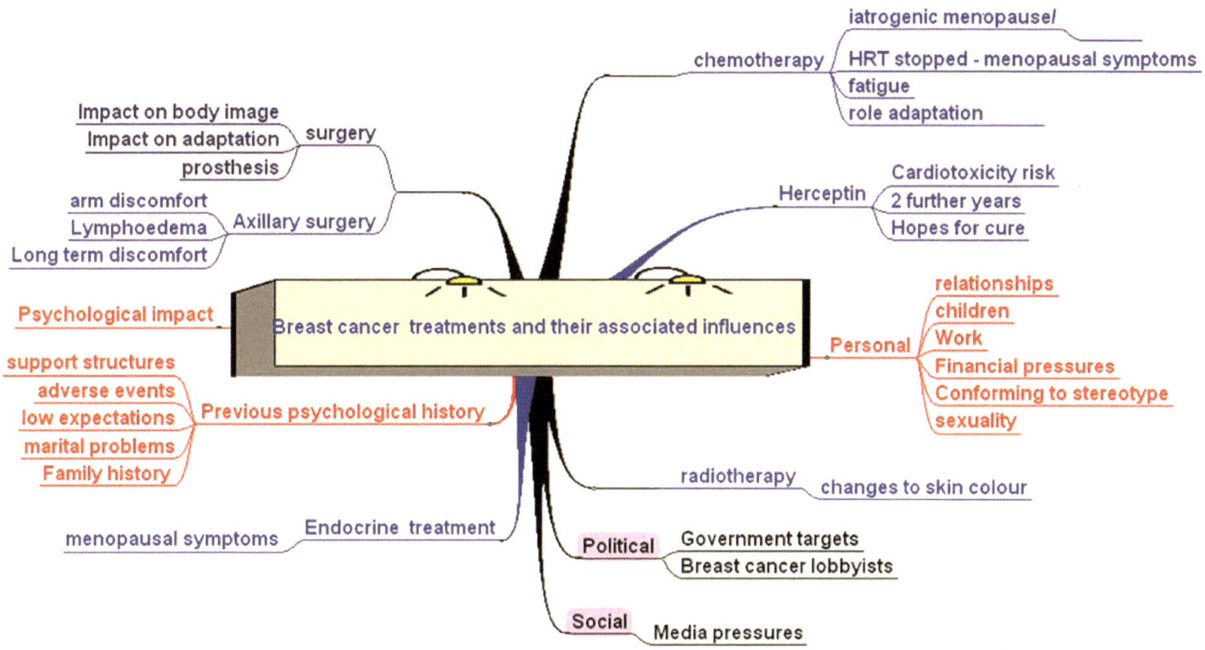

FIGURE 12.1
Mind map of breast cancer.

Source: **Courtesy of Susanne Cruickshank.**

BOX 12.1 SUMMARY OF RECOMMENDATIONS FOR RISK COMMUNICATION TO PATIENTS (SEE FURTHER REF. 9).

1. Use plain language to make written and verbal materials more understandable
2. Present data using absolute risks
3. Present information in pictographs if you are going to include graphs
4. Present data using frequencies
5. Use an incremental risk format to highlight how treatment changes risks from preexisting baseline levels
6. Be aware that the order in which risks and benefits are presented can affect risk perceptions
7. Consider using summary tables that include all of the risks and benefits for each treatment option
8. Recognise that comparative risk information (e.g. What the average person's risk is) is persuasive and not just informative
9. Consider presenting only the information that is most critical to the patients' decision making, even at the expense of completeness
10. Repeatedly draw patients' attention to the time interval over which a risk occurs

In younger women under 50 years old the impact of a diagnosis can be an extreme shock.[2] Three trajectories have been highlighted that impact on psychological response in this age group: clinical psychological risks, feminine-specific concerns (i.e. sexuality, body image, fertility/pregnancy), and resources between individual and relational aspects. Together they reflect the complexity of the impact on this younger group of women.

12.1 Communication

Communication is key; from a cancer patient's perspective, communication can be the most important aspect of care, in part because of its capacity to exacerbate or allay the fear that accompanies the disease. Communication also allows more informed consent and decision-making regarding information related

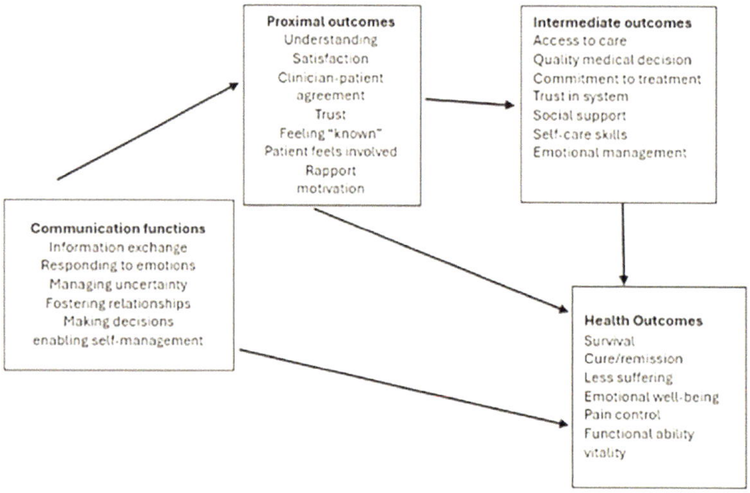

FIGURE 12.2
Relationships between communication and outcomes.

Source: **Ref. 10, with permission.**

to treatment and has implications on a patient's adherence to treatment regimens.

Communication encompasses three areas of activity:

1. Cognitive—giving and receiving information
2. Emotional—the feeling and expression of psychological response
3. Spiritual—the expression of feelings and thoughts in relation to existential issues beyond the self

The entire multi-professional team is responsible for communicating with people affected by breast cancer and understanding each other's role in a team can improve the consistency and quality of information people receive.

When a patient is diagnosed with breast cancer, there are many challenges. These include:

- Managing difficult emotions, such as shock, fear, anger
- Navigating logistical challenges, such as work, finance, and medical appointments
- Keeping up to date with monitoring tests
- Having productive clinical appointments
- Building a medicine management routine
- Learning about the cancer, treatment, prognosis, and potential adverse effects of treatment
- Deciding who and what to tell friends, family, and colleagues and how to ask for help

All these can interfere with a patient's ability to understand information delivered by the healthcare team, and thus bring unwanted confusion and misunderstanding. It is vital that healthcare professionals assess the patient at every opportunity regarding their understanding of the next step of care and that support services are dovetailed to bolster the patient and combat any unmet need they may have.

Cancer treatments and outcomes are complex and require different communication strategies depending on the interaction. Figure 12.2 illustrates some important functions of communication and their pathways to improved health-related outcomes.[10]

12.2 Definitions of Risk Communication and Risk Perception

Risk communication can be defined as an 'interactive process of exchange of information and opinion among individuals, groups, and institutions. It involves multiple messages about the nature of risks or about the legal and institutional arrangements for risk management'.[9]

Risk perception should be considered in association with risk-reducing behaviour or as an outcome of risk communication; it is also a key contributing factor of health behaviour models. Perception of risk is a multifaceted concept, comprising the potential degree of harm attributable to an event (in this case, reducing risk post breast cancer diagnosis of a recurrence), on its controllability, on the number of people simultaneously exposed, on the familiarity of consequences and effects and on the degree of subjective control over the risk. Risk perception is also dependent on the individual's defensive responses to health communication. Heightening risk perception without adequately addressing specific concerns or maximising their ability to self-manage their risk reduction may increase distress and induce behavioural inaction.

12.3 Effective Risk Communication

Knowledge is empowering for people and can promote a person's sense of control over their life including decisions relating to their lifestyle, family environment, and self-management of their disease. Imparting knowledge requires an individual to have reasonably good levels of health literacy. Health literacy is described as a 'set of knowledge and skills that enables individuals to obtain, communicate, process and understand information, and services to make appropriate health decisions and to successfully navigate the health care system'. Cancer literacy presents a unique set of challenges compared to other conditions/diseases because there are several time critical decisions to be made by both the patient and clinicians.[11]

Coughlin[12] reported that up to 16% of cancer survivors had low levels of health literacy, with the prevalence higher among Hispanic and Black patients, and those with poor health status, low income, and poor levels of educational attainment. Indeed, in the USA, it is suggested that this figure may be as high as 27%. Practitioners caring for people with breast cancer must consider a person's health literacy when endeavouring to optimise cancer education.

12.4 Supportive Care

Nurses can do much to alleviate a patient's fears and anxieties and help render the experience at diagnosis, during treatment, and post treatment more tolerable. Nowadays we use the term 'supportive care', which arose from the medical oncology literature when managing toxicities of cancer-related treatment. It is not unidimensional, but rather multidimensional, and encompasses all symptoms experienced from the perspective of the patient.[13]

There is growing evidence that using Patient Reported Outcome Measures (PROMS), and Patient Reported Experience Measures (PREMS) enables better patient centred care, enhances patient-provider satisfaction, and improves monitoring of treatment response.[14] Basch et al.[14] reported improved survival in the group of patients with advanced cancer who used PROMs to report their symptoms to health professionals and the information was acted upon. There are several systematic reviews that report the effectiveness of implementing PROMs into routine cancer practice[15–17] the use of PROMs to assess the effectiveness of interventions in specific patient groups,[18,19] and the barriers and facilitators to enable successful implementation of PROMs in routine cancer care.[20–22] Van Egdom et al.[18] reported that PROMs provide a positive impact on patients (e.g. symptom distress, quality of life, and satisfaction) and outcomes for providers (clinical decision-making, symptom management) and care processes/systems (referrals, hospital visits). These studies add to our understanding of using PROMs in routine clinical care, but they frequently allude to a lack of inclusion from under-served groups and/or diversity in populations.

There are several PROMS used specifically in clinical practice by nurses. One of these is the Concerns Checklist, which was introduced as part of a recovery package[23] and is a series of key interventions, which, when delivered together, can improve outcomes for people living with and beyond cancer. It specifically focuses on holistic needs assessment[24] and tailoring support packages to address the needs reported by the person with cancer. As numbers increase and resources are stretched, this approach enables nurses to focus on what is important to the patient rather than important to the service. It identifies those who need help and those who can self-manage effectively.

12.5 Fear of Recurrence, Anxiety, and Depression

Earlier diagnosis and improved targeting of treatments have led to improved survival outcomes. A consequence of this is an increasing number of people living with not only the short, medium, and late physical side effects of treatment but also fears that their cancer will recur, described as fear of cancer recurrence (FCR). Some level of FCR is normal and reflects the reality that cancers do recur in subtypes of breast cancer at 1, 5, and 10 years plus. However, what is apparent is that 50% of survivors experience moderate to high levels of FCR.[25]

Fear, worry, and concern about the cancer returning is not only cited widely within the literature as a principal cause of distress for people recovering from cancer treatment, but is witnessed daily in clinical consultations with cancer patients. A certain degree of worry and sadness is to be expected but healthcare workers should be alert to signs of disabling anxiety (somatic stress symptoms, lack of concentration, feelings of panic) or depression (a 'flat' mood, an exaggerated feeling of guilt and self-blame, suicidal ideation). If these are noted, refer the patient to a psychologist or psychiatrist. A course of anxiolytic and antidepressant medication and various forms of psychological therapy may be required before other forms of counselling therapy can be effective.

Several psychological interventions have predominantly been developed for severe or disabling FCR in breast and colorectal cancer patients. The majority focus on cognitive behavioural approaches, with studies demonstrating these are effective and can prevent escalation of mild-moderate FCR to debilitating FCR. Tools such as the 'mini-AFTERc' have been shown to be an efficient 'minimal intervention'.[26,27] Some of the new approaches refer to a stepped care approach, intervening early to reduce the long-term sequalae.[28,29]

These 30-minute telephone interventions can be delivered by specialist nurses and would be applicable to multiple tumour types. Addressing and reducing FCR with a short, low-resource intensity tool would be an important strategy for personalising and optimising care for cancer survivors. This chimes with a priority highlighted within the NHS Long-Term Plan and the Living With and Beyond Cancer work that has received attention in recent years.[30]

12.6 Motivational Interviewing

There may be several interactions with breast cancer survivors whereby the outcome may require a change in behaviour of that person.

Motivational interviewing (MI) is a counselling approach initially described when attempting to support behaviour change in problem drinking.[31] Subsequently the concepts of MI and associated approaches were further expanded upon by Rollnick and Miller.[32] Because of positive results from alcohol addiction, use of MI was extended to include substance abuse[20] and smoking.[33] It is nowadays employed extensively across different fields of medicine, including diabetes, cancer, rheumatological conditions and obesity. MI focuses on various objectives, such as increasing medication adherence,[34] self-efficacy, physical activity, and reducing depressive symptoms, emotional distress, blood pressure, HbA1c levels, chronic pain, etc. These expanded applications of MI have generally had positive effects.[35–40]

MI encompasses a method of communication where individuals are *guided* to express their thoughts and feelings through *following* (good listening) and *directing* (giving information and advice). The key aim of MI is to *empower* people to change by prompting them to discover the meaning, importance, and capacity for change themselves. MI is characterised by a respectful, non-judgemental, and curious way of interacting with people that facilitates the natural process of change and ensures a person's autonomy.

The process of exchange of information and ultimately behaviour change requires patience and ensuring that the person is ready to change. The skills which are implemented to achieve this are encapsulated in the abbreviation OARS (see Figure 12.3 and Table 12.1).

Open questions are questions that cannot be answered with a simple yes or no; rather, they encourage the client to provide more information about what they are being asked. The aim is to draw out and explore the person's experiences, perspectives, and ideas through reflection on how change may be meaningful or possible along with an exploration of possibilities and options.

Affirmations are important to support the person in reinforcing their hope and confidence in their ability to change. The practitioner here will acknowledge and praise the person's strengths, efforts, and past successes.

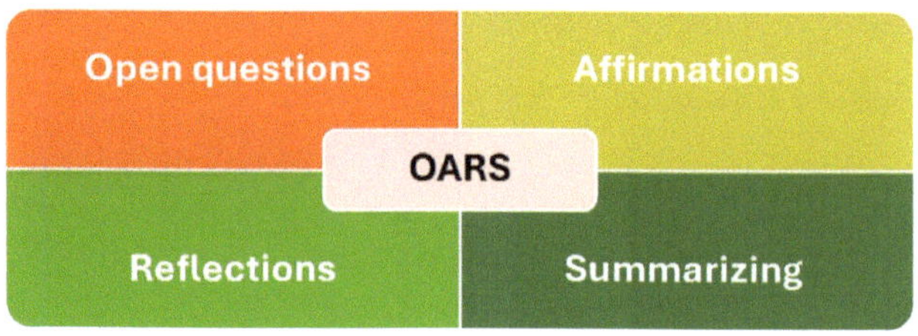

FIGURE 12.3
OARS skills.

Source: **See further ref. 32.**

TABLE 12.1

Examples of OARS

Skill	Examples
Open-ended questions	*How are you feeling today?* *How have you been getting on with the treatment?* *What do you want to do next?*
Affirmations	*You have had a very challenging time recently, but you have shown tremendous strength coping with everything.* *If I were in your shoes, I don't know if I could have managed nearly so well.* *That is an excellent suggestion.*
Reflections	*So, you mentioned that. . .* *It sounds like you. . .* *You're wondering if. . .*
Summarising	*Let me see if I understand so far. . .* *Here is what I have heard. Tell me if I have missed anything.* *To sum up. . .*

Reflections refer to repeating, rephrasing, or offering a deeper guess about what the person is trying to communicate. Reflections rely on careful listening and trying to understand what the person is saying which is an important in expressing empathy.

Summarising what has been discussed between patient and clinician ensures that both are aligned, while reinforcing key points made by the patient.

12.7 Cancer Survivorship

As treatments become more successful and mortality rates for cancers fall, an increasing number of people living in the community have completed cancer treatment; this group, along with those living with manifestations of cancer, are often referred to as 'cancer survivors'. Many cancer survivors experience long-term side effects from previous treatment or from the cancer itself and have to overcome a number of psychological and medical issues.[41] In recent years, interest and expert resource has shifted towards supporting the process of a patient returning to normal or a new normal (normalisation).[42] It is therefore important that healthcare professionals sharpen the tools of treatment and more accurately assess individual patient risk and associated benefits of treatment for that patient.

12.8 Risk Prognostic and Prediction Tools

Several tools have been developed with the aim of personalising treatments according to subtype of breast cancer. This tool can potentially save patients from unpleasant and lasting adverse effects of treatment (namely, chemotherapy) that may not have had much effect on reducing their chance of breast cancer recurrence. Either computer prognostication models can be used or a sample of breast cancer tissue can be analysed in a multigene assay. Benefits of these tools are information regarding the likelihood of benefit from a treatment with calculation of absolute benefit. This information can better arm healthcare professionals and steer the conversation and shared decision-making with patients that relates to the relative risks versus benefits of adjuvant treatment.[43]

12.9 PREDICT

The *PREDICT* breast cancer prognostication and treatment benefit prediction model (v1) was developed in 2010 using data from the UK East Anglia Cancer Registration and Information Centre (ECRIC) for model fitting and data from the West Midlands Cancer Intelligence Unit for model validation. It has since been refitted using a national data set of patients diagnosed from 2000 to 2017 with the aim of refining the hazard ratio estimates for the variables in the current model and to estimate the effect of the year of diagnosis on prognosis to be able to recalibrate the model for contemporary patients.[44] The authors believe this will provide a more accurate absolute treatment benefit prediction for individual patients.

In clinical settings, the tool is primarily designed to help patients and clinicians see how different treatments for early invasive breast cancer might improve survival rates after surgery. It only asks for certain information about the cancer, questions such as size of breast cancer, HER2 status, ER status, etc. This information enables the online tool to predict survival rates. It does not differentiate between the types of surgery (for example, mastectomy or breast-conserving surgery) nor does it ask for lifestyle factors such as smoking or exercise.

12.10 Endopredict (Myriad Genetics)[43]

The EndoPredict is a CE marked assay designed to predict the likelihood of distant recurrence within 10 years of primary diagnosis and benefit of chemotherapy. It is intended for use in both pre-and post-menopausal patients with early breast cancer that are:

- ER-positive
- HER2-negative
- Lymph-node-negative or lymph-node-positive (up to 3 positive nodes)

This test measures 12 genes: 3 proliferation-associated genes, 5 hormone receptor-associated genes, 3 reference (normalisation) genes, and 1 control gene. Together this information produces a 12-gene molecular score (EP score).

- Below 3.3 indicates low risk of distant recurrence in next 10 years (less than 10%), less benefit from chemotherapy
- 3.3 or higher indicates high risk

12.11 MammaPrint (Agendia)[43]

MammaPrint is a CE-marked microarray designed to predict the likelihood of distant recurrence within 10 years of primary diagnosis and predict the benefit of chemotherapy. Test is intended for pre- and post-menopausal women with primary stage 1 or 2, or operable stage 3 cancer, with the following features:

- ER- or PR-positive
- HER2-negative
- Tumour less than or equal to 5 cm
- Lymph node-negative or lymph node-positive (up to 3 positive nodes)

The test measures the expression of 70 cancer-related genes and 465 control genes. Together this information calculates a MammaPrint result on a scale –1 to +1

- A result of 0 or below indicates high risk of metastases in 10 years
- Above 0 indicates low risk (10% or less) of metastases at 10 years
- Above 0.355 indicates ultra-low risk (more than 99% breast cancer-specific survival at 8 years and 97% at 20 years with 2 to 5 years of tamoxifen treatment)

12.12 Oncotype DX (Exact Science)[43]

The Oncotype DX is a CE-marked assay to quantify 9-year risk of distance recurrence and identify those patients who will derive benefit from chemotherapy. It also reports tumour biology: ER, PR, and HER2 status. It is intended for pre-or post-menopausal people with early breast cancer that is:

- ER- or PR-positive
- HER2-negative
- Lymph-node-negative or lymph-node-positive (up to 3 positive nodes)

The test quantifies the expression of 21 genes. Sixteen are cancer-related correlated with distant recurrence-free survival and 5 reference genes. Together this information calculates the Oncotype DX Breast Recurrence Score (RS) of between 0 and 100.

- RS up to 13 predicts 2.3% chemotherapy benefit at 5 years.
- RS between 14 and 25 predicts 2.9% chemotherapy benefit at 5 years.
- For post-menopausal women with LN-positive cancer, the instructions for use state that an RS of up to 25 predicts no apparent chemotherapy benefit (less than 1%) at 5 years. In both groups, the instructions for use state that guidelines recommend chemotherapy in addition to hormone therapy for people with an RS between 26 and 100

12.13 Prosigna (Veracyte)[43]

Prosigna is CE-marked assay designed to provide information on breast cancer subtype and to predict distant recurrence-free survival at 10 years. It is intended for post-menopausal women with early breast cancer that is:

- ER- or PR-positive
- HER2- negative
- Lymph-node-negative or lymph-node-positive (up to 3 positive nodes)

The test measures the expression of 50 genes (PAM50) used for intrinsic subtype classification, 8 housekeeping genes used for signal normalisation, 6 positive controls, and 8 negative controls. Prosigna classifies the risk of recurrence within 10 years after 5 years of endocrine therapy, based on PAM50 gene signature, breast cancer subtype, tumour size, nodal status, and proliferation score.

Together the information gives an overall risk of recurrence score between 0 and 100. For LN-positive cancer (up to 3 positive nodes):

- 0–15: low risk
- 16–40: intermediate risk
- 41–100: high risk
- 4 positive nodes or more, any score assigned high risk

These tumour profiling tests can be used as part of a shared decision-making process. As anxiety can be increased using these tests, some people may benefit from additional support or counselling to help manage this anxiety—indeed, ongoing fears of the cancer returning can impede recovery post-treatment.

12.14 Pregnancy and Infertility

Breast cancer is one of the most prevalent cancers affecting women worldwide. Its relationship with reproductive factors, particularly pregnancy and infertility, has been a subject of extensive research. Numerous studies have demonstrated that pregnancy can have a protective effect against breast cancer. Full-term pregnancy, especially at a younger age, has been associated with a reduced lifetime risk of breast cancer. Breastfeeding also has a protective effect against breast cancer and is not only associated with the number of times a woman breastfeeds but also the duration of breastfeeding.

12.15 Pregnancy-Associated Breast Cancer

Pregnancy does not appear to influence the prognosis of pregnancy-associated breast cancer, but the diagnosis may be more difficult due to breast changes during pregnancy that can make imaging more difficult to interpret. These women should always be referred to a specialised breast centre and undergo triple assessment; clinical examination, imaging, and a biopsy if a lump is present. Ultrasound is a valuable diagnostic tool and mammography is not undertaken in pregnant women. Each case should be discussed within the breast multidisciplinary team, the obstetric team, and family doctor.

Surgery can be offered to a woman during any trimester of pregnancy. When breast-conserving surgery is offered, it needs to be close to the delivery date so as not to delay adjuvant radiation treatment. When surgery is conducted earlier on in the pregnancy and delay to radiotherapy deemed excessive, a mastectomy may be recommended. Any breast reconstruction should be delayed until after completion of pregnancy, to avoid exposure of the foetus posed to a prolonged anaesthetic.

Chemotherapy is not recommended at all in the first trimester of pregnancy due to the increased risk to the foetus in terms of organogenesis, but can be safely delivered from the second trimester onwards without serious adverse effects upon the foetus. Neoadjuvant chemotherapy may be offered, to allow downsizing of a breast cancer during pregnancy, with the aim of performing less extensive surgery—to either the breast or axilla.

Endocrine therapies are not recommended during pregnancy, nor are targeted treatments such as trastuzumab. Most women who have treatment for breast cancer during pregnancy continue to full-term and deliver normally. There may be a lasting inability to feed from the ipsilateral breast due to major ducts being excised at the time of surgery and breastfeeding during chemotherapy should be avoided.[45]

12.16 Infertility and Breast Cancer

Adjuvant modalities of treatment for breast cancer can cause both temporary and often irreversible damage to ovarian function, and breast cancer patients have a 3% chance of pregnancy post treatment: equating to 40% lower than the general population.[46]

There are also issues regarding childbearing for those with a BRCA1 and BRCA2 gene mutation, along with a general recommendation that women wait at least two years following treatment for breast cancer before attempting to conceive. This latter point is based on a relatively high likelihood of recurrence occurring within this time frame.[45] Fertility preservation prior to starting any treatment may provide women with the opportunity of having children in the future despite any infertility issues that may arise from treatment of breast cancer.

To overcome the effects of treatment-induced infertility, women can choose to bank oocytes or embryos after medically managed ovarian stimulation.

Many younger female patients fail to understand the role of fertility preservation prior to commencing treatment. This has been shown to affect their level of decision-making conflict and decision regret, future sexual relationships; thus, it is a vital area for healthcare professionals to address with patients being supported and referred on for fertility treatment to potentially enrich their quality of life in the longer term.[47,48] Multidisciplinary team working can streamline scheduling of treatments if fertility preservation is sought.

12.17 Clinical Implications

The relationships between pregnancy, infertility, and breast cancer risk are complex multifaceted and have clinical implications. While pregnancy (and breastfeeding) confers long-term protection against breast cancer, the timing of pregnancies and the use of fertility treatments can modulate this effect.

Healthcare providers should consider reproductive history, including timing of pregnancy, when assessing an individual's breast cancer risk. Women of childbearing age undergoing treatment for breast cancer should be offered comprehensive information on treatment-related fertility effects, with appropriate access to fertility specialists and counselling. These younger patients should also be informed of the importance of remaining breast aware, reporting any persistent changes or aberrations to the norm and attending any regular cancer screening invitations.

As our understanding of these complex interactions improves, healthcare providers will be better equipped to offer personalised risk assessments and management strategies to women concerned about breast cancer risk, as well as those undergoing treatment for breast cancer in the context of their reproductive health.

References

1. Brown T, et al. Specialist breast care nurses for support of women with breast cancer. Cochrane Database Syst Rev. 2021;2:CD005634.
2. Martino ML, et al. A review of psychological impact of breast cancer in women below 50 years old. Health Care Women Int. 2021;42:7–9, 1066–85.
3. Maguire GP, et al. Psychiatric problems in the first year after mastectomy. Br Med J. 1978;1(6618):963–5.
4. Humphris G, Ozakinci G. The AFTER intervention: a structured psychological approach to reduce fears of recurrence in patients with head and neck cancer. Br J Health Psychol. 2008;13:223–30.
5. Mutsaers B, et al. Identifying the key characteristics of clinical fear of cancer recurrence: an international Delphi study. Psycho-oncology. 2020;29(2):430–6.
6. Lebel S, et al. From normal response to clinical problem: definition and clinical features of fear of cancer recurrence. Support Care Cancer. 2016;24:3265–8.
7. Thewes B, et al. Fear of cancer recurrence in an era of personalized medicine. J Clin Oncol. 2017;35:3275–8.
8. Séguin Leclair C, et al. The relationship between fear of cancer recurrence and health behaviors: a nationwide longitudinal study of cancer survivors. Health Psychol. 2019;38(7):596–605.
9. Fagerlin A, et al. Helping patients decide: ten steps to better risk communication. J Natl Cancer Inst. 2011; 103:1436–43.
10. Jiang S, Pathway linking patient-centred communication to emotional well-being: taking into account patient satisfaction and emotion management. J Health Commun. 2017;22(3):234–42.
11. Sorensen K, et al. The call for a strategic framework to improve cancer literacy in Europe. Arch Public Health. 2020;78:60.
12. Coughlin SS, et al. Health literacy among cancer survivors: results from the 2016 behavioral risk factor surveillance system survey. Medicine. 2022;101(9):e29010.
13. Olver I, et al. Supportive care in cancer-a MASCC perspective. Support Care Cancer. 2020;28(8):3467–75.
14. Basch E. New frontiers in patient-reported outcomes: adverse event reporting, comparative effectiveness, and quality assessment. Annu Rev Med. 2014;65:307–17.
15. Graupner C, et al. Patient outcomes, patient experiences and process indicators associated with the routine use of patient-reported outcome measures (PROMs) in cancer care: a systematic review. Support Care Cancer. 2020;2:1–21.
16. Chen J, et al. A systematic review of the impact of routine collection of patient-reported outcome measures on patients, providers and health organisations in an oncologic setting. BMC Health Serv Res. 2013;13(1):1–24.
17. Adam R, et al. Can patient-reported measurements of pain be used to improve cancer pain management? A systematic review and meta-analysis. BMJ Support Palliat Care. 2017;7:373–82.
18. van Egdom LS, et al. Implementing patient-reported outcome measures in clinical breast cancer care: a systematic review. Value Health. 2019;22(10):1197–226.
19. Bouazza YB, et al. Patient-reported outcome measures (PROMs) in the management of lung cancer: a systematic review. Lung Cancer. 2017;113:140–51.
20. Antunes B, et al. Euroimpact: implementing patient-reported outcome measures in palliative care clinical practice: a systematic review of facilitators and barriers. Palliat Med. 2014;28(2):158–75.
21. Foster A, et al. The facilitators and barriers to implementing patient reported outcome measures in organisations delivering health related services: a systematic review of reviews. J Patient Rep Outcomes. 2018;2(1):1–16.
22. Greenhalgh J, et al. How do patient-reported outcome measures (PROMs) support clinician-patient communication and patient care? A realist synthesis. J Patient Rep Outcomes. 2018;2(1):1–28.
23. Macmillan Cancer Support. The recovery package [internet], 2018. Available at: https://be.macmillan.org.uk/be/s-1086-additional-resources-and-archived-material.aspx.

24. Williamson S, et al. The patient needs assessment in cancer care: identifying barriers and facilitators to implementation in the UK and Canada. Support Care Cancer. 2021;29:805–12.
25. Luigjes-Huizer YL, et al. What is the prevalence of fear of cancer recurrence in cancer survivors and patients? A systematic review and individual participant data meta-analysis. Psychooncology. 2022;31(6):879–92.
26. Cruickshank S, et al. Specialist breast cancer nurses' views on implementing a fear of cancer recurrence intervention in practice: a mixed methods study. Support Care Cancer. 2020;28(1):201–10.
27. McHale C, et al. Mini-AFTERc: a controlled pilot trial of a nurse-led psychological intervention for fear of breast cancer recurrence. Pilot Feas Stud. 2024;10:3.
28. Shaw J, et al. Setting an international research agenda for fear of cancer recurrence: an online delphi consensus study. Front Psychol Psycho-Oncol. 2021;12:596682.
29. Pradhan P, et al. Towards a stepped care model for managing fear of cancer recurrence or progression in cancer survivors. Cancer Manag Res. 2021;13:8953–65.
30. NHS long-term plan [Internet], 2019. Available at: https://www.longtermplan.nhs.uk/wp-content/uploads/2019/08/nhs-long-term-plan-version-1.2.pdf (accessed September 2024).
31. Miller WR. Motivational interviewing with problem drinkers. Behav Cogn Psychother. 1983;11(2):147–72.
32. Rollnick S, Miller WR. What is motivational interviewing? Behav Cogn Psychother. 1995;23:32534.
33. Saunders B, et al. The impact of a brief motivational intervention with opiate users attending a methadone programme. Addiction. 1995;90:415–24.
34. Butler CC, et al. Motivational consulting versus brief advice for smokers in general practice: a randomized trial. Br J Gen Pract. 1999;49:611–6.
35. Papus M, et al. Motivational interviewing to support medication adherence in adults with chronic conditions: systematic review of randomized controlled trials. Patient Educ Counsel. 2022;105(11):3186–203.
36. Bilgin A, et al. The effect of motivational interviewing on metabolic control and psychosocial variables in individuals diagnosed with diabetes: systematic review and meta-analysis. Patient Educ Counsel. 2022;105(9):2806–23.
37. Çakmak HSG, Kapucu S. The effect of educational follow-up with the motivational interview technique on self-efficacy and drug adherence in cancer patients using oral chemotherapy treatment: a randomized controlled trial. Semin Oncol Nurs. 2021;37(2): 151140.
38. Borsari B, et al. A pilot trial of collaborative care with motivational interviewing to reduce opioid risk and improve chronic pain management. Addiction. 2021;116(9):2387–97.
39. Berhe KK, et al. Effect of motivational interviewing intervention on HgbA1C and depression in people with type 2 diabetes mellitus (systematic review and meta-analysis). PLoS One. 2020;15(10):e0240839.
40. Huffman JC, et al. A positive psychology-motivational interviewing program to promote physical activity in type 2 diabetes: the BEHOLD-16 pilot randomized trial. Gen Hosp Psychiatr. 2021;68:65–73.
41. Harmer V. Helping survivors to adjust after cancer. Nurs. Times. 2012;108(6):12, 14, 16.
42. Harmer V, Hughes C. Nursing issues. In: Verhoeven D, Kaufman CS, Mansel R, Siesling S, Breast Cancer Global Quality Care, Oxford University Press, 2020:211–7.
43. National Institute for Health and Care Excellence, Tumour profiling tests to guide adjuvant chemotherapy decisions in early breast cancer (Diagnostics guidance [DG58]), 2024. Available at: https://www.nice.org.uk/guidance/dg58/chapter/2-The-diagnostic-tests (accessed September 2024).
44. Grootes I, et al. An updated PREDICT breast cancer prognostic model including the benefits and harms of radiotherapy. Breast Cancer. 2024;10: 6.
45. Royal College of Obstetrics and Gynaecologists, Pregnancy and Breast Cancer Green-top Guideline 12 [internet], 2011. Available at: https://www.rcog.org.uk/guidance/browse-all-guidance/green-top-guidelines/pregnancy-and-breast-cancer-green-top-guideline-no-12/ (accessed September 2024).
46. Slepicka PF, et al. Pregnancy and breast cancer: pathways to understand risk and prevention. Trends Mol Med. 2019;25:866–81.
47. Xiao Y, et al. Qualitative study of the fertility information support experiences of young breast cancer patients. Eur J Oncol Nurs. 2023;62:102275.
48. Montañés-Muro P, et al. Psychosocial care needs of women with breast cancer: body image, self-esteem, optimism, and sexual performance and satisfaction. Health Soc Work. 2023;48(2):115–23.

13

Surgical Oncology of Breast Cancer

John R. Benson and Ismail Jatoi

13.1 Principles of Breast Surgery

13.1.1 Surgical Paradigms

Halstedian paradigm: William Stewart Halsted (1852–1922) postulated that breast cancer is a loco-regional disease and metastatic dissemination occurs by centrifugal and contiguous spread of the primary tumour with progressive involvement of adjacent tissue and the lymphatic system of the breast.[1] The operation of radical mastectomy aimed to remove en bloc the breast, pectoral musculature, and the axillary lymph nodes (up to level III). This operation is eponymously known as the Halsted mastectomy and was adopted as routine surgical practice for breast cancer patients in the first half of the 20th century. This procedure was undertaken for all operable tumours irrespective of clinical features and its rationale underpinned by the so-called Halstedian paradigm that maximal efforts at local control would prolong survival. Breast cancer was considered to originate as a localised disease with the belief that cure rates could be improved by a meticulous and comprehensive surgical approach with thorough resection of loco-regional tissues. Local recurrence was considered to be the cause of distant metastases, and the aim was to minimise rates of local relapse. Many patients treated with initial radical mastectomy developed local recurrence before they succumbed from distant metastatic disease. The operation of radical mastectomy dramatically reduced rates of local recurrence but had no impact on overall survival. Hence, this frequently mutilating operation did not yield any additional years of life for patients implying a problem with the existing paradigm.

Fisherian paradigm: An alternative hypothesis was proposed by Bernard Fisher (1918–2019) and termed biological predeterminism. This paradigm was a polar opposite to the aforementioned paradigm and contended that any tumour within the breast is a local manifestation of a systemic disease with complex interactions between the host, the primary tumour and distant micrometastases.[2] According to this paradigm, breast cancer was able to access the circulation at an early stage in carcinogenesis with cancer cells breaking away from the tumour bolus and entering the bloodstream via gaps between endothelial cells in the neovasculature. Moreover, an additional route for haematogenous dissemination was via lymphatico-venous communications in the regional (axillary) lymph nodes. It followed that surgery could only achieve local control of disease and some form of systemic treatment was necessary to improve overall survival—the latter was predetermined by the presence of micrometastases at the time of presentation (Figure 13.1).

Intermediate paradigm: A spectrum or intermediate paradigm is emerging which encompasses this variable capacity to form distant metastatic disease, with more indolent, slower growing tumours (luminal subtypes) behaving according to the Halstedian paradigm and more aggressive tumours (triple-negative and HER2-positive cancers) disseminating early on consistent with the Fisherian paradigm.[3] Molecular profiling of tumours has revealed a dichotomy of gene expression patterns that permits assignment of tumours to one or other group based on predicted biological behaviour with appropriate intensities of loco-regional and systemic treatments (Figure 13.2).

13.1.2 Breast-Conserving Surgery

The National Institutes of Health consensus conference in 1991 endorsed breast conserving surgery (BCS) as the preferred standard of care for management of women with early-stage breast cancer.[4] Several seminal trials of BCS have demonstrated equivalent survival outcomes for BCS compared with mastectomy procedures involving extirpation of all breast tissue (Figure 13.1).

Trials of BCS: The paradigm of biological predeterminism was supported by results of six randomised trials allocating breast cancer patients to either a breast-conserving procedure (lumpectomy, wide local excision, quadrantectomy) or total mastectomy. These included the Milan I trial conducted by Umberto Veronesi (1925–2016) and the large National Surgical Adjuvant

DOI: 10.1201/9781003394785-13

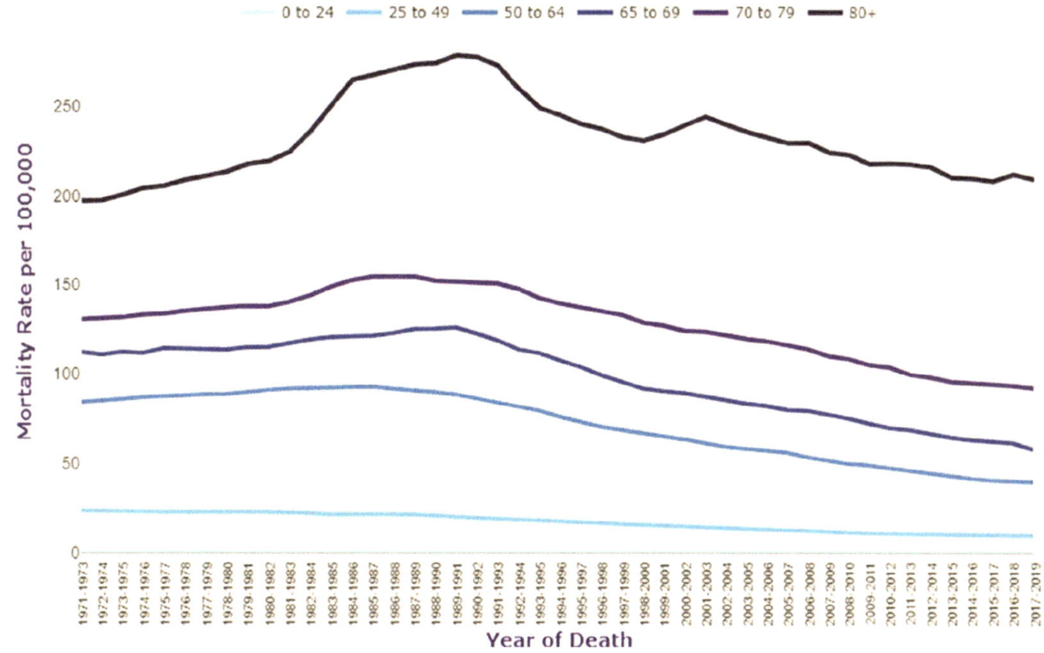

FIGURE 13.1
European age-standardised breast cancer mortality rates in UK by age from 1971 to 2019. Rates have decreased in the age groups 35–49s (58%), 50–64s (53%), 65–69s (48%), and 70–79s (29%) but have increased in the over 80s age group (6%).

Source: **Cancer Research UK, https://www.cancerresearchuk.org/health-professional/cancer-statistics/statistics-by-cancer-type/breast-cancer/mortality#heading-Two.**

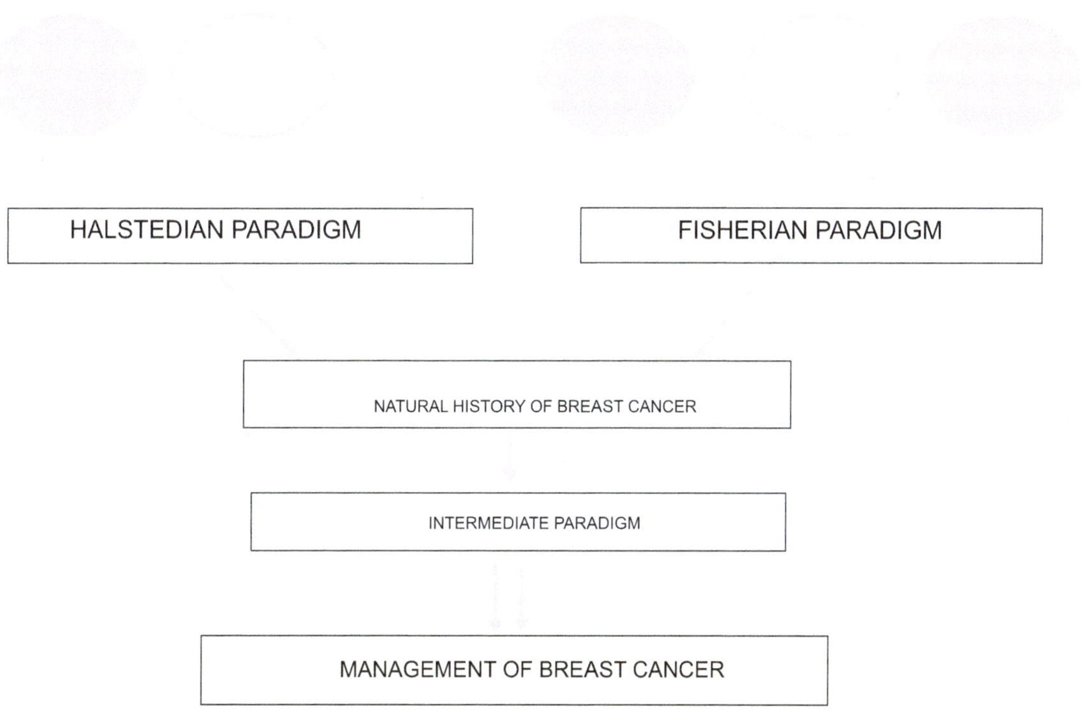

FIGURE 13.2
The natural history of breast cancer is increasingly explained by an intermediate paradigm that encompasses elements of both the Halstedian and Fisherian paradigms. It is now acknowledged that some tumours behave more in accordance with the Halstedian paradigm and tend to be slow growing and indolent, whilst others are intrinsically more aggressive and Fisherian in behaviour with early spread in the bloodstream.

Breast and Bowel Project (NSABP B-06) trial.[5–7] Results of the Milan I trial provided level I evidence demonstrating survival equivalence for breast conservation therapy compared with radical or modified radical mastectomy.[6] An update of the NSABP B-06 trial with 20-year follow-up confirms that post-operative irradiation improves local recurrence-free survival after breast-conserving surgery (BCS) with similar distant disease-free and overall survival for modified radical mastectomy, wide local excision and radiotherapy or wide local excision alone.[7] Hence, permutations of breast surgery seemingly have no impact on breast-cancer-specific mortality and BCS was deemed to be a safe surgical procedure for patients with tumours <5 cm in size.[4] This heralded the start of a trend for de-escalation of breast surgical procedures and a move away from the radical mastectomy and modified radical mastectomy. The latter operation is attributed to David Patey of the Middlesex Hospital who advocated preservation of the pectoralis major muscle unless directly infiltrated by tumour[8] [Figure 13.3]. Nonetheless, resection of the pectoralis minor muscle remained an essential component of surgery, allowing access to higher-echelon axillary nodes. Residual cancer cells following lumpectomy (wide local excision) are a determinant of local failure but not of distant metastatic disease and lead to a finite rate of ipsilateral breast tumour recurrence (IBTR) after BCS that is halved with breast irradiation. Contemporary rates of IBTR are very low (<1% per annum) with combined multimodality treatments; systemic therapies reduce IBTR by approximately one-third and anti-HER2-directed treatments halve rates of in-breast recurrence. An intriguing population-based observational study comparing survival outcomes for BCS and mastectomy was published in 2016 and involved a primary cohort of almost 40,000 patients who were treated between January 1st 2000 and December 31st 2004.[9] There was a statistically significant overall survival advantage for BCS compared with mastectomy [HR 0.81; 95% CI 0.78–0.85 ($p<0.001$)] at a median follow-up of 11.3 years. This study was subject to confounding with BCS patients tending to be younger with smaller tumours on average. Nonetheless, evidence has emerged from even larger studies supporting improved survival outcomes associated with BCS.

Surgical margins: BCS represents a balance between oncological mandates and cosmetic outcomes with the aim of removing the tumour and a narrow margin of surrounding breast tissue such that negative margins are achieved. The closer ink is to tumour, the narrower are margins with a positive margin associated with ink on cancer cells [Figure 13.4]. Margin status is a predictor of local recurrence and therefore an adequate width of surgical margins is important.

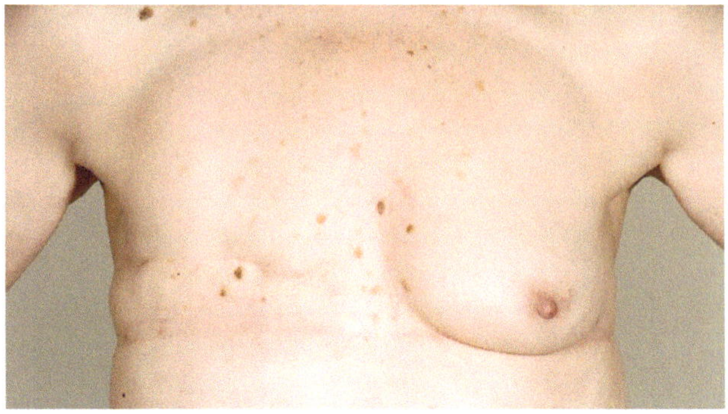

FIGURE 13.3
A patient who has undergone a modified radical mastectomy with preservation of the pectoralis major muscle—the anterior axillary fold is evident.

Careful selection of patients for BCS is essential with an inverse relationship between oncological demands for surgical radicality on the one hand and optimal cosmesis on the other. There is now international consensus that an adequate margin exists when invasive tumour is not touching ink and wider margins do not reduce rates of local recurrence.[10] Nonetheless, the Association of Breast Surgery (UK) have decreed that a negative margin requires tumour to be no closer than 1 mm from the inked margin for invasive and 2 mm for non-invasive breast cancer. It should be appreciated that a negative margin does not imply absence of any residual disease within the remaining breast tissue, but indicates a residual tumour burden sufficiently low to be controlled with adjuvant treatments. Local surgery does not completely eliminate residual disease with local recurrence determined by a combination of surgery, tumour biology, radiation, and systemic therapies.[8] A retrospective cohort study involving more than 50,000 patients treated with BCS for either invasive or non-invasive disease within the

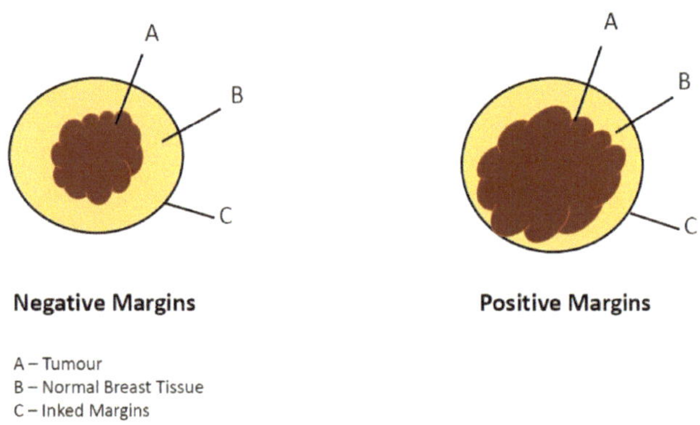

FIGURE 13.4
A positive margin after breast-conserving surgery is defined as tumour at the inked margin whilst a negative margin is defined by international consensus as 'no ink on tumour'; hence a margin width of just 0.1 mm would be negative.

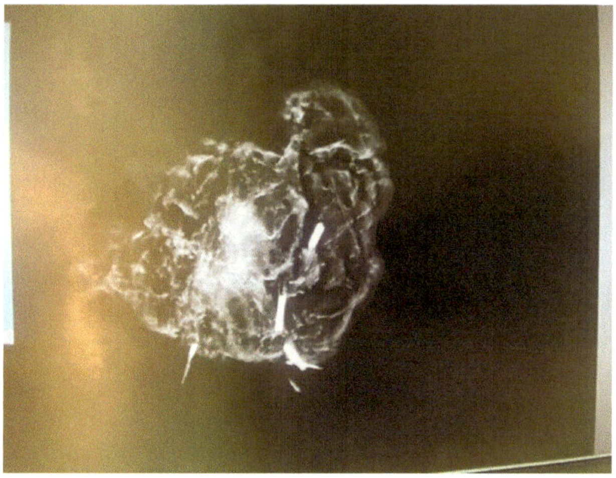

FIGURE 13.5
A specimen radiograph after a wide local excision of a breast tumour. The tumour is a dense central opacity and surrounded by a macroscopic margin of normal fibroglandular breast tissue.

UK National Health Service revealed an overall re-operation rate of 20% with rates of 18% for invasive disease and 29.5% for DCIS[11]; it is often the presence of coexisting DCIS extending beyond the invasive component in breast cancer specimens that prompts re-excision. It is perhaps ironic that higher rates of re-excision might imply careful margin assessment by pathologists coupled with a more rigorous margin re-excision policy. Re-excision constitutes an additional workload for the pathologist and generates much anxiety and psychological distress for patients. Furthermore, the need for re-excision can delay commencement of adjuvant therapies and worsen the final cosmetic outcome from removal of additional tissue and re-opening of the breast incision. Some discretion can be applied with any decision to re-excise; for example, an elderly patient with a single positive radial margin or any single margin that is focally positive irrespective of age could avoid re-excision. It remains unclear whether focally positive margins should be managed differently from involvement of a margin across a broad front (>5 mm). Oncoplastic surgical resections (especially therapeutic mammoplasty) lead to wider margins of resection and permit resection of tumours typically measuring up to 70 mm in maximum extent in large breasted patients. Most patients who are deemed eligible for BCS will have a favourable tumour-to-breast-size ratio and be suitable for conventional wide local excision (lumpectomy); the surgeon will aim to resect 1–2 cm of macroscopically normal tissue around the tumour with no attempt to formally remodel the breast, although mobilisation of breast parenchyma with limited undermining of tissues will facilitate closure of the cavity. Despite the need for re-excision in some patients, the majority should attain an optimal cosmetic outcome after breast irradiation. Many surgeons are now electing to access tumours through a peri-areolar incision rather than making a curvilinear incision in a natural skin crease directly overlying the tumour. These remote incisions avoid scars in exposed areas of the breast mound but can be more challenging for guided resection of impalpable lesions and in the event of margin re-excision [Figure 13.5]. Skin should not be routinely excised with conventional BCS, but any zones of skin tethering clinically can be incorporated into a narrow crescent-shaped ellipse of skin.

13.1.3 Skin-Sparing Forms of Mastectomy

The modified radical mastectomy much reduced the morbidity of the traditional radical operation. With the rapid development of breast reconstructive techniques over the past three decades, the modified radical mastectomy has evolved into the skin-sparing (SSM) and nipple-sparing (NSM) forms of mastectomy that are now being applied to both prophylactic and therapeutic breast surgical procedures[12,13] [Figure 13.6]. Initial concerns that greater skin preservation with SSM and NSM might lead to higher rates of local recurrence have not been justified. Several studies have now confirmed low rates of local recurrence (<5%) for skin-sparing procedures that are not significantly higher than for conventional forms of mastectomy when patients are matched for stage of disease. Skin-sparing types of mastectomy represent forms of conservative mastectomy whereby much of the breast skin envelope is preserved. Meticulous surgical technique is essential for these skin-sparing forms of mastectomy with careful distraction of mastectomy flaps during surgery and ensuring that surgical dissection is confined to the oncological plane between the breast parenchyma and subcutaneous tissues (the anterior lamella of the superficial fascia). Current studies are attempting to define those breast cancer patients for whom NSM can be safely performed as a therapeutic procedure without adversely affecting oncological outcomes (especially recurrence within the territory of the nipple). An important aspect of NSM is to ensure that ductal tissue within the nipple is 'cored' out without compromising the vascular supply to the nipple-areola complex.[14] There is now better appreciation of how tissue can be excised from the central core of the nipple without risk to its blood supply and without compromising oncological safety of the procedure. A sample of retro-areolar tissue can be taken at the time of surgery with a delayed resection of the nipple-areola complex if malignancy is confirmed histologically (paraffin sections).

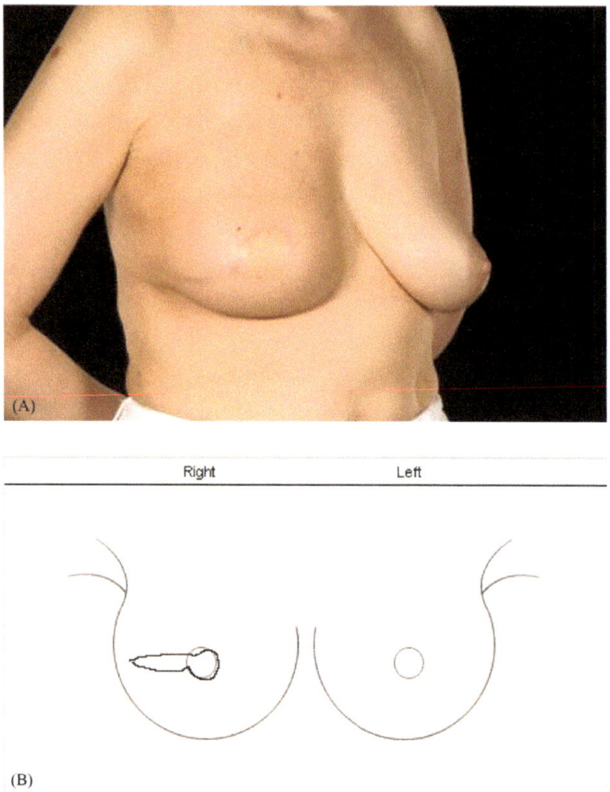

FIGURE 13.6
(A, B) A skin-sparing mastectomy preserves most of the skin envelope but removes the nipple areola complex. The breast tissue is removed through a peri-areolar incision, which is closed either with inset of disc of a skin from a transposed flap or as a linear incision in the case of implant-based breast reconstruction.

13.1.4 Axillary Surgery

Surgical staging of the axilla is an integral component of breast cancer surgery and has undergone a revolutionary change with progressive de-escalation of nodal resection. The operations of both radical and modified radical mastectomy implied concomitant axillary lymph node dissection (ALND). The latter can be associated with considerable morbidity; thus, within two years of ALND, patients report a variety of symptoms, including the following:

1. Axillary pain (39%)
2. Ipsilateral numbness or paraesthesia (68%)
3. Restriction of arm mobility (21%)
4. Dissatisfaction with the appearance of the axillary scar (15%)
5. Some degree of arm swelling (lymphedema) (75%)

Sentinel lymph node (SLN) biopsy is Halstedian and relies on the sequential spread of cancer cells from the lower to the higher-echelon nodes—a false negative rate occurs with the technique because the hypothesis is not pure—some cancer cells will bypass the sentinel node to reach nodes at a higher level in the axilla [Figures 13.7a and b]. The SLN biopsy procedure can substantially reduce these untoward effects, but does not completely eliminate them [Figures 13.8a, b, and c]. The morbidity of ALND and its adverse impact on quality-of-life has been a major impetus for reduction in the extent of axillary surgery (or omission thereof) without compromising patient safety. With the advent of SLN biopsy, formal ALND is now much less commonly performed (as either a primary or secondary procedure); the NSABP B-32 trial randomised more than 5000 patients to either SLN biopsy plus ALND

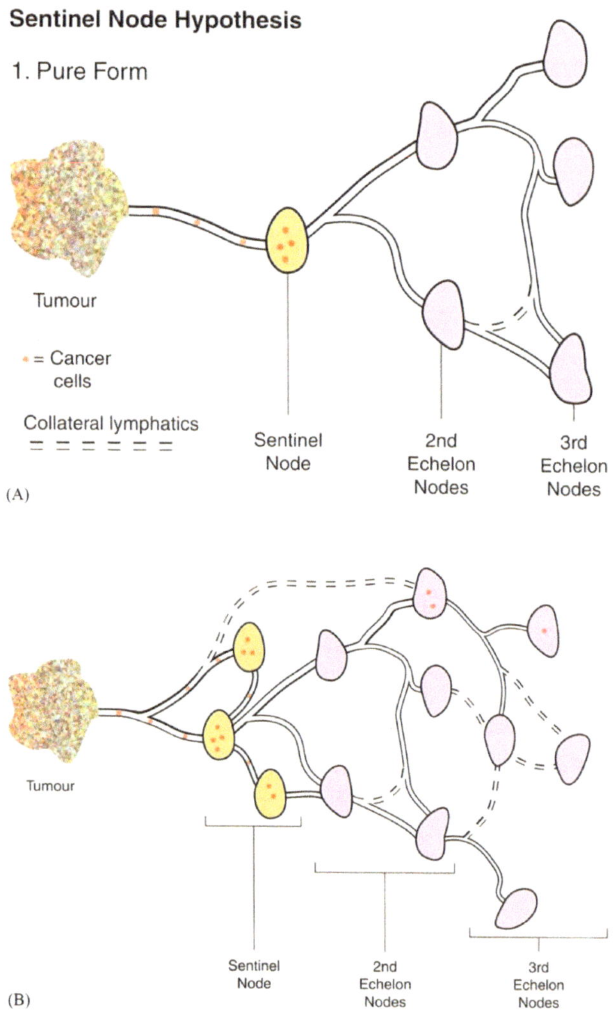

FIGURE 13.7
The sentinel lymph node hypothesis. (A) In the pure form of this hypothesis, cancer cells spread to 7 single nodes in the lower axilla from the primary tumour and then move on to higher-echelon nodes. (B) In reality, cancer cells spread to 2–3 sentinel nodes and can even bypass the sentinel node to reach nodes at a higher level—hence resulting in a false negative result.

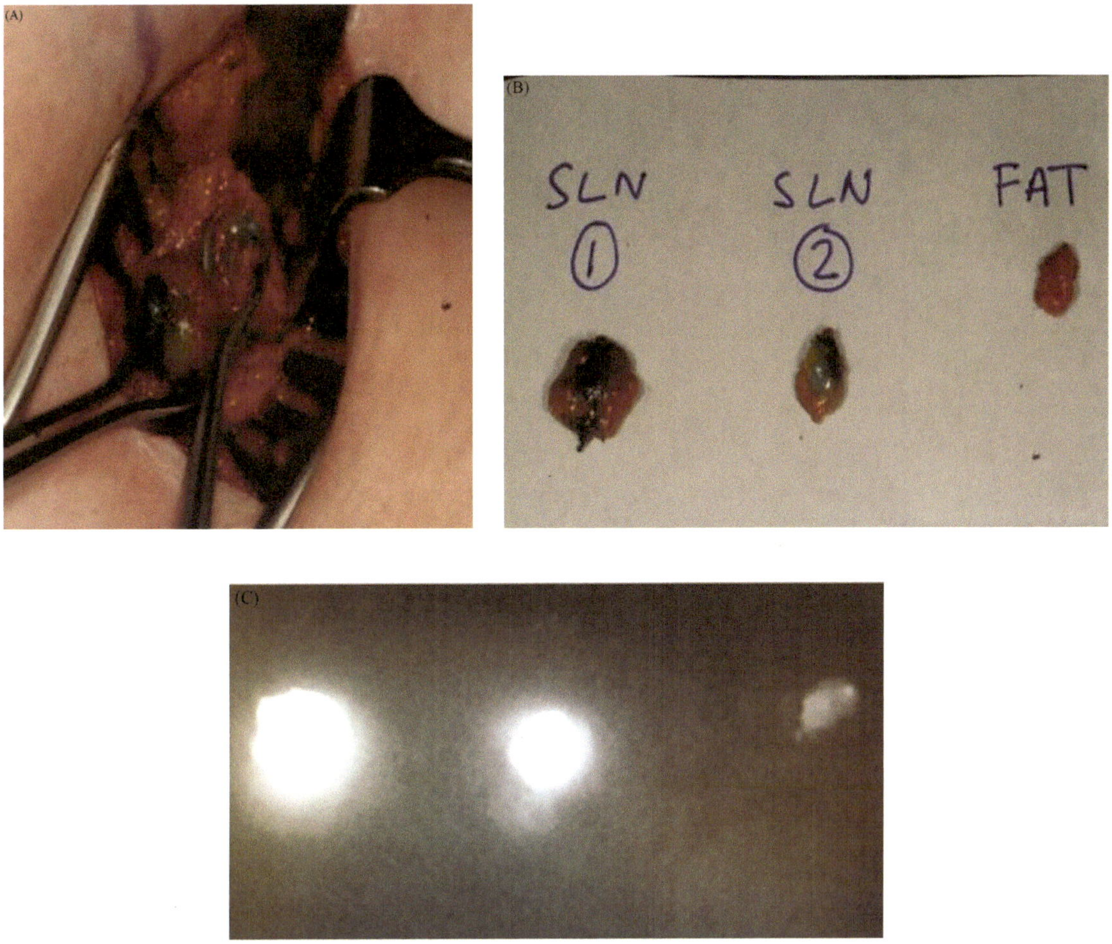

FIGURE 13.8
The sentinel node is usually localised with a combination of tracer agents—blue dye and radioisotope. (A, B) The nodes appear blue, and a radioactive signal can be detected with a gamma probe. (C) Alternative methods include fluorescent mapping using indocyanine green that emits a fluorescent signal that is detected with a photodynamic eye and camera.

or SLN biopsy alone.[15,16] At a median follow-up of 96 months, there were no significant differences in disease-free or overall survival with similar rates of regional control in both arms of the trial. These results supported SLN biopsy as a safe, appropriate, and effective management option for clinically node negative early-stage breast cancer patients. The latter includes those patients without palpable nodes, with palpable nodes that appear normal on imaging or abnormal nodes on imaging for which needle biopsy reveals no evidence of malignancy.

A notable change in axillary management following introduction of routine SLN biopsy for clinically node-negative patients has been omission of completion ALND in selected sentinel node positive cases with reliance on adjuvant non-surgical treatment modalities for eradication of low burden axillary disease in non-sentinel lymph nodes.[17] The ACOSOG Z0011 study examined omission of completion ALND in SLN biopsy-positive patients presenting with clinically node negative breast cancer.[18] Patients with no more than 2 positive sentinel nodes containing either macro- (>2 mm) or micro-metastases (44%) were randomised to completion ALND or observation only. All patients underwent BCS and were scheduled to receive whole breast radiotherapy and adjuvant systemic treatment with about 50% of patients receiving irradiation with high tangent fields. An updated analysis of this trial at 10 years has reaffirmed low rates of axillary relapse (0.5% in the completion ALND arm and 1.5% in the SLN biopsy arm). There were no significant differences in outcomes for regional recurrence ($p = 0.28$) or overall survival ($p = 0.02$).[19] The majority of patients nowadays undergo initial SLN biopsy, be this in the context of conventional mastectomy without reconstruction, SSM, NSM, or BCS. Thus, patients are more likely to undergo simple mastectomy combined with SLN biopsy rather than mastectomy and ALND—the modified radical mastectomy. If SLN biopsy reveals no axillary nodal involvement or a low burden of tumour (≤2 positive nodes with micro- [≤2 mm] or macro-metastases [>2 mm]), then further axillary treatment can usually be avoided in the context of primary conservation surgery. Conversely, evidence of more than 2 nodes with macrometastases should prompt ALND or possibly axillary irradiation for both BCS and mastectomy patients.

13.2 Oncoplastic Breast Surgery

Historical development: Oncoplastic breast surgery (OPBS) and partial breast reconstruction is a natural evolution in the application of BCS to management of breast cancer. Most patients who are considered eligible for BCS have a favourable tumour to breast size ratio and are suitable for conventional forms of wide local excision with local glandular readjustment without formal remodelling of the breast. Even when re-excision of margins is required (in up to one-quarter of cases), an optimal cosmetic outcome should be attainable in the long term after irradiation of the breast. There is a 'grey area' where the limits of BCS are being approached, and the patient may be better served with a skin-/nipple-sparing mastectomy and immediate breast reconstruction at the outset. It becomes progressively more difficult to achieve a good cosmetic outcome as the proportion of breast tissue removed increases. When more than 10–20% of breast tissue is removed, there is a risk of an unsatisfactory result, but relatively modest losses of 5–10% of breast volume from tumours in cosmetically sensitive areas (medial and inferior quadrants) can adversely affect cosmesis.[20] Oncoplastic breast surgery provides the opportunity for enhancing quality of life by improving cosmetic outcomes and psychological well-being after larger resections for unifocal and some multifocal breast cancers [Figures 13.9a, b, and c]. OPBS can facilitate wide surgical clearance of a tumour and improve a patient's cosmetic outcome when larger volumes of resected tissue are required.[21]

OPBS techniques: These include volume replacement and volume displacement techniques.[22] The former imports additional tissue in the form of a flap and attempts to compensate for loss of volume from surgical excision. By contrast, the latter rearranges the remaining breast tissue using methods of glandular advancement that serve to redistribute the parenchyma and minimise the impact of wide local excision [Figures 13.10 and 13.11]. Volume displacement techniques absorb volume loss over a wider area and do not incur donor site morbidity from harvesting of any local tissue flaps. The term 'oncoplastic surgery' was coined by Werner Audretsch from Dusseldorf in Germany and refers to incorporation of plastic surgery techniques into routine breast surgery for purposes of partial breast reconstruction after extirpative procedures for breast cancer. Krishna Clough from Paris is another oncoplastic pioneer who has contributed greatly to the establishment of OPBS techniques and defining indications for their use based on tumour size, location in the breast and whether uni- or multifocal.[23] The advent of these OPBS techniques has shaped current approaches to breast surgery and acknowledgment within the breast surgery community that a good cosmetic result should be standard of care for all patients without compromise of oncological safety.

Selection of patients for OPBS: A particular challenge is integration of adjuvant treatments into management pathways for breast cancer patients with determination of optimum sequencing and timing of chemotherapy and radiotherapy. Careful selection of patients is crucial and partial breast reconstruction should not be attempted in patients who are not amenable to BCS from an oncological perspective and for whom mastectomy is warranted.[24] These techniques of OPBS must be appropriately integrated with ablative breast surgery to avoid emergence of a 'breast cripple'. Cross-specialty training opportunities are fostering increasing numbers of oncoplastic breast surgeons, and those without relevant experience should work cooperatively with plastic surgeons to provide a comprehensive service. Notwithstanding availability of surgical expertise, these OPBS techniques are appropriate for a relatively small proportion of patients (10–15%) and should only be offered in units managing large numbers of breast cancer patients.[25] These newer techniques of OPBS have undoubtedly presented greater opportunity for conservation whilst satisfying oncological mandates. More extensive oncoplastic resections reduce the chance of a 'positive' or 'close' margin [12% v 21%; $p < 0.0001$] and the need for re-excision as a secondary procedure [14.6% v 4%]. However, there is no clear evidence that excision of tumours with a very wide surgical margin (e.g. therapeutic mammoplasty) is associated with lower rates of breast local recurrence. This might partly be related to tumours being significantly larger for oncoplastic resections compared with conventional wide local excision [average tumour size 2.7 cm v 1.2 cm].[26] It is perhaps ironic that a minimal margin mandate for BCS ('no tumour on ink' or 1 mm) now prevails and surgeons no longer need to strive for wide margins of resection that are associated with OPBS. Nonetheless, published material to date does support OPBS providing local control

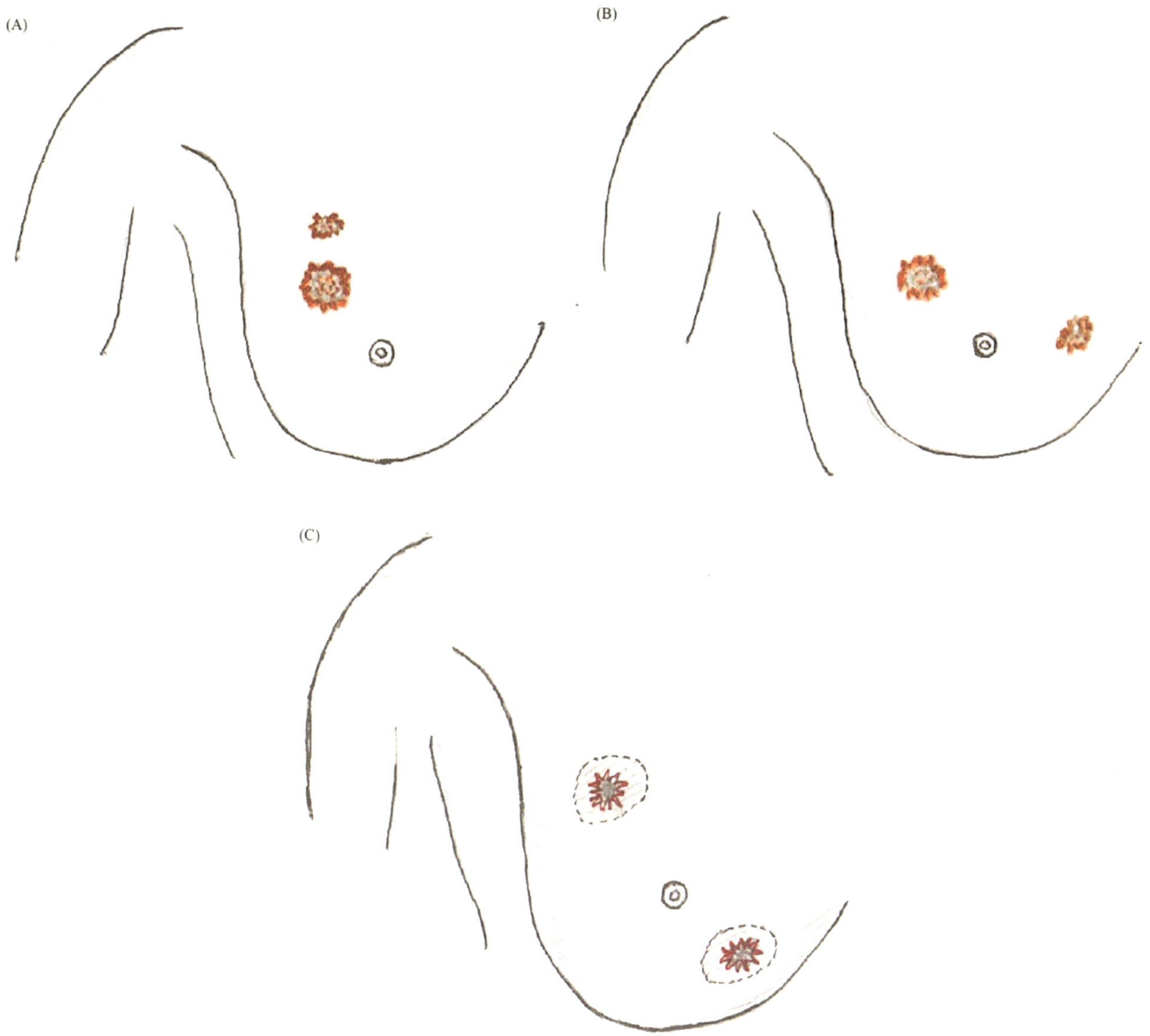

FIGURE 13.9
Multiple foci of cancer can occur in either (A) the same or (B) different quadrants of the breast, and this influences approaches to surgery. (C) Two wide local excisions can be performed for distant tumours in a relatively large breast.

of disease, good cosmetic outcomes, and improved quality of life.[27] One advantage of having a minimal margin mandate is that this may facilitate excision of multiple ipsilateral cancers with clear surgical margins using an adaptive surgical approach.

Outcomes of OPBS: It is often a challenge collecting high quality comparative evidence for surgical procedures. There are many confounding factors and lack of surgical equipoise often thwarts attempts to obtain robust evidence from randomised controlled trials.[28] Furthermore, many non-randomised cohort studies of OPBS have methodological shortcomings with results not being generalisable. Nonetheless, there is much retrospective data from meta-analyses that supports the safety of OPBCS with no evidence for increased rates of local recurrence or poorer patient reported outcome measures.[21] Judicious clinical judgement is essential and surgeons need to know when it is best to recommend mastectomy and whole breast reconstruction rather than an ambitious attempt at OPBS that might be associated with a relatively high rate of in-breast recurrence as well as poor cosmetic and patient reported outcomes. Prospective observational studies with parallel design may be more realistic in an age of shared decision-making and patient-centred care.

Goals of OPBS: Breast surgeons must work cooperatively with plastic surgeons to ensure that the mix

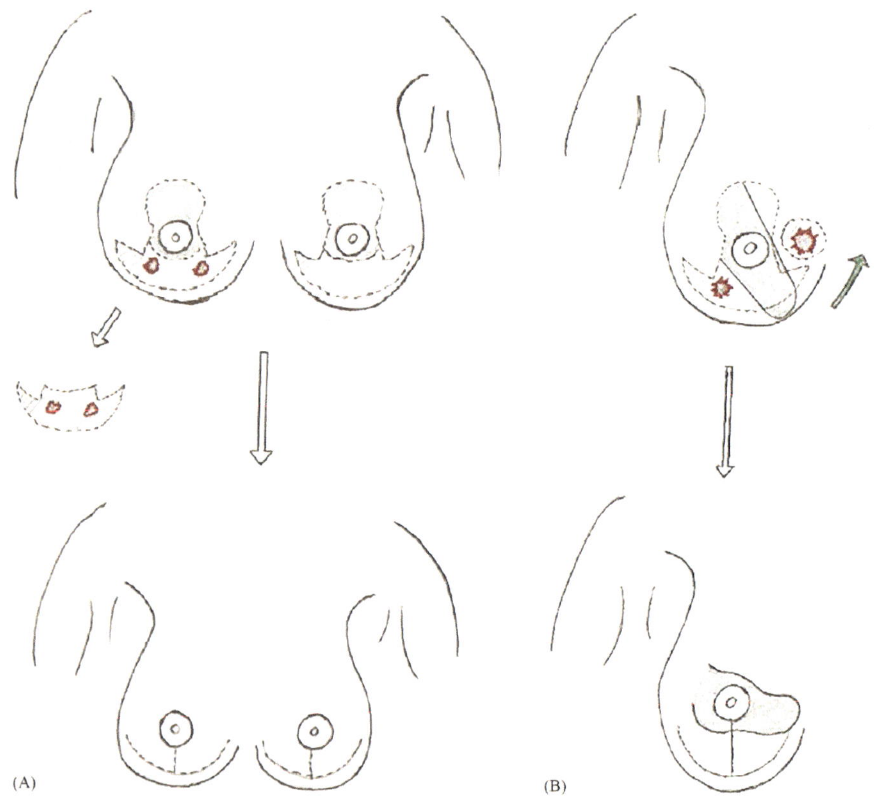

FIGURE 13.10
Oncoplastic surgery advances the limits of breast-conserving surgery and permits resection of large volumes of breast tissue as part of either a volume displacement or displacement technique. (A) A therapeutic mammoplasty is ideally suited to tumours in the inferior aspect of larger breasts but (B) secondary pedicles can be created for resection of tumours above the breast meridian.

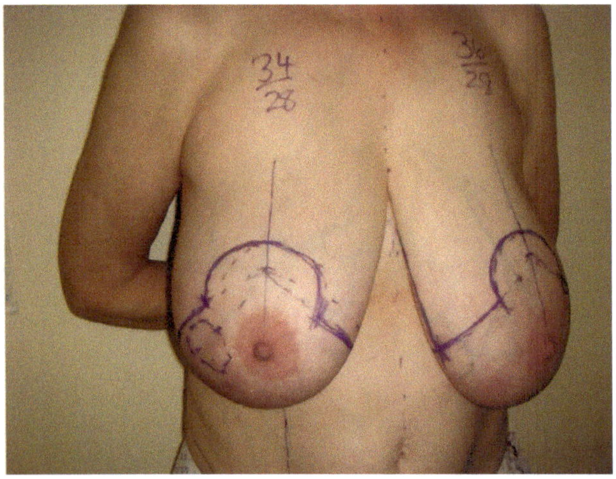

FIGURE 13.11
A patient with large breasts has been marked up for a therapeutic mammoplasty that will incorporate resection of a tumour in the lower outer quadrant of the right breast.

of surgical skills can be optimally applied to maximise oncological, aesthetic and patient-reported outcomes. By restoring the size, shape, and appearance of the breast, reconstruction improves a patient's gender identity and quality of life across multiple domains—psychological, social, sexual, emotional, and functional. There is enhanced aesthetic satisfaction from immediate reconstruction compared with mastectomy alone, and patients with borderline conservable tumours may opt for mastectomy and whole breast reconstruction rather than BCS with partial breast reconstruction.[29,30] It is imperative that patients make fully informed decisions and are aware of reconstructive options early on in discussions of surgical management of their breast cancer. Breast surgical oncologists have a key role as gatekeepers in ensuring that patients have access to reconstructive surgeons and referral to plastic surgery colleagues is made as soon as possible following diagnosis of breast cancer—including patients managed with primary chemotherapy. Decisions made in terms of breast reconstruction are very much 'preference sensitive' and must be individualised and made jointly between a patient and her surgeon(s). They should take account not only of a patient's wishes, but also her personality, self-perception, and socio-economic circumstances. Outcomes of breast cancer surgery are better when clinical decision-making integrates information giving, shared decision-making and patients' personal values.

Patient-reported outcomes and expectations: There is now greater appreciation of a patient's perspective and issues such as quality-of-life and patient choice. More subjective outcomes relating to psychological, emotional, and functional aspects of reconstruction can be formally measured with validated questionnaire-based instruments such as BREAST-Q.[31] Incorporation of patient reported outcomes (PROMS) with more objective clinical parameters will inform future patient choice and lead to improvements in clinical care. Patients' expectations must be realistic, and they should appreciate that the reconstructed breast is a facsimile of and not identical to a normal breast. A patient's expectations of the final cosmetic result will be determined by any relevant prior knowledge and influenced by information derived from friends, other patients, the media, and increasingly the Internet. Any misperceptions must be corrected and fully informed consent obtained before proceeding with any form of breast reconstruction. Patients must be given sufficient time to assimilate all information and reach a decision that feels right for them; sometimes they will change their mind and this has to be accommodated. Surgeon preference should not dominate discussions, and patients should be offered a full repertoire of reconstructive options and not compelled to accept a reconstructive method that is especially favoured by their surgeon. Higher levels of patient satisfaction are associated with immediate breast reconstruction compared with mastectomy alone in terms of psychosocial, sexual, and physical well-being.[32,33] Nonetheless, a desire to complete adjuvant cancer treatments prior to reconstructive surgery is a frequently cited reason for patients deliberately opting for a delayed breast reconstruction.[34]

The range of OPBS options in the modern era are considerable and the potential choice of options available to a woman with a newly diagnosed breast cancer can be overwhelming. There is arguably no longer a primary decision of BCS versus mastectomy with or without reconstruction. Instead, two key questions are whether the patient is a candidate for conventional BCS and if not, can she be spared mastectomy with either pre-operative chemotherapy or an oncoplastic procedure?[35] Addressing these questions may involve complex surgeon-patient discussions with viewing of MRI images and anonymised before and after former patient photographs. These discussions will involve patient tailoring measurements and conceptualised diagrams. The possibility of retaining or improving shape whilst replacing or displacing breast tissue with OPBS may be an option. Alternatively, there will always be the option of removing all breast tissue with preservation of much of the skin envelope and whole breast reconstruction with prosthetic material, autologous tissue, or a combination thereof.

There are three key aspects that need to be addressed for a patient being considered for oncoplastic and reconstructive surgery of the breast:

1. *Optimal oncological outcome:* performing an extirpative procedure that minimises the chance of recurrence by removing the tumour with a clear margin of normal surrounding breast tissue as part of either a partial or complete mastectomy.
2. *Optimal aesthetic outcome:* reconstituting the breast with either partial or whole breast reconstruction to provide satisfactory symmetry and shape in relation to the native breast.
3. *Timing of adjuvant treatments:* avoidance of delays in commencement of adjuvant treatments attributable to post-operative complications such as infection, haematoma, seroma formation, or fat necrosis that adversely impact on delivery of chemotherapy and radiotherapy.

13.3 Conclusions

The Halsted radical mastectomy was predicated on the observation that many patients developed local recurrence before manifestation of any distant metastasis or death from breast cancer. This operation prevailed for much of the 20th century but was challenged by the concept of biological predeterminism proposed by Bernard Fisher. A spectrum paradigm now prevails with recognition that some tumours have a propensity to spread to loco-regional tissues whereas others disseminate early on through the bloodstream. Genetic profiling of tumours has now revealed a dichotomy with luminal tumours behaving in a more Halstedian fashion with TNBC/HER2-positive tumours being intrinsically more aggressive with increased likelihood of haematogenous spread. Improved overall survival from radiotherapy accords with Halstedian principles and has reinforced the link between local control and survival and emphasised the importance of adequate loco-regional treatments. In theory, a relatively high proportion of smaller (and especially screen-detected) invasive cancers will be cured by surgery alone—they have an excellent prognosis without pre-existing micrometastases at diagnosis and hence modest absolute benefits from adjuvant treatments. Newer techniques of oncoplastic breast surgery have presented exciting opportunities for conservation whilst satisfying oncological mandates. However, there is no clear evidence that excision of tumours with a very wide surgical margin is associated with lower rates of breast local recurrence. It is perhaps ironic that although oncoplastic procedures do permit wide resection of tissue with tumour-free margins, we finally have some degree of consensus on the definition of 'negative' surgical resection margin for BCS—with a minimal margin mandate. Nonetheless, published material to date does support OPBS providing local control of disease, good cosmetic outcomes, and improved quality of life.

It is often a challenge collecting high quality comparative evidence for surgical procedures. There are many confounding factors and lack of surgical equipoise often thwarts successful randomised controlled trials. The apparent lack of high-quality evidence doesn't mean that the basis for oncoplastic surgery is unsound; judicious clinical judgement is essential and surgeons need to know when it is best to recommend mastectomy and whole breast reconstruction than attempt an ambitious oncoplastic procedure that might be associated not only with a relatively high rate of in-breast recurrence but also poor cosmesis and PROMS. Sometimes a well-performed conventional lumpectomy with level I oncoplastic adjustment will suffice without the need for more complex level II procedures that often involve surgery to the opposite breast to achieve symmetry.[36] There is ongoing interest in sampling of the tumour bed in so-called exceptional responders for whom there is evidence of minimal residual disease clinically and on imaging. The main impediment to elimination of surgery after primary systemic therapy is the limitation of standard and functional breast imaging. It is now possible to integrate percutaneous needle biopsy of the breast tumour bed and axillary nodes so as to complement imaging and more accurately predict residual disease. The questions that need addressing are firstly, what is the least morbid method to confirm or exclude residual disease in the breast and axillary nodes? Secondly, what are the consequences in terms of clinical outcomes if any minimal residual disease is missed and a 'watch and wait' policy is adopted? It remains unclear whether minimal residual disease can be controlled with a combination of breast RT and systemic treatment or even systemic treatment alone. Hence, it is likely that most patients will continue to require surgical resection of malignant breast disease for the foreseeable future, but there remains potential for further de-escalation as more effective systemic therapies become available.

References

1) Halsted W. The results of operations for the cure of cancer of the breast performed at the Johns Hopkins hospital from June, 1889, to January, 1894. Ann Surg (1894) 20(5):497–555.
2) Fisher B, Anderson S, Fisher ER, et al. Significance of ipsilateral breast tumour recurrence after lumpectomy. Lancet (1991) 338(8763):327–31.
3) della Rovere GQ, Benson JR. Ipsilateral local recurrence of breast cancer: determinant or indicator of poor prognosis? Lancet Oncol (2002) 3(3):183–7.
4) NIH Consensus Conference. Treatment of early breast cancer. JAMA (1991) 265:391–5.
5) Conservative treatment of breast cancer: a trial in progress at the National Cancer Institute of Milan. Cancer (1977) 39:2822–6.
6) Veronesi U, Cascinelli N, Mariani L, et al. Twenty-year follow-up of a randomized study comparing breast conserving surgery with radical mastectomy for early breast cancer. N Engl J Med (2002) 347(16):1227–32.
7) Fisher B, Anderson S, Bryant J, et al. Twenty-year follow-up of a randomized trial comparing total mastectomy, lumpectomy, and lumpectomy plus irradiation for the treatment of invasive breast cancer. N Engl J Med (2002) 347(16):1233–41.
8) Patey DH, Dyson WH. The prognosis of carcinoma of the breast in relation to the type of operation performed. Br J Cancer (1948) 2(1):7–13.
9) van Maaren M, de Munck L, de Bock GH, et al. 10 Year survival after breast conserving surgery plus radiotherapy compared with mastectomy in early breast cancer in the Netherlands: a population-based study. Lancet Oncol (2016) 17(8):1158–70.
10) Moran MS, Schnitt SJ, Giuliano AE, et al. Society of Surgical Oncology-American Society for Radiation Oncology consensus guideline on margins for breast-conserving surgery with whole-breast irradiation in stages I and II invasive breast cancer. Int J Radiat Oncol Biol Phys (2014) 88(3):553–64.
11) Jeevan R, Cromwell DA, Trivella M, et al. Reoperation rates after breast conserving surgery for breast cancer among women in England: retrospective study of hospital episode statistics. BMJ (2012) 245:e4505.
12) Joo JH, Ki Y, Kim W, et al. Pattern of local recurrence after mastectomy and reconstruction in breast cancer patients: a systematic review. Gland Surg (2021) 10(6):2037046.
13) Vaughan A, Dietz JR, Aft R, et al. Patterns of local breast cancer recurrence after skin-sparing mastectomy and immediate breast reconstruction. Am J Surg (2007) 194(4):438–43.
14) Rusby JE, Smith BL, Gui GPH. Nipple-sparing mastectomy. Br J Surg (2010) 97(3):305–16.
15) Krag DN, Anderson SJ, Julian TB, et al. Sentinel-lymph-node resection compared with conventional axillary-lymph-node dissection in clinically node-negative patients with breast cancer: overall survival findings from the NSABP B-32 randomised phase 3 trial. Lancet Oncol (2010) 11(10):927–33.
16) Benson JR. An alternative to axillary lymph node dissection. Lancet Oncol (2010) 11(10):908–9.
17) Jatoi I, Benson JR. Surgical management of the axilla in early breast cancer. Curr Probl Surg (2018) 55(2):47–65.
18) Giuliano AE, Hunt KK, Ballman KV, et al. Axillary dissection vs no axillary dissection in women with invasive breast cancer and sentinel node metastasis: a randomized clinical trial. JAMA (2011) 305(6):569–75.
19) Giuliano AE, Ballman KV, McCall L, et al. Effect of axillary dissection vs no axillary dissection on 10-year overall survival among women with invasive breast cancer and sentinel node metastasis: the ACOSOG Z0011 (alliance) randomized clinical trial. JAMA (2017) 318(10):918–26.
20) Cochrane RA, Valasiadou P, Wilson ARM, et al. Cosmesis and satisfaction after breast-conserving surgery correlates with the percentage of breast volume excised. Br J Surg (2003) 90(12):1505–9.
21) Losken A, Dugal CS, Styblo TM, Carlson GW. A meta-analysis comparing breast conservation therapy alone to the oncoplastic technique. Ann Plast Surg (2014) 72(2):145–9.

22) Benson JR, Absar MS. Volume replacement and displacement techniques in oncoplastic surgery. Adv Breast Cancer (2008) 5(1):3–10.
23) Clough KB, Kaufman GJ, Nos C, et al. Improving breast cancer surgery: a classification and quadrant per quadrant atlas for oncoplastic surgery. Ann Surg Oncol (2010) 17(5):1375–91.
24) Rocco N, Catanuto G, Cinquini M, et al. Should oncoplastic breast conserving surgery be used for the treatment of early stage breast cancer? Using the GRADE approach for development of clinical recommendations. Breast (2021) 57:25–35.
25) Clough KB, Meredith I. The oncoplastic frenzy: beware the swing of the pendulum. Ann Surg Oncol (2019) 26(12):3792–3.
26) Chakravorty A, Shrestha AK, Sanmugalingam N, et al. How safe is oncoplastic breast conservation? Comparative analysis with standard breast conserving surgery. Eur J Surg Oncol (2012) 38(5):395–8.
27) Down SK, Burger A, Hussein M. Oncological advantages of oncoplastic breast conserving surgery in treatment of early breast cancer. Breast J (2013) 19(1):5–63.
28) Ingram J, Beasant L, Benson J, et al. The challenge of equipoise: qualitative interviews exploring the views of health professionals and women with multiple ipsilateral breast cancer on recruitment to a surgical randomised controlled feasibility trial. Pilot Feasibility Stud (2022) 8(1):46.
29) Alderman AK, Hawley ST, Waljee J, et al. Correlates of referral practices of general surgeons to plastic surgeons for mastectomy reconstruction. Cancer (2007) 109(9):1715–20.
30) Jagsi R, Li Y, Morrow M, et al. Patient-reported quality of life and satisfaction with cosmetic outcomes after breast conservation and mastectomy with and without reconstruction: results of a survey of breast cancer survivors. Ann Surg (2015) 261(6):1198–206.
31) Pusic AL, Klassen AF, Scott AM, et al. Development of a new patient-reported outcome measure for breast surgery: the BREAST-q. Plast Reconstr Surg (2009) 124(2):345–53.
32) Eltahir Y, Werners LLCH, Dreise MM, et al. Quality-of-life outcomes between mastectomy alone and breast reconstruction: comparison of patient-reported BREAST-q and other health-related quality-of-life measures. Plast Reconstr Surg (2013) 132(2):201e–9e.
33) Atisha DM, Rushing CN, Samsa GP, et al. A national snapshot of satisfaction with breast cancer procedures. Ann Surg Oncol (2015) 22(2):361–9.
34) Kim C, Muktar S, Malata C, Benson JR. Reasons for choosing delayed rather than immediate contralateral prophylactic mastectomy in patients with unilateral breast cancer. Cancer Res (2022) 83:P6-05. doi: 10.1158/1158-7445. (SABCS22-P6-05-44)
35) Kronowitz S, Benson J, Nava M, eds. Oncoplastic and Reconstructive Management of the Breast, Third Edition. CRC Press, Boca Raton, 2020.
36) Morrow M, Harris JR, Schnitt SJ. Surgical margins in lumpectomy for breast cancer; bigger is not better. N Engl J Med (2012) 367(1):79–82.

14

Techniques for Partial and Whole Breast Reconstruction

John R. Benson and Dorin Dumitru

Reconstructive breast cancer surgery refers to mastectomy and whole breast reconstruction, as well as partial breast reconstruction, employing a variety of oncoplastic techniques that have been developed by breast surgeons and often drawn from plastic surgery principles.

14.1 Partial Breast Reconstruction after Breast-Conserving Surgery

Oncoplastic breast surgery (OPBS) encompasses both volume replacement and volume displacement techniques; the former imports additional tissue with a flap to compensate for loss of volume from surgical ablation. By contrast, volume displacement rearranges the remaining breast tissue using methods of glandular advancement that serve to redistribute parenchyma and minimise the cosmetic impact of tumour excision. In effect, the volume loss is absorbed over a wider area with concomitant reshaping of the breast. Volume displacement surgery is less complex than autologous tissue transfer methods without associated donor site morbidity. The reconstructed breast is notably of smaller volume and surgery on the contralateral side is often required for symmetrisation [Figure 14.1]. This applies especially to therapeutic mammoplasty where tumour excision is incorporated into a standard or modified reduction procedure. Volume replacement represents the simplest option for partial breast reconstruction and is usually preferred over techniques for volume displacement that involve more extensive surgery with harvesting a myocutaneous or subcutaneous perforator flap. Volume displacement techniques are only possible in patients with medium to large breasts, while volume replacement techniques are suited to women with small breasts. Techniques for OPBS have been formally classified by Krishna Clough and are divided into two categories based on the extent of breast tissue resection and degree of surgical complexity for reconstruction of the conserved breast:

Level 1: These techniques involve resection of at least 20% of total breast volume and require relatively straightforward volume displacement techniques to achieve an acceptable cosmetic result. These surgical procedures consist of reshaping the breast through advancement, rotation or transposition of existing parenchyma and skin with a resultant decrease in overall breast volume.

Level 2: These techniques involve resection of between 20% and 50% of total breast volume with restoration using methods for either displacement or replacement of breast tissue that may be combined with skin reduction or transfer.

14.1.1 Level 1 OPBS Techniques

When up to 20% of breast volume is resected without any attempt to mobilise and remodel the adjacent glandular tissue, a significant defect in breast contour, shape, and size is likely to ensue. Resection of breast tissue in the upper outer or lower outer quadrants is less likely to result in a noticeable defect compared with resections in more cosmetically sensitive areas such as the upper inner quadrant. The cosmetic outcome after removal of a relatively small volume of tissue can be enhanced by simple mobilisation of breast tissue adjacent to the surgical cavity. The extent of mobilisation required will depend on the size of the defect but may necessitate undermining the whole breastplate. Extensive mobilisation of breast tissue can sometimes threaten the blood supply to both the glandular tissue and overlying skin. This can lead to post-operative necrosis and secondary infection with impairment of aesthetic outcomes and quality of life.[1] Therefore, mobilisation and displacement of glandular tissue using advancement or rotational flaps to fill a defect requires detailed knowledge of breast

DOI: 10.1201/9781003394785-14

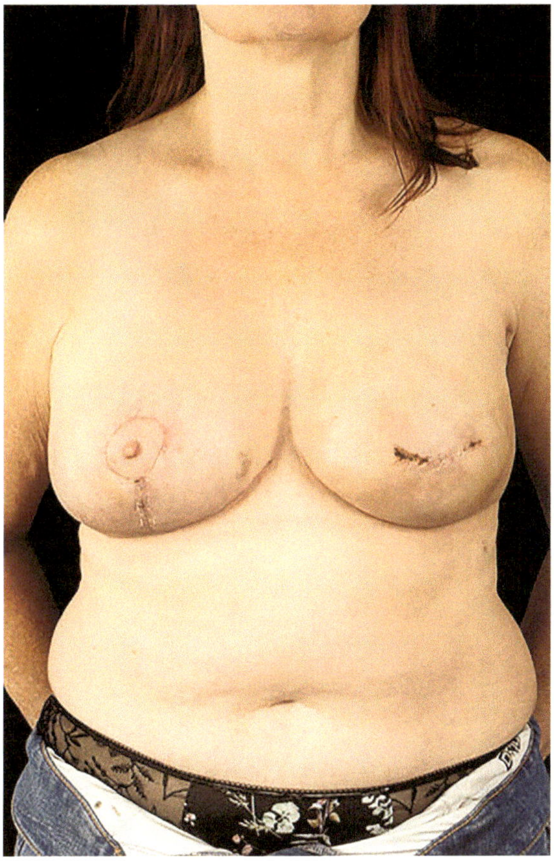

FIGURE 14.1
Surgery on the opposite breast is often necessary for symmetrisation due to loss of overall breast volume whether following mastectomy and whole breast reconstruction or breast-conserving surgery with partial breast reconstruction. The opposite breast can be operated on at the same time as the cancer surgery or at a later date when breast irradiation has been completed and the final size and shape of the breast is apparent (about 10% shrinkage occurs with radiotherapy).

anatomy and appreciation of variations in patterns of vascular supply.[2]

14.1.2 Level 2 OPBS Techniques

Volume displacement techniques: These can be employed to adjust for loss of larger breast volumes (20–50%) and usually involve some form of mammoplasty. The latter include a variety of techniques, such as Wise pattern, batwing, Benelli, round block, and vertical.

These various mammoplasty techniques involve resecting the tumour and a predetermined volume of tissue and skin with rearrangement of the glandular tissue to reform the breast. The refashioned breast is often smaller and less ptotic than the native breast and contralateral breast surgery is frequently indicated for symmetrisation (especially for high percentage excision of breast volume). Depending on tumour location and disease extent, it may be feasible to preserve the nipple-areola complex on a defined pedicle, but otherwise, this structure may need to be sacrificed. An inferior pedicle technique preserves a pyramid of tissue in the inferior portion of the breast to maintain perfusion of the nipple. This can potentially compromise the oncological resection volume for a tumour in the inferior portion of the breast and therefore a superior pedicle is more appropriate [Figure 14.2]. The batwing and hemibatwing mammoplasty are used for tumours in the superior breast that are relatively close to the nipple-areola complex and involve less mobilisation of glandular tissue yet permit excision of tumours with an adequate margin and a good cosmetic result. A symmetrising procedure on the contralateral breast can be undertaken simultaneously with the therapeutic procedure or at a later date following completion of adjuvant treatments, such as chemotherapy and radiotherapy. It is important to allow time for radiotherapy changes to settle before undertaking these complex breast surgical manoeuvres.

Volume replacement techniques: These have previously been reliant on use of the latissimus dorsi flap harvested as either a myo-cutaneous or myo-subcutaneous flap but are increasingly based on local flaps such as chest wall perforator and Grisotti flaps. Chest wall perforator flaps have become popular in recent years as a method for partial breast reconstruction when larger volumes of tissue are resected in the inferior and lateral aspects of the breast. These highly specialised volume replacement techniques include the lateral intercostal artery perforator flap (LICAP), anterior intercostal artery perforator flap (AICAP), medial intercostal artery perforator flap (MICAP), and the thoracodorsal artery perforator (TDAP) [Figure 14.3]. These techniques are often employed in women with smaller breasts and a relatively low body mass index (BMI).[3–6]

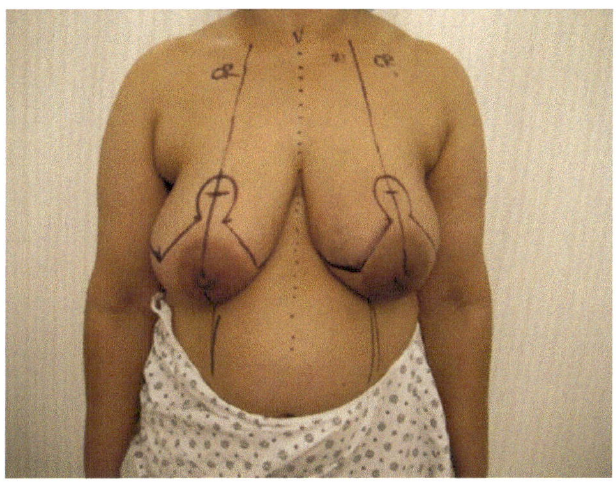

FIGURE 14.2
A therapeutic mammoplasty is best performed using a superior pedicle as an inferior pedicle can potentially restrict the volume of tissue that is resected for extirpation of the cancer.

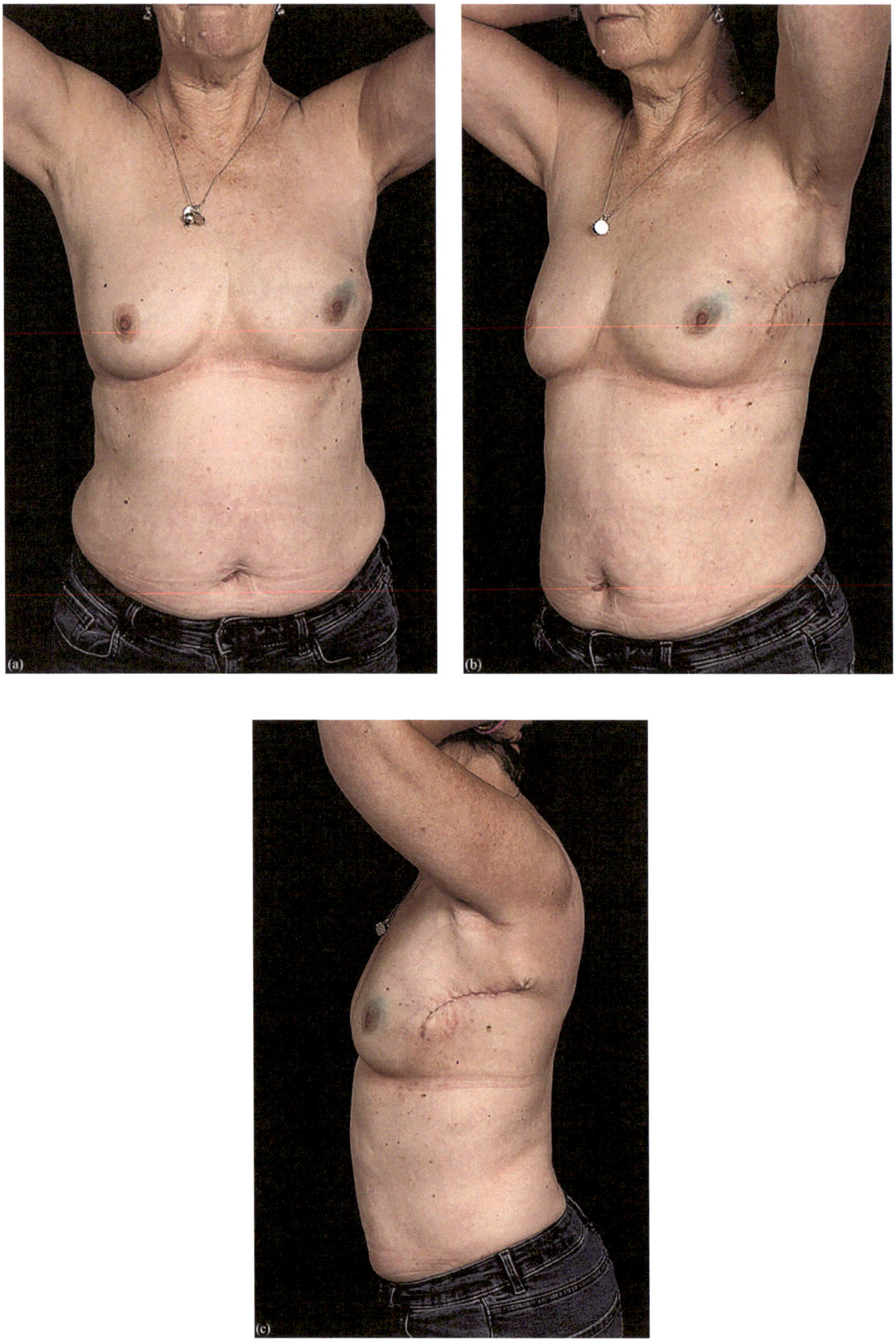

FIGURE 14.3
(a, b, c) Chest wall perforator flaps are especially well-suited to partial breast reconstruction following resection of tumours in the upper outer quadrant of the left breast. The thoracodorsal perforator flap (TDAP) is based on the same vascular pedicle as the latissimus dorsi myocutaneous flap. The lateral row of perforators does not penetrate the muscle and allows for mobilisation of the TDAP flap. Note the relatively long scar associated with this surgical procedure.

Other methods for enhancing breast volume include lipo-modelling that has recently had a renaissance in the context of breast cancer surgery. This is especially useful as an adjunctive technique to 'plump up' mastectomy skin flap thickness around implants and restoring volume following breast conservation. Lipo-modelling involves harvesting fat from a donor site, such as the lateral thigh, hip, lower back, buttocks, or abdomen, filtering the fat and injecting into the breast to improve volume, shape, and symmetry. It can also be used to fill localised mastectomy flap defects after whole breast reconstruction. The benefits of fat grafting relate to its biocompatibility, availability, versatility, and ability to integrate into host tissues and survive. Lipo-modelling can result in improved aesthetic outcomes but has some notable disadvantages, especially pertaining to the donor site where there may be a defect or cellulite like appearance in the long term. Moreover, short-term bruising can be associated with significant morbidity for patients. Only about half of the injected fat is likely to be retained at the recipient site with significant local absorption of grafted fat tissue a persistent problem.[7,8] In addition, there are risks of fat necrosis and oil cyst formation as well as a necessity for multiple courses of lipo-modelling that require general anaesthesia. Nonetheless, lipo-modelling has permitted correction of intractable breast deformities and minor asymmetries that were previously difficult to ameliorate surgically.

A wide range of OPBS techniques are now available and selection of the optimal method for any individual patient is dependent on breast size, degree of ptosis, tumour location (quadrant) and patient preference. In terms of patient satisfaction, it is important that expectations are realistic and patients understand that their overall breast size may be reduced and scarring can be more extensive than anticipated for some level II OPBS techniques (especially chest wall perforator flaps).

Careful planning of skin incisions and appropriate orientation of the nipple-areola complex pedicle is essential when performing more complex volume displacement techniques that demand detailed knowledge of the blood supply of the breast and appreciation of plastic surgery principles. This applies particularly to transposition of glandular tissue when there has been extensive undermining from both chest wall and skin and secondary pedicles have been created during a classical Wise-pattern (therapeutic) mammoplasty. The nipple-areola complex must be preserved on a robust pedicle—be this superior or inferior. These more complex cases of OPBS often demand a multidisciplinary approach involving collaboration between plastic and breast surgeons for optimal outcomes.

It is important to take account of adjuvant treatment effects upon surgical outcomes for OPBS; any reduction in final breast volume and shape can be unpredictable following radiotherapy. The ultimate aesthetic result may fall short of patient and surgeon expectations even in the absence of any technical challenges during surgery or complications thereafter.

14.2 Whole Breast Reconstruction

Breast reconstruction can be performed at the time of mastectomy (immediate breast reconstruction [IBR]) or at any time after mastectomy (delayed breast reconstruction [DBR]). In recent years, IBR has gained wider acceptance with improved cosmetic results and reassuring evidence that reconstruction does not mask detection of recurrent disease.[9–13] Furthermore, there are documented psychological benefits from IBR and patients awake from anaesthesia with two breasts. By contrast, patients must endure being flat for a period of time whilst awaiting DBR. Nowadays, patients most frequently request IBR and studies with PROMS have shown high levels of satisfaction for IBR (although some studies report higher scores for DBR as patients may compare the reconstructed breast with a flat chest rather than a native breast).

For some patients, mastectomy is mandated for breast cancer treatment based on factors such as the tumour: breast ratio, multifocal/centric tumours, or perhaps failed attempts at BCS. A decision for mastectomy may also relate to age, genetic predisposition, and availability of IBR. Not all patients seek IBR and this may be contraindicated for some patients based on co-morbidities, BMI, and smoking history. When proceeding with IBR, one of the most important early decisions is whether the nipple-areola complex should be preserved, and this will be determined on grounds of oncological safety, aesthetic benefit, and patient wishes. If pre-operative imaging reveals no direct involvement of the nipple by tumour, then nipple preservation is usually feasible and several studies have confirmed the safety of NSM in terms of local recurrence.[14,15] Nonetheless, some surgeons prefer to take nipple biopsies either pre-operatively with a needle or intra-operatively with frozen section examination of the specimen.

Many breast units have strict selection criteria for IBR with smoking status and BMI being of paramount importance. A BMI in excess of 30 is associated with a fourfold increase in major complications following IBR, but in reality, most breast units set a BMI threshold between 32 and 35 for IBR.[16,17] It is essential that patients understand the relative risks and benefits associated with IBR, especially for autologous tissue reconstruction and show compliance with post-operative guidance/instruction.

Skin incisions for skin- and nipple-sparing mastectomy should be discussed between the surgeon and patient, but a peri-areolar incision (+/− medial/lateral extensions) and infra-mammary fold (IMF) incision, respectively, are conventionally used. The IMF incision is generally used for smaller breasts with no pre-operative ptosis, but a radial incision can be employed for more central access to the breast parenchyma [Figure 14.4].

The technique for performing either skin- or nipple-sparing mastectomy should respect the oncological plane and ensure that dissection is confined to the plane between the anterior lamella of the superficial fascia and the subcutaneous tissue. It is crucial that subcutaneous blood vessels are preserved and flaps are not too thin as this will compromise viability and lead to areas of flap necrosis. Adequate access is imperative to ensure that dissection continues to the extreme medial and superior limits of the breast; a separate axillary incision can be made if necessary to approach the ligament of Spence and axillary contents. Some patients require reduction of the breast skin envelope, and this will usually be undertaken with a Wise pattern incision and an inferior dermal sling can be created to support the reconstruction.

14.2.1 Autologous Tissue- or Implant-Based Reconstruction

Breast reconstruction can be performed using either prosthetic material or autologous tissue whether this is IBR or DBR. It is recommended that patients meet with a plastic surgeon early on to discuss options for reconstruction and be fully informed about these,

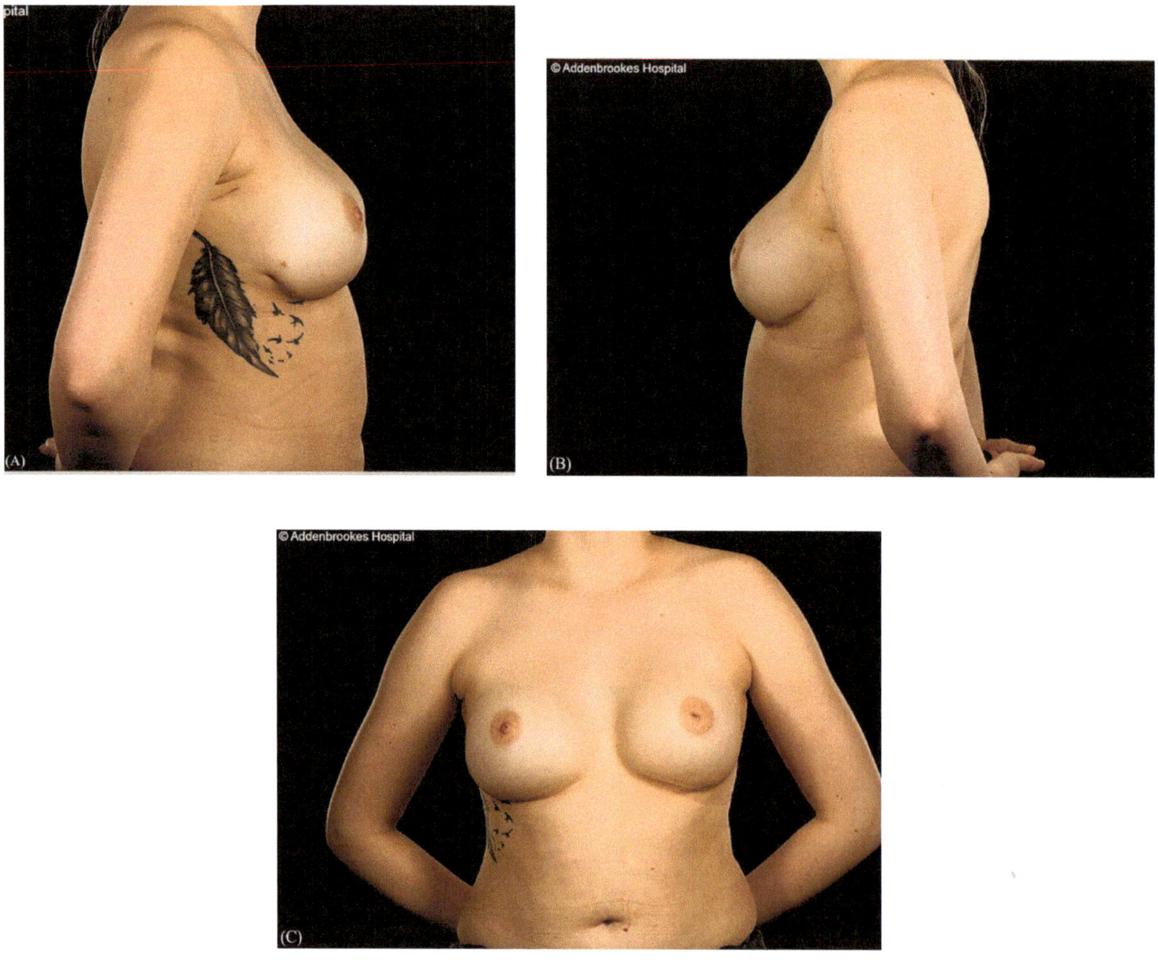

FIGURE 14.4
Nipple-sparing mastectomy preserves the entire breast skin envelope and is usually undertaken with an infra-mammary fold incision. High-risk patient (BRCA1 gene mutation) having undergone bilateral risk-reducing mastectomy and immediate reconstruction with pre-pectoral implants and acellular dermal matrix: (A) frontal view, (B) right lateral, (C) left lateral. Skin incisions are within the infra-mammary fold and not visible in the frontal image but just discernible in the lateral views.

especially with regards to various types of autologous reconstruction; patients may underestimate the complexity and risks of surgery involving tissue transfer techniques.

Autologous tissue reconstruction most commonly involves one of three types of flaps:

1. Latissimus dorsi (LD) flap
2. Transverse rectus abdominis myocutaneous (TRAM) flap
3. Deep inferior epigastric artery perforator flap (DIEP)

Interestingly, the use of the LD flap in conjunction with an implant (implant-assisted LD flap) for breast reconstruction has dramatically fallen in recent years with the advent of acellular dermal matrices that provide alternative coverage and support for an implant.[18,19] Similarly, a totally autologous LD flap is now less frequently performed with emergence of pre-pectoral approaches to implant-based breast reconstruction that minimise animation and reduce post-operative pain. The TRAM flap provides generous tissue bulk for reconstruction purposes and supplementation with an implant is unnecessary. These abdominal flap-based reconstructions have pedicle and free-flap variants and are more technically challenging with a greater risk of complications, especially when a microvascular anastomosis is involved. The free-TRAM flap necessitates harvesting of some anterior abdominal wall musculature with associated morbidity. The DIEP flap involves dissection and isolation of vascular perforators that pass from the inferior epigastric artery to the rectus muscle fibres. The latter therefore remain intact without compromise of abdominal wall integrity but retaining viability of a large infra-umbilical pannus of skin and subcutaneous tissue for reconstruction of the breast. The evolution of the free-TRAM into the DIEP flap has helped reduce donor site morbidity, but there remains a finite risk of complete flap failure. This is generally between 3% and 5% and surgeon-specific rates should be made available to patients who may prefer not to embark on these higher-risk reconstructive procedures. Preoperative CT angiography has helped predict the likelihood of a successful DIEP flap reconstruction by identifying candidate perforators and conversely indicating those patients who are technically unsuitable for this procedure.[20]

14.2.2 Implant-Based Reconstruction

Implant-based procedures are the most commonly performed type of reconstruction worldwide and constitute about 70% of breast reconstructions in the UK (and an increasing proportion of cases in the United States). This represents a simpler reconstructive option and has a more acceptable risk profile for many patients than autologous tissue reconstruction. A particular advantage of implant-based IBR is a more rapid return to work and daily activities, including domestic responsibilities and other social commitments. Most women prefer to retain the same breast size, but bilateral mastectomy and implant reconstruction provide the option for either downsizing or upsizing.

Implant-based reconstruction is technically easier and faster to perform but can be associated with an overall complication rate of 25% and a recent national audit done in the UK revealed a mean implant loss rate of almost 10%.[21]

Key issues with implant-based reconstruction relate to type of implant (fixed volume or expander), anatomical site (sub-pectoral or pre-pectoral), shape (bidimensional or round), and implant size.

Type of implant: Round implants provide uniform projection all around and especially in the upper pole. Rotation of such implants has minimal consequence in terms of cosmetic appearance. By contrast, bi-dimensional implants are teardrop in shape and more closely mimic the natural anatomical shape of the breast. Fixed-volume implants are exactly as their name implies and have an immutable size and volume compared with expander implants whose volume is adjustable via a port that is tunnelled subcutaneously. A low fill-volume can be employed initially to relieve any pressure on the mastectomy flaps/wound during healing and then slowly inflated. Expanders can be temporary or permanent and ports can be removed separately if required.

Positioning of implant: Fixed-volume implants and tissue expanders can be placed in a sub-muscular location with either complete muscle coverage (beneath a pocket formed from the pectoralis major and serratus anterior muscles) or partial coverage in a dual-plane setting. In the latter scenario, a piece of ADM is sutured between the lateral border of pectoralis major superiorly, and the chest wall inferiorly to complete the implant pocket. Increasingly, the implant is placed in a pre-pectoral location without disruption of the pectoralis major muscle. In consequence, there is no muscle animation, less post-operative pain, and evidence of less capsular contracture.[22] A potential disadvantage of pre-pectoral implants is rippling, which is more apparent in patients with a lower BMI (<24) and hence thinner flaps. Lipo-filing can subsequently be employed to 'plump up' and improve overall contour of the flaps. Emerging data including a meta-analysis suggests there is no difference in patient reported outcome measures (BreastQ scores) between pre-pectoral and sub-pectoral implant reconstruction, but there are significant differences in rates of capsular contracture, animation deformity, and prosthesis failure that favour pre-pectoral placement of implants. In addition to issues such as pain and animation, dissection of a sub-pectoral pocket with elevation of the pectoralis major muscle in a dual-plane approach with ADM can cause significant upper limb morbidity with associated arm weakness.[23]

Complications of implants: The current (fifth) generation of implants are composed of material that is unlikely to cause an issue with longevity and necessitate routine replacement. Capsular contracture is an individual response of the host and exacerbated by exposure to radiation that may require further surgery with capsulotomy and implant exchange. Breast-implant-associated anaplastic large-cell lymphoma (BIA-ALCL) and breast-implant-related illness are well-publicised conditions and remain poorly understand, but explanation of associated risks is part of the standard consent process. The risk of BIA-ALCL is commonly quoted as 1 in 28,000, but figures vary widely. This rare form of lymphoma arises in an effusion or scar capsule and patients are warned that any sudden breast swelling occurring more than 8–10 years from the time of original surgery should be investigated to exclude BIA-ALCL. Fluid aspirated from around the implant can be tested for CD30 and the disease-specific marker ALK (anaplastic lymphoma kinase), reflecting a translocation in the tyrosine kinase receptor gene. Treatment in most cases is local and involves excision of the capsule and removal of the implant with later stages sometimes requiring systemic treatment with chemotherapy that is more effective for ALK positive cases.[24]

Radiotherapy has a major impact on aesthetic outcomes following irradiation of skin and remaining breast parenchyma after OPBS and in the context of post-mastectomy radiotherapy (PMRT) with whole breast implant-based reconstruction. Although all cases of breast conservation will require radiotherapy, often a final decision on PMRT is made post-operatively when results of definitive histopathology are available. Nonetheless, PMRT may be anticipated, and this will be factored into the decision-making process in terms of surgical approach. Reports to date suggest that ADM offers some protection from radiotherapy effects and pre-pectoral reconstruction is not associated with significantly higher rates of capsular contracture following PMRT.[25,26]

14.3 Complications of Oncoplastic Surgery

Complications relating to breast surgery patients are generally of mild to moderate severity and lie somewhere between grade 1 and grade 3b based on the Dindo classification system.[27] Nonetheless, these levels of complication can cause significant harm to a patient's physical and mental well-being as well as trust in their surgeon. Neoadjuvant chemotherapy (NACT) patients often require some form of oncoplastic or reconstructive surgery on completion of induction chemotherapy and are more susceptible to surgical complications. The latter may lead to delays in either radiotherapy (breast, chest wall, regional nodes) or systemic adjuvant treatments; the latter are increasingly being used in patients with residual disease following NACT (e.g. capecitabine, CDK 4/6 inhibitors, immunotherapy). Major complications and problems with wound healing can impact significantly on breast cancer outcomes in terms of disease-free and overall survival. Therefore, efforts should be made to minimise the incidence of any adverse surgical events, and patients carefully selected for more complex reconstructive procedures with cessation of smoking at least 6 weeks before surgery and optimal BMI. In addition, there should be judicious use of surgical adjuvant materials with administration of antibiotics and thromboembolic prophylaxis where indicated (Figure 14.5).

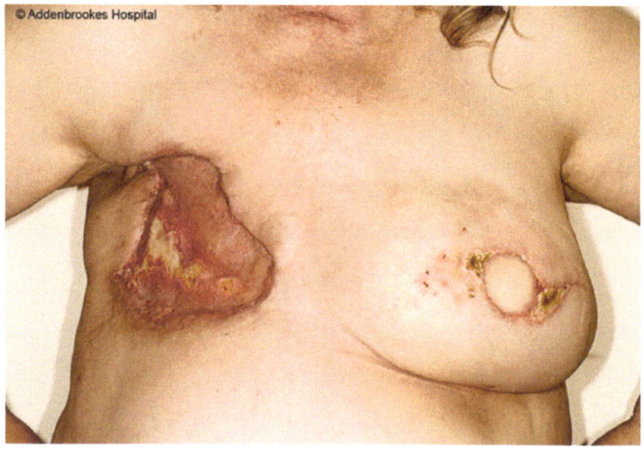

FIGURE 14.5
A patient with a failed deep inferior epigastric perforator flap reconstruction secondary to thrombosis within the venous anastomosis. The entire flap became necrotic and required debridement with chest wall coverage using a meshed split-skin graft.

References

1) Blok YL, Verduijn PS, Corion LUM, et al. An analysis of complication rates and the influence on patient satisfaction and cosmetic outcomes following oncoplastic breast surgery. J Plast Reconstr Aesthet Surg (2022) 75(11):4152–9.
2) Massey EJD, Gouveia PF, Nos C, et al. A new level 1 oncoplastic technique for breast conserving surgery: rotation glandular flap. Breast (2013) 22(2):186–9.
3) Hamdi M, Van Landuyt K, Monstrey S, Blondeel P. Pedicled perforator flaps in breast reconstruction: a new concept. Br J Plast Surg (2004) 57(6):531–9.
4) Hamdi M, Van Landuyt K, de Frene B, et al. The versatility of the inter-costal artery perforator (ICAP) flaps. J Plast Reconstr Aesthet Surg (2006) 59(6):644–52.
5) Hamdi M, Spano A, Landuyt KV, et al. The lateral intercostal artery perforators: anatomical study and clinical application in breast surgery. Plast Reconstr Surg (2008) 121(2):389–96.
6) McCulley SJ, Schaverien MV, Tan VKM, Macmillan RD. Lateral thoracic artery perforator (LTAP) flap in partial breast reconstruction. J Plast Reconstr Aesthet Surg (2015) 68(5):686–91.
7) Sowa Y, Inafuku N, Tsuge I, et al. Patient-reported outcomes after autologous fat grafting in prosthetic breast reconstruction: prospective cohort study using a multivariate analysis. Ann Plast Surg (2023) 90(2):123–7.
8) Groen JW, Negenborn VL, Twisk JWR, et al. Autologous fat grafting in cosmetic breast augmentation: a systematic review on radiological safety, complications, volume retention, and Patient/Surgeon satisfaction. Aesthet Surg J (2016) 36(9):993–1007.
9) Siotos C, Naska A, Bello RJ, et al. Survival and disease recurrence rates among breast cancer patients following mastectomy with or without breast reconstruction. Plast Reconstr Surg (2019) 144(2):169e–77e.
10) Bargon CA, Young-Afat DA, Ikinci M, et al. Breast cancer recurrence after immediate and delayed postmastectomy breast reconstruction: a systematic review and meta-analysis. Cancer (2022) 128 (19):3449–69.
11) Nedumpara T, Jonker L, Williams MR. Impact of immediate breast reconstruction on breast cancer recurrence and survival. Breast (2011) 20(5):437–43.
12) Costeira B, da Silva FB, Oom R, et al. Locoregional recurrence in skin-sparing and nipple-sparing mastectomies. J Surg Oncol (2022) 125(3):352–60.
13) Langstein HN, Cheng MH, Singletary SE, et al. Breast cancer recurrence after immediate reconstruction: patterns and significance. Plast Reconstr Surg (2003) 111(2):712–20.
14) De La Cruz L, Moody AM, Tappy EE, et al. Overall survival, disease-free survival, local recurrence, and nipple-areolar recurrence in the setting of nipple-sparing mastectomy: a meta-analysis and systematic review. Ann Surg Oncol (2015) 22(10):3241–9.
15) Smith BL, Tang R, Rai U, et al. Oncologic safety of nipple-sparing mastectomy in women with breast cancer. J Am Coll Surg (2017) 225(3):361–5.
16) Srinivasa DR, Clemens MW, Qi J, et al. Obesity and breast reconstruction: complications and patient-reported outcomes in a multicenter, prospective study. Plast Reconstr Surg (2020) 145(3):481E–90E.
17) Panayi AC, Agha RA, Sieber BA, Orgill DP. Impact of obesity on outcomes in breast reconstruction: a systematic review and meta-analysis. J Reconstr Microsurg (2018) 34(5):363–75.
18) Kankam HKN, Hourston GJM, Fopp LJ, et al. Trends in post-mastectomy breast reconstruction types at a breast cancer tertiary referral centre before and after introduction of acellular dermal matrices. J Plast Reconstr Aesthet Surg (2018) 71(1):21–7.
19) Leff DR, Bottle A, Mayer E, et al. Trends in immediate postmastectomy breast reconstruction in the United Kingdom. Plast Reconstr Surg Glob Open (2015) 3(9):e507.
20) Ngaage LM, Oni G, Di Pace B, et al. The effect of CT angiography and venous couplers on surgery duration in microvascular breast reconstruction: a single operator's experience. Gland Surg (2018) 7(5):44048–448.
21) Potter S, Conroy EJ, Cutress RI, et al. Short-term safety outcomes of mastectomy and immediate implant-based breast reconstruction with and without mesh (iBRA): a multicentre, prospective cohort study. Lancet Oncol (2019) 20(2):254–66.
22) Ostapenko E, Nixdorf L, Devyatko Y, et al. Prepectoral versus subpectoral implant-based breast reconstruction: a systemic review and metaanalysis. Ann Surg Oncol (2023) 30(1):126–36.
23) Le NK, Persing S, Dinis J, et al. A comparison of BREAST-q scores between prepectoral and subpectoral direct-to-Implant breast reconstruction. Plast Reconstr Surg (2021) 148(5):708E–14E.
24) Turton P, El-Sharkawi D, Lyburn I, et al. UK guidelines on the diagnosis and treatment of breast implant-associated anaplastic large cell lymphoma on behalf of the medicines and healthcare products regulatory agency plastic, reconstructive and aesthetic surgery expert advisory group. Br J Haematol (2021) 192(3): 444–58.
25) Craig ES, Clemens MW, Koshy JC, et al. Outcomes of acellular dermal matrix for immediate tissue expander reconstruction with radiotherapy: a retrospective cohort study. Aesthet Surg J (2019) 39(3):279–88.
26) Sobti N, Weitzman RE, Nealon KP, et al. Evaluation of capsular contracture following immediate prepectoral versus subpectoral direct-to-implant breast reconstruction. Sci Rep (2020) 10(1):1–11.
27) Dindo D, Demartines N, Clavien PA, Clavien PA. Classification of surgical complications a new proposal with evaluation in a cohort of 6336 patients and results of a survey. Ann Surg (2004) 240(2):205–13.

15

Risk-Reducing Surgery, Ductal Carcinoma In Situ, Neoadjuvant Chemotherapy

John R. Benson

15.1 Risk Reducing Surgery

Genetic predisposition to breast cancer: In recent years there has been an upsurge of interest in identifying women with genetic predisposition and this has been facilitated by enhanced understanding of the genetic basis for breast cancer susceptibility derived from genome-wide linkage analysis and mutational screening. The focus has shifted from high-penetrance genes to intermediate- and low-penetrance mutations that confer lower levels of risk individually but collectively are more significant. Genetic counselling and testing for breast cancer predisposition has been formally implemented in many countries and the number of women seeking genetic testing continues to rise. Nonetheless, despite these advances in genetics, approximately 30% of familial breast cancer risk remains unaccounted for by mutations in currently known genes. Moreover, genetic changes do not necessarily have a causative association with a diseased state and phenotypic manifestations of cancer are variable. The clinical management of women with an asymptomatic mutation in BRCA1 or BRCA2 and those with carriage of a mutation in other high-risk genes, such as TP53, PALB2, or pTEN, is increasingly complex. Approaches include screening, chemoprevention, and risk-reducing surgery, but the outcomes of these different interventions for risk reduction remain variable in terms of accuracy of data and levels of certainty. In particular, although an intervention may reduce the chance of developing breast cancer, this may not translate into a reduction in mortality with gains in both breast-cancer-specific and overall survival. No randomised trials have addressed the impact of these risk-reducing strategies on either incidence or survival outcomes with much of the evidence for efficacy derived from observational studies that are prone to systematic biases. It important that women with a hereditary predisposition are fully informed about the limitations of the existing knowledge base relating to risk-reducing interventions for breast cancer.

Risk reduction strategies: Once an asymptomatic woman has been identified as a carrier of a documented high-risk gene mutation (BRCA1, BRCA2, PALB2, p53), options for management include screening, chemoprevention, and risk-reducing surgery. Decision-making for these high-risk individuals can be challenging, and sometimes a woman may choose a combination of more than one option depending on personal circumstances and estimated levels of risk. For instance, a BRCA1 mutation carrier may elect to undergo breast cancer screening until she has had her children and completed breastfeeding. She may subsequently opt for risk-reducing surgery with initial bilateral mastectomy, followed by bilateral salpingo-oophorectomy (BSO) in her early 40s.

For women with a genetic predisposition to breast cancer, risk-reducing surgery likely offers the greatest potential benefit in terms of decreasing the chance of developing breast cancer. Bilateral prophylactic mastectomy (BPM) reduces the expected risk of breast cancer by more than 90% among carriers of a gene mutation. In a retrospective study of more than 600 women at moderate to high risk who had undergone bilateral prophylactic mastectomy, the incidence of breast cancer was reduced by 89.5% ($p < 0.001$).[1] An established Gail model for risk estimation was used to predict the number of breast cancer cases expected in these two groups without surgical intervention. This seminal study along with several smaller ones has validated bilateral BPM as a management option for women at increased risk for development of breast cancer. It is claimed that BSO not only reduces ovarian cancer risk but also decreases breast cancer risk by 50% among mutation carriers when undertaken during the pre-menopausal years.[2] This effect is presumably due to oestrogen deprivation and epidemiological studies have shown that for unselected patients, ovarian ablation reduces the risk of breast

DOI: 10.1201/9781003394785-15

cancer in pre-menopausal women by up to two-thirds. When risk-reducing surgery is combined (BPM and BSO), the net reduction in risk of developing breast cancer is 95%.[3] Once again, these estimates of benefit should be interpreted with caution and recent analyses have suggested that much of the apparent benefit of BSO on breast cancer risk might be accounted for by selection bias rather than being a true reduction in risk. It has been argued that oophorectomy should not be recommended as a procedure to specifically reduce breast cancer risk (in conjunction with surveillance imaging) and risk-reducing mastectomy should remain the optimal approach for minimising risk of developing breast cancer in BRCA1 and BRCA2 mutation carriers. The effect of risk-reducing surgery (both BPM and BSO) on breast cancer survival has been difficult to evaluate with much reliance on modelling studies using simulated cohorts. To date, there is no clear evidence that BPM improves breast-cancer-specific or overall survival, but data more strongly supports a breast cancer survival benefit for BSO.[4] Nipple-sparing mastectomy is usually the preferred type of mastectomy for prophylaxis and preservation of the nipple does not attenuate the magnitude of risk reduction [Figure 15.1]. It is important that all breast tissue is excised in the vicinity of the nipple-areola complex with coring out of the nipple but care taken not to compromise the viability of this structure [Figure 15.2].

Notwithstanding these limitations of observational studies, it is highly unlikely that there will ever be randomised evidence available to assess the efficacy of

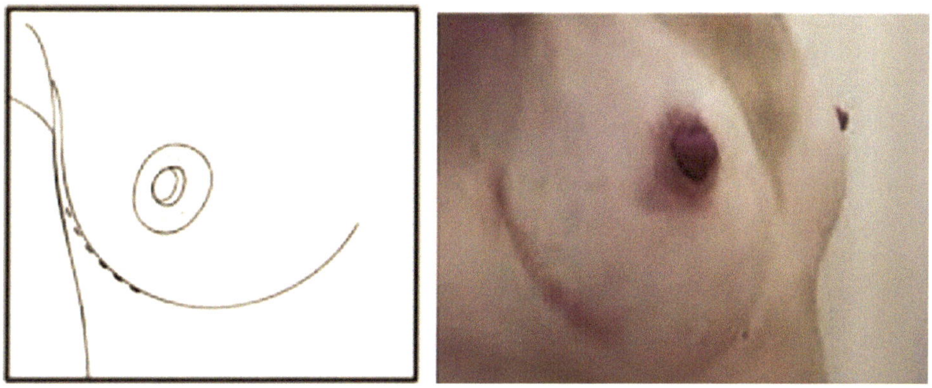

FIGURE 15.1
An infra-mammary fold incision is usually employed for nipple-sparing mastectomy in patients with small to moderate-sized breasts. This avoids any interference with blood supply to the nipple-areola complex but can impede access to the peripheral zones of the breast tissue (especially superiorly) and lead to inadvertent retention of breast tissue.

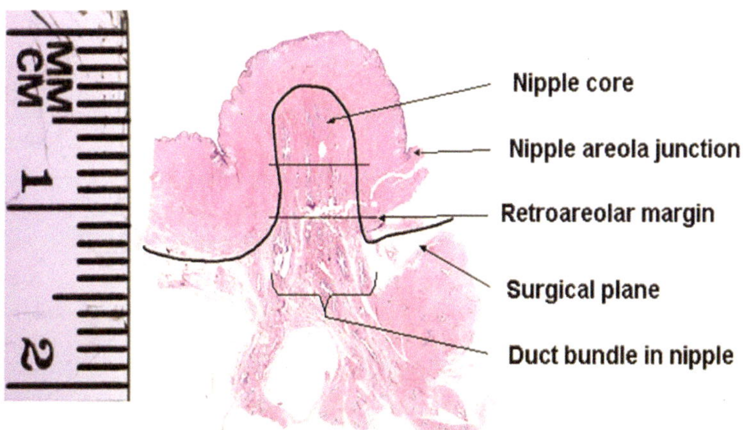

FIGURE 15.2
Section-through tissues of the nipple to show the plane of dissection for safely performing nipple-sparing mastectomy with the removal of the central core of breast tissue but also the preservation of an adequate blood supply to the nipple-areola complex.

Source: **Image courtesy of Miss Jenny Rusby.**

risk-reducing surgery in mutation carriers. The decision to proceed with risk-reducing surgery is greatly influenced by an individual's personal beliefs and values and a woman is unlikely to relinquish her right to self-destiny in this respect. Therefore, future management strategies will be based on observational studies that have consistently shown highly significant benefits in terms of risk-reduction from surgical ablation. An updated Cochrane systematic review examined data on more than 15,000 women undergoing risk-reducing mastectomy with a range of risk factors for breast cancer including a personal history of the disease and carriage of BRCA1 and BRCA2 predisposing genes. In terms of BPM, this procedure was found to be most effective for reducing breast cancer incidence and disease-specific mortality among women with BRCA1 and BRCA2 mutations. Nonetheless, the 21 studies included in this analysis were observational with some methodological limitations and the authors emphasised the need for more rigorous prospective studies (albeit non-randomised).[5]

Interestingly, although rates of BPM have increased in recent years, most women do not opt for prophylactic mastectomy even when good-quality immediate breast reconstruction is available. There can be profound psychological sequela from this radical form of intervention and studies have shown that a small minority (3–6%) of women regretted their decision to choose a surgical option for risk reduction. This is more likely when women have been 'talked into' the operation. Health professionals should inform rather than 'sell' this option; there is a difference between offering and recommending BPM, and the final decision must be left to the patient. Women should be allowed plenty of time to reach a final decision and must fully understand the risks, benefits, and limitations of bilateral risk-reducing surgery; this procedure should probably not be undertaken under the age of 25 years and carefully considered in women over the age of 60 years for whom the mean years of life gained is minimal.

Several of these issues relating to BPM are pertinent to patients with a proven BRCA1/2 gene mutation who develop unilateral breast cancer and seek contralateral risk-reducing surgery in addition to a therapeutic mastectomy. If a BRCA1 or BRCA2 mutation carrier without any personal history of breast cancer is considered eligible for BPM, then a CPM in the same individual must be easier to justify on statistical probability for breast cancer development. The risk of developing contralateral breast cancer in mutation carriers appears to be three or four times greater than that of average risk cohorts. Estimates for the latter are typically between 0.1% and 0.6% per annum (1–6% at 10 years), and hence, the risk of contralateral breast cancer in a BRCA mutation carrier is up to 2% per annum or 20% at 10 years. Moreover, age at diagnosis of the first breast cancer is a significant predictor of contralateral breast cancer risk in BRCA1 and BRCA2 mutation carriers.

There would appear to be a compelling argument for offering CPM in patients with proven hereditary predisposition and/or a strong family history of breast cancer combined with a diagnosis of unilateral breast cancer.[6] Additional factors to consider are dense breast parenchyma, problems with radiological surveillance/recall fatigue, florid benign changes, and fear of cancer (risk aversion). These would strengthen any decision-making process in favour of prophylactic surgery for mutation carriers and perhaps justify contralateral risk-reducing surgery in the absence of any strong family history or genetic predisposition. Although CPM is more readily justified in BRCA mutation carriers with unilateral breast cancer, surgical complications are increased with bilateral surgery. However, these are not simply doubled when CPM with reconstruction is undertaken; the overall rate of complications has been reported to be significantly higher in the cancerous breast group (24.4%) compared with the prophylactic non-cancerous breast group (10%) with notably more major complications in the cancerous group (8.1% versus 3.1%) ($p < 0.05$).[7] Patients should be informed of a *lower* incidence of complications in the non-cancerous group as this may influence their decision to undergo contralateral risk-reducing surgery. Hitherto there has been an assumption that complication rates are doubled for patients who opt for contralateral risk-reducing surgery and bilateral breast reconstruction, but this may be rather simplistic and no studies have previously analysed cancerous and non-cancerous breasts separately.

15.1.1 Ductal Carcinoma In Situ

Unlike many cases of invasive disease, ductal carcinoma in situ (DCIS) is not considered to be a systemic disease and commonly presents as a localised screen-detected malignancy that is amenable to BCS. Management of DCIS is intended to minimise both local recurrence and treatment-related morbidities. Surgery, radiotherapy, and endocrine therapy are treatment modalities that are each utilised either alone or in combination to reduce the risk of local recurrence. Moreover, systemic therapies administered for treatment of DCIS aim to reduce local recurrence, and none of the trials that have assessed various permutations of treatment for DCIS have shown a mortality reduction for one treatment option over another. Clinical trials have shown differences in local recurrence rates for various therapeutic combinations and results thereof have determined management recommendations that have been widely implemented into routine clinical practice. Approximately two-thirds of cases of DCIS detected in the NHS breast-screening programme are high-grade forms of the disease with a greater potential to either progress to invasion if left untreated, or recur after treatment [Figure 15.3a and b]. Ductal carcinoma in situ often presents as microcalcification detected on screening mammography. This tends to be a linear or branching pattern or is more punctate in character. This represents dystrophic calcification in the necrotic centre of ducts. The incidence of DCIS has increased dramatically since introduction of breast cancer screening and now represents approximately one-quarter of newly diagnosed cases of breast cancer [Figure 15.4].

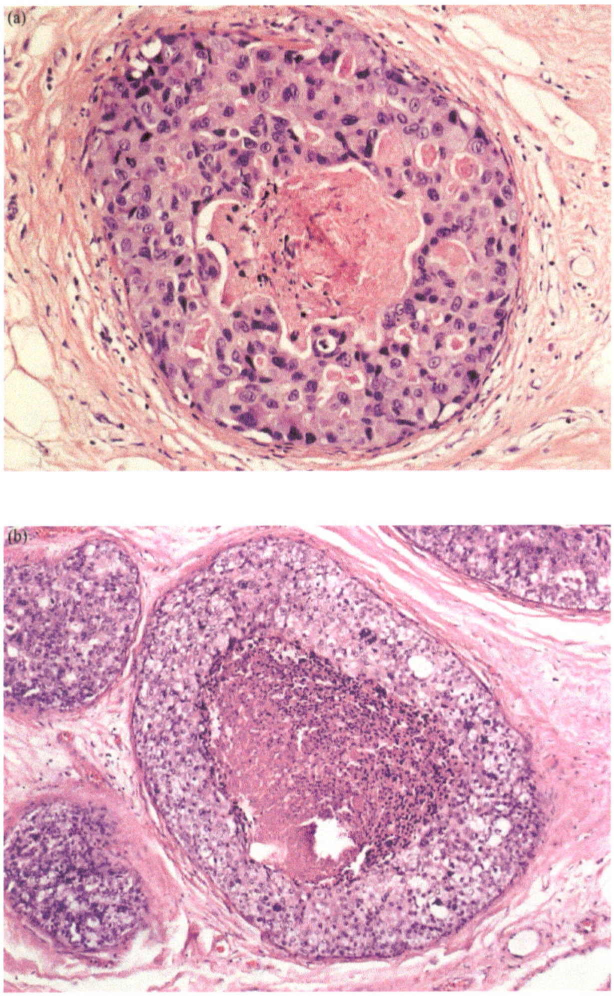

FIGURE 15.3
High-nuclear-grade ductal carcinoma in situ showing typical comedonecrosis in the centre of the ducts. Cells are characterised by enlarged nuclei with marked variation in nuclear size and shape, prominent nucleoli, and scattered mitoses. (a) 20× magnification; (b) 10× magnification.

DCIS that is localised to one quadrant of the breast is generally amenable to some form of BCS. It is important that DCIS is completely excised with clear surgical margins around the lesion. There is persistent controversy as to what constitutes a 'clear margin' for DCIS. The issue of margin width after surgical excision for localised DCIS may be different than invasive carcinoma; DCIS typically has a discontinuous growth pattern and may demand special consideration in terms of surgical clearance. It is estimated that up to 40% of DCIS is associated with skip lesions that can potentially be separated by a distance exceeding a designated negative margin.[8] Therefore, a wider surgical margin may be warranted for optimal resection of DCIS for which up to half of local recurrences following BCS are invasive disease. A meta-analysis of more than 4000 patients in various clinical trials who underwent BCS with radiotherapy for DCIS found that a margin threshold of ≥2 mm was associated with a lower risk of IBTR than <2 mm (i.e. 1 mm or no tumour on ink) with an odds ratio of 0.53 (95% CI 0.26–0.96).[9] It was concluded that a margin width of 2 mm was adequate when breast radiotherapy is administered as adjuvant therapy, and this was echoed by a study-level meta-analysis of local recurrence and threshold widths for negative margin status amongst 7883 patients undergoing BCS with irradiation for DCIS.[10]

Despite clear resection margins after lumpectomy, there is a 25% risk of local recurrence with half these cases being DCIS and the remainder invasive disease. Adjuvant radiotherapy may be administered and reduces risk of local recurrence by about 50% for all age groups. Moreover, radiotherapy has a similar magnitude of effect for invasive breast cancer and DCIS (about 50% reduction in risk of local recurrence for each). Long-term follow-up of the National Surgical Adjuvant Breast and Bowel Project (NSABP) B-17 trial has shown a risk reduction for local recurrence of 43% at 15 years with rates of local recurrence for wide local excision only versus breast irradiation after surgery of 35% and 19.8%, respectively.[11] The proportional reduction in risk was slightly higher for invasive disease with a hazard ratio of 0.48 [95% CI 0.33–0.69 ($p < 0.01$)], thus representing a 52% decrease in the chance of invasive disease recurrence. Nonetheless, despite these dramatic effects upon rates of IBTR, there was no difference in disease-free or overall survival. These findings were echoed by results of the European Organisation for Research and Treatment of Cancer (EORTC) trial that likewise showed a halving of local recurrence but no impact of radiotherapy on distant disease-free or overall survival.[12]

Following surgery and radiotherapy, the risk of local recurrence can be reduced even further by the

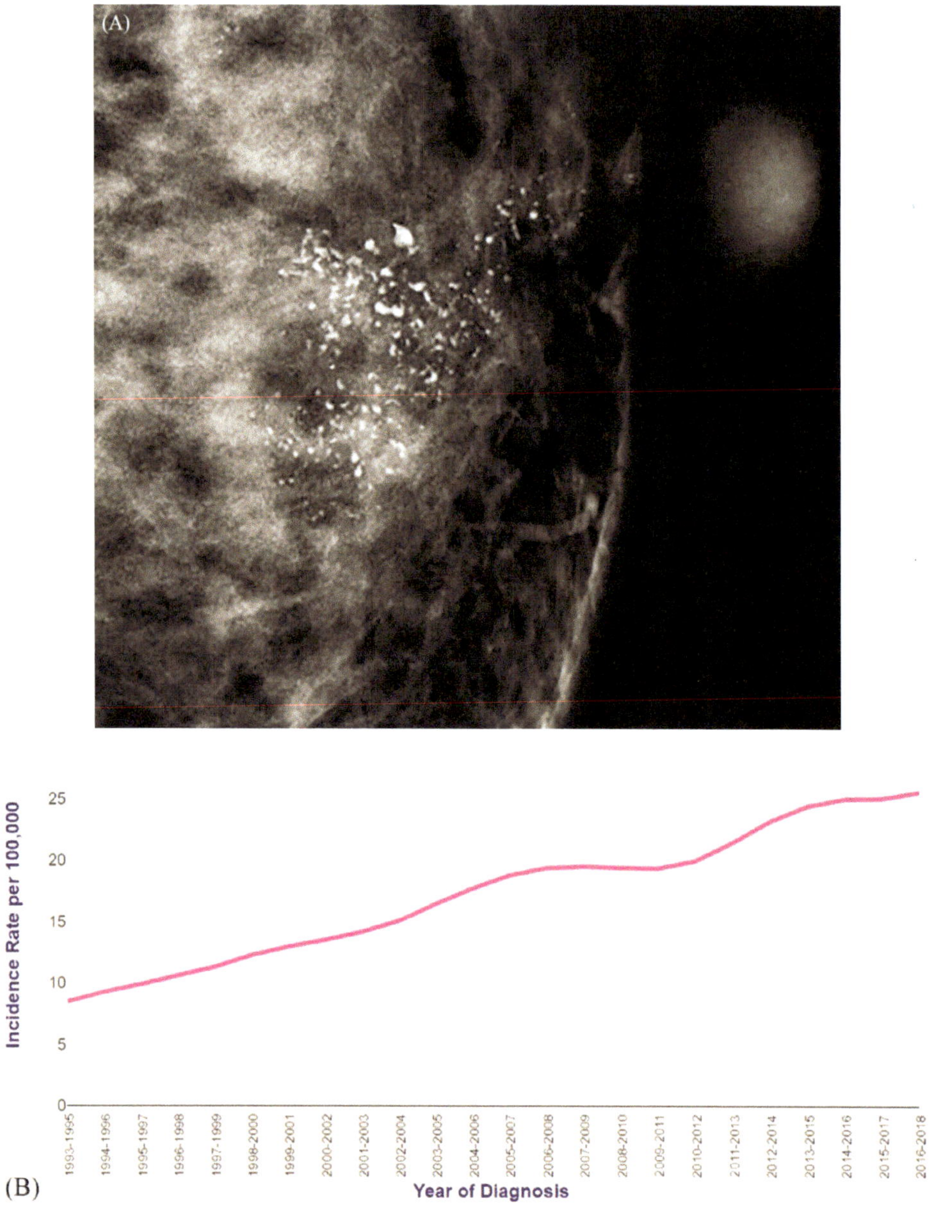

FIGURE 15.4

(A) Ductal carcinoma in situ often presents as microcalcification detected on screening mammography. This either has a linear and branching pattern or is pleiomorphic in character. (B) The incidence of ductal carcinoma in situ has increased threefold in the United Kingdom over the period 1993–2018.

Source: **Cancer Research UK Statistics, with permission, https://www.cancerresearchuk.org/health-professional/cancer-statistics/statistics-by-cancer-type/breast-cancer/incidence-in-situ#heading-Two.**

administration of endocrine therapy (5 years) for patients with hormone receptor (HR)-positive DCIS. Approximately 70–80% of all DCIS cases are positive for oestrogen receptor (ER) and/or progesterone receptor (PR). Tamoxifen is a selective oestrogen receptor modulator and can be used in either pre-menopausal or post-menopausal women. By contrast, aromatase inhibitors are effective only for post-menopausal women for whom peripheral synthesis in fatty tissue is the principal source of oestrogens. The NSABP B-24 trial randomised patients undergoing BCS combined with radiotherapy for localised DCIS to either 5 years of tamoxifen (20 mg daily) or placebo. Rates of local relapse at 15 years follow-up were slightly lower for the group receiving endocrine therapy (13.2% versus 16.6%). These results were only statistically significant for patients with invasive recurrence [HR 0.68 95% CI 0.49–0.95; (p = 0.025)], and there were no differences in breast cancer-specific or overall survival between the tamoxifen and placebo groups. A further analysis of this trial has concluded that there are no statistically significant differences between tamoxifen and placebo groups with minimal benefits from tamoxifen and concerns about overusage of adjuvant endocrine therapy in DCIS patients managed with BCS.[13]

For patients with multi-centric DCIS, total mastectomy is usually mandatory, but a very wide excision with partial breast reconstruction may be possible; oncoplastic surgical procedures permit resection of DCIS measuring up to 70–80 mm in maximum extent. Radiotherapy is usually not required following mastectomy for DCIS, but endocrine therapy might be recommended after unilateral total mastectomy to reduce the risk of a new breast cancer in the contralateral breast. For patients treated with bilateral mastectomy, there is rarely any indication for either radiotherapy or endocrine therapy.

Sentinel lymph node biopsy: This is not usually indicated for most cases of (impalpable) screen-detected DCIS. However, if a patient presents with a palpable lump in the breast and core biopsy reveals DCIS alone, then SLN biopsy should be considered. In such cases, failure to detect invasion might be attributable to under-sampling of the breast mass with needle biopsy, and invasive cancer may subsequently be evident on definitive histology after examination of the entire breast mass. If core biopsy reveals DCIS with micro-invasion, then SLN biopsy should be considered alongside lumpectomy in the event of upstaging from DCIS to invasive disease.

Sentinel node biopsy should be considered for patients with extensive DCIS who undergo mastectomy. There is about a 15% chance that DCIS diagnosed on core biopsy will be upstaged to invasive breast cancer following histological examination of the surgical specimen. As the lymphatic connections between the breast and axillary lymph nodes are abrogated following extirpation of all breast tissue, it may not be possible to subsequently identify the sentinel node and either blind sampling or formal ALND would be indicated.

15.2 Neoadjuvant Chemotherapy

Multimodality approaches to breast cancer management integrate surgery, radiotherapy, and systemic treatments. Increasingly breast cancer is being treated initially with upfront or neoadjuvant systemic therapies followed by surgery. Combination and sequencing of therapies in a shared decision-making process optimises management and avoids over- and under-treatment. There are advantages of neoadjuvant chemotherapy (NACT) for stage III and some larger stage II lesions. These include in vivo determination of tumour sensitivity with a possible change of chemotherapy regimen in the event of a poor response or progressive disease. In theory early administration of systemic therapy can eradicate micrometastatic disease with improvement of distant disease-free and overall survival. Finally, NACT can downstage both the breast tumour and axillary nodes to facilitate surgical resection. It is essential to obtain core biopsy confirmation of invasive carcinoma before commencing induction chemotherapy.[14,15] Moreover, the receptor profile of the tumour (ER, PR, and HER2 status) will determine the likelihood of response to chemotherapy—and in particular the chance of a complete pathological response (pCR) [Figure 15.5].

The role of NACT has expanded from downsizing and down-staging inoperable tumours to treatment of operable early breast cancer.[16] Nonetheless, there have been limited reductions in the extent of surgery following successful response to NACT.[17] This may relate to difficulties in determining the exact pattern of disease response after completion of chemotherapy; there remains poor radio-pathological correlation despite improvements in imaging technologies. The main benefit of down-staging the primary tumour in the context of operable breast cancer is reduction in the tumour: breast size ratio that potentially increases eligibility for BCS if there is *concentric* shrinkage of the tumour and no evidence of multi-centricity, extensive in situ component, lymphovascular invasion, and a non-lobular phenotype. Improvements in the efficacy of chemotherapy and targeted therapies over the past decade have increased rates of pCR for

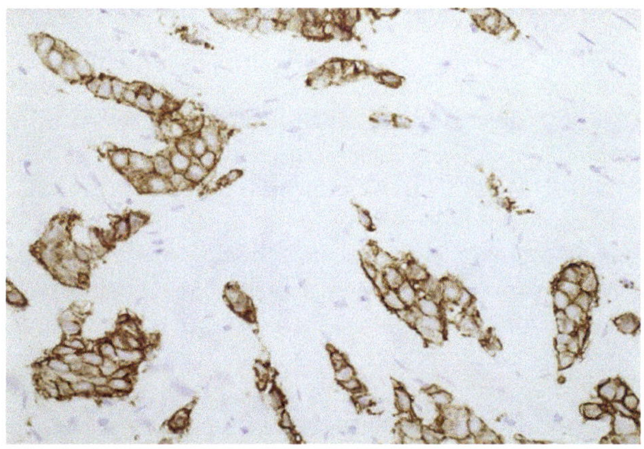

FIGURE 15.5
Invasive carcinoma showing positive membranous (3+) for HER2 on immunohistochemistry. For tumours with less intensive staining (2+), fluorescent in situ hybridisation is performed as a supplementary test to assess HER2 status. About one-quarter of invasive cancers are HER2 positive and eligible for anti-HER2 treatments (20× magnification).

phenotype appropriate early stage breast cancer.[18] Thus, invasive and sometimes non-invasive disease can be completely eliminated in the breast and axilla in those patients with specific phenotypes, namely, triple-negative cancers lacking expression of both hormone receptors and HER2 receptors as well as HER2-positive tumours (irrespective of ER and PR levels) [Figure 15.6]. The rate of pCR for triple-negative tumours is between 40% and 50 % whilst rates of up to 60–65% can be achieved for HER2 positive tumours.[19] A complete pathological response rate renders patients more amenable to BCS and reduces the chance of local relapse after either mastectomy or BCS. Moreover, this subgroup of patients with a pCR in both the breast and axilla have improved longer term survival.[16,18] Therefore, pCR is a powerful prognostic factor and correlates with improved disease-free survival at 3 years; it can be viewed as a surrogate biomarker for effects of chemotherapy on distant micrometastases.

Typically, two-thirds of NACT patients overall have residual disease post-chemotherapy and require surgical excision for local control. The majority of patients previously underwent mastectomy following chemotherapy but can now be safely offered breast conservation therapy if strict selection criteria are applied. Surgical resection has hitherto been necessary to determine pathological response and confirm the presence or absence of residual disease. Between one-half and two-thirds of patients with a complete radiological response will be found subsequently to have a pCR. Conversely, one-third of patients with a pCR will have radiological evidence of residual disease, and there is much variation in reported rates of diagnostic accuracy for various imaging modalities in terms of negative predictive value (NPV) and false negative rate (FNR). There is generally poor clinico-radiological/pathological correlation for combined modality treatment.[20] It remains a challenge to consistently identify residual tumour with any imaging modality be that ultrasound, magnetic resonance imaging (MRI), PET-CT, or dynamic imaging with F-FDG PET. The sensitivity of MRI is about 90%, but its accuracy depends on the type of tumour and neoadjuvant chemotherapy schedule; sensitivity is highest for ER-negative, HER2-positive, and triple-negative tumours and lowest for luminal subtypes. MRI has high sensitivity for detection of residual cancer provided this is not scattered microscopic foci, but there is much heterogeneity for specificity. A radio-opaque titanium clip should be placed at the start of chemotherapy under ultrasound guidance and will permit identification of the tumour bed in the event of a complete radiological response. This ensures accuracy of surgical resection by acting as a target for localisation (using a conventional guide-wire or one of several novel technologies such as paramagnetic steel or radioactive seeds and radiofrequency/radar localisation devices). *Patterns of response:* Tumours do not necessarily shrink in a symmetric and concentric fashion but may reduce in volume and bulk in a honeycomb fashion with viable cancer cells persisting throughout the initial tumour area. It is often difficult to assess both the extent and pattern of tumour regression in response to chemotherapy from radiological imaging. The pattern of response is related to tumour subtype with triple-negative cancers and non-luminal HER2-positive tumours exhibiting concentric shrinkage or volume reduction with an early response and few residual histological changes when a pCR occurs [Figure 15.7a]. By contrast, luminal tumours (ER/PR positive; HER2 negative) are characterised by diffuse cell loss and have different stromal characteristics with lower proliferative activity [Figure 15.7b]. There is an increased risk of local recurrence that is likely attributable to incomplete resection of residual disease post-chemotherapy. It is safe to proceed with BCS if selection criteria are satisfied and the radiological appearances at the end of chemotherapy are consistent with concentric shrinkage of a unifocal lesion. A localised wide excision of impalpable residual tumour is performed that aims to remove any residual tumour together with 1–2 cm of normal surrounding breast tissue or 2 cm of breast tissue around a clip if there has been a complete radiological response and no residual lesion is detectable. The minimum margin of clearance for wide local excision post-NACT is 'no ink on tumour' and special immuno-histochemical staining is necessary to exclude the presence of scattered tumour cells. When there is an extensive area of residual DCIS even if in the absence of residual invasive disease, then re-excision or mastectomy is indicated.

Omission of surgery: Several ongoing and upcoming trials are evaluating the safety of eliminating breast (and axillary) surgery following chemotherapy in phenotype appropriate cases (TNBC and HER2 positive). These include stage T1-2, N0-1 tumours measuring less than 5 cm at presentation with a complete or partial/near complete radiological response. Patients undergo needle biopsy of the tumour bed with either large gauge vacuum-assisted or standard core biopsy. Those patients with no residual disease on biopsy do not proceed to breast surgery but have the option of breast irradiation. Patients with residual disease undergo standard loco-regional treatment with lumpectomy and breast irradiation. Results of trials to date suggest that breast surgery might safely be omitted for phenotype-appropriate stage T1-2N0 tumours without any residuum on imaging and a negative vacuum-assisted needle biopsy of the tumour bed. Breast surgery with

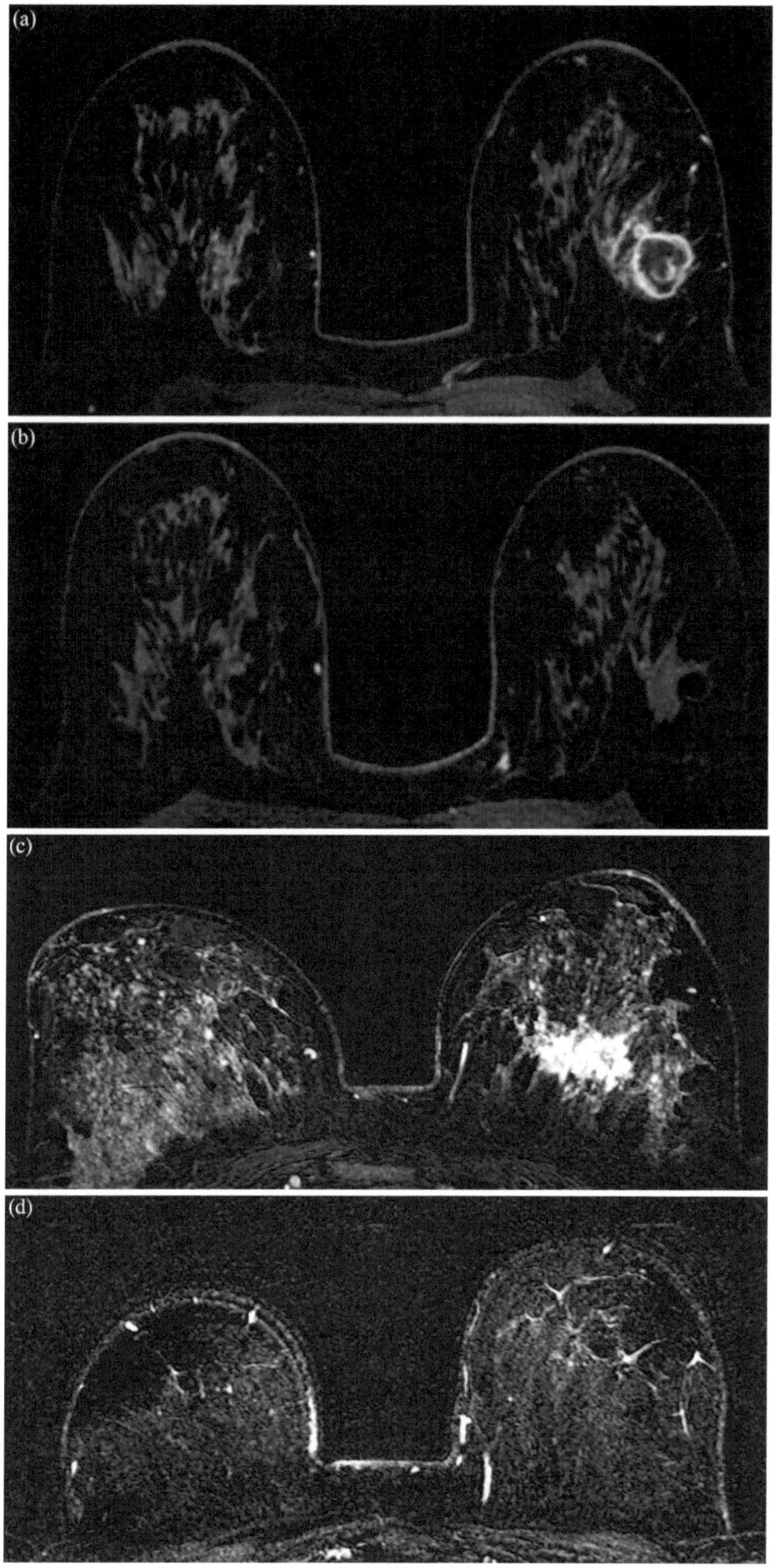

FIGURE 15.6
Two cases (a, b and c, d) of invasive breast cancers that has responded to primary chemotherapy with complete radiological response (rCR). Tumours characteristically demonstrate rapid uptake of contrast material (type III curve) and can be distinguished from benign entities that have a slower uptake. Surgery cannot be omitted in these cases, and the tumour bed with a margin of surrounding breast tissue must be excised. A clip is placed in the tumour before the first cycle of chemotherapy.

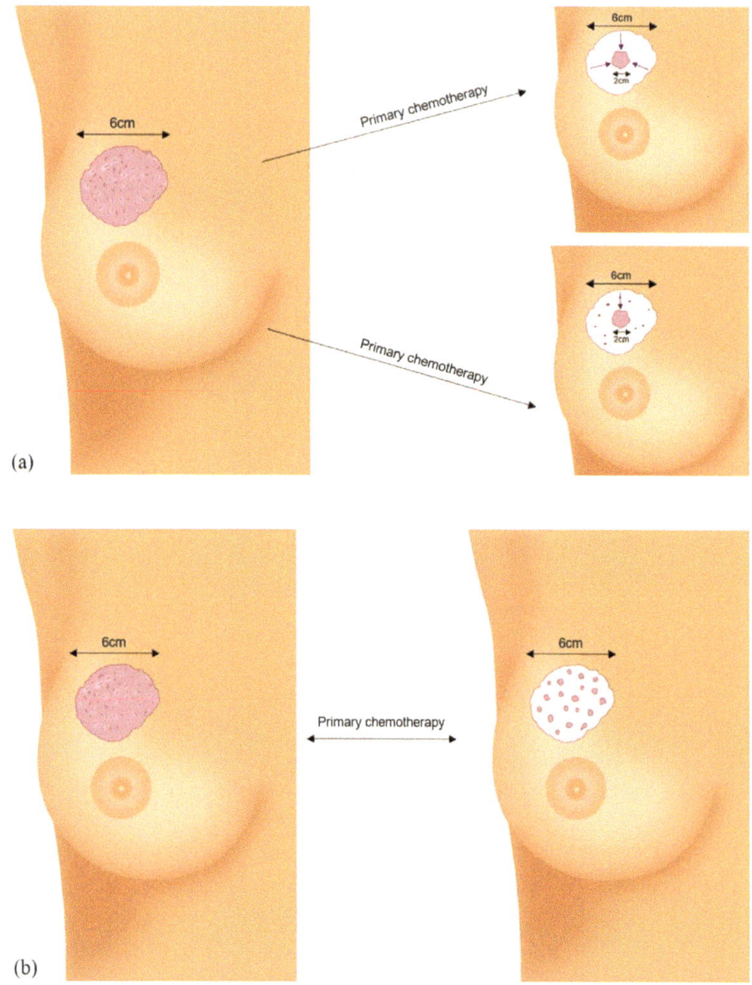

FIGURE 15.7
Tumours respond to primary chemotherapy in one of two patterns. There is either concentric shrinkage of the tumour (a) or a diffuse loss of tumour with reduction in tumour bulk but maintenance of the original footprint (honeycomb or Swiss cheese response) (b).

irradiation remains standard treatment for all tumours that are hormone-receptor-positive and HER2-negative as well as higher-stage triple-negative and HER2-positive tumours (T3N1).[21]

Axillary management: Neoadjuvant chemotherapy downstages nodal disease in patients with either clinically node negative (cN0) or node positive (cN1) disease. A dichotomy of practice initially emerged in attempts to define how SLN biopsy should be incorporated into the neoadjuvant setting. Thus, for cN0 patients, an upfront SLN biopsy prior to NACT can be helpful if negative and indicates that no further axillary treatment is necessary. Moreover, this can reinforce any decision to withhold radiation therapy after definitive surgical treatment (chest wall or regional [supraclavicular fossa, internal mammary] nodes (RNI)). Current practice favours SLN biopsy after NACT that can take advantage of nodal staging, especially for triple-negative and HER2-positive tumours, thus avoiding ALND in up to 60% of patients.[22] Recent studies have confirmed the accuracy of SLN biopsy post-NACT for both clinically node-negative and node-positive patients with pooled estimates for identification rates, sensitivity, and false negative rates similar for primary surgical procedures.[23] For cN0 patients with pathologically negative sentinel nodes after NACT (ypN0), no further local treatment to the axilla is required. For those with residual disease, further axillary treatment is mandatory and usually consists of completion ALND although irradiation of the axilla may suffice for patients with only micrometastases (≤2 mm) or isolated tumour cells (ITCs) (≤0.2 mm). Axillary radiotherapy should be considered for patients without viable tumour but evidence of nodal fibrosis (suggestive of previous sub-clinical nodal involvement at presentation). Biopsy-proven clinically node-positive patients should have normalised axillary nodes on ultrasound/MRI imaging following NACT before proceeding to SLN biopsy. There is now greater confidence in declaration of a 'negative' SLN biopsy after chemotherapy (ypN0) for node positive disease (cN1) and withholding further axillary treatment in selected cases.[24] It is important in these circumstances to remove at least 3 sentinel nodes and use dual localisation with two tracer agents (usually blue dye and radioisotope). Targeted forms of ALND are being evaluated which rely on strategies for marking the biopsied node and ensuring its subsequent guided retrieval at operation.[25,26] This can reduce false negative rates for SLN biopsy post-NACT to <10%, and several technologies are available for marking and localising the node confirmed to be pathologically positive on needle biopsy. These include paramagnetic steel or radioactive seeds, radiofrequency/radar localisation devices, and charcoal and ink; alternatively, the clip deployed at the time of node biopsy can be localised with a conventional guide-wire and this avoids the need for placement of an additional localisation device alongside the standard biopsy clip [Figure 15.8]. However, wire-free devices can be inserted days or weeks in advance of surgery and can be more convenient and comfortable for patients. There is an option to withhold any further axillary treatment for ypN0 patients and prospectively audit outcomes in a registration study. Alternatively, these patients can be entered into a randomised trial evaluating no further treatment versus either completion ALND or axillary radiotherapy (NSABP B-51[27]; ATNEC trial[28]). Any evidence of tumour deposits on H&E staining (including ITCs) in cN1 patients should prompt completion ALND although it may be safe to omit ALND for residual ITC's (ICARO).[29] Indeed, the ALLIANCE (A11202) and NSABP B-51 studies together aim to determine whether (i) chest wall radiotherapy should be based on axillary status before or after NACT, (ii) axillary radiotherapy (and RNI) is non-inferior to completion ALND (and RNI) for ypN1 disease (ALLIANCE), and (iii) the combination of chest wall irradiation and RNI or addition of RNI to breast radiotherapy after BCS increases invasive breast cancer recurrence-free interval in cN1 patients converting to yN0 after NACT (NSABP B-51).

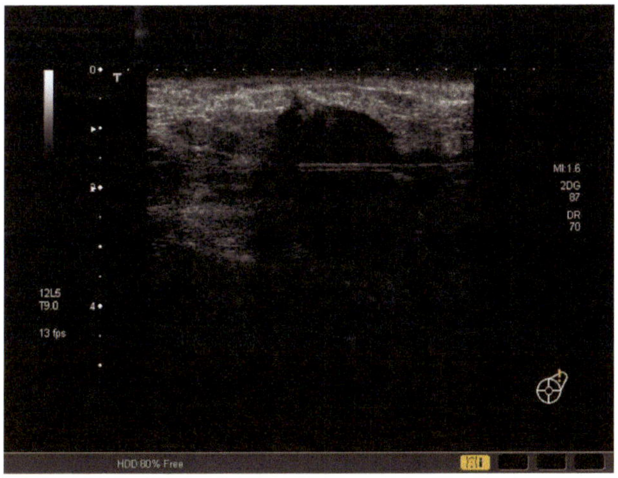

FIGURE 15.8
Several technologies are available for marking and localising the node confirmed to be pathologically positive on needle biopsy. A marker device should ideally be placed at the time of initial node biopsy but can be done after histological confirmation of node positivity.

References

1) Hartmann LC, Schaid DJ, Woods JE, et al. Efficacy of bilateral prophylactic mastectomy in women with a family history of breast cancer. N Engl J Med 1999; 340: 77–84.
2) Rebbeck TR, Lynch HT, Neuhausen SL, et al. Prophylactic oophorectomy in carriers of BRCA-1 or BRCA-2 mutations. N Engl J Med 2002; 346: 1616–1622.
3) Domchek SM, Friebel TM, Singer CF, et al. Association of risk-reducing surgery in BRCA1 or BRCA2 mutation carriers with cancer risk and mortality. JAMA 2010; 304(9): 967–975.
4) Eleje GU, Eke AC, Ezebialu IU, et al. Risk-reducing bilateral salpingo-oophorectomy in women with BRCA1 or BRCA2 mutations. Cochrane Database Syst Rev 2018; 8(8): CD012464.
5) Carbine NE, Lostumbo L, Wallace J, et al. Risk-reducing mastectomy for the prevention of primary breast cancer. Cochrane Database Syst Rev 2018; 4: CD002748.
6) Van Sprundel TC, Schmidt MK, Rookos MA, et al. Risk reduction of contralateral breast cancer and survival after contralateral prophylactic mastectomy in BRCA-1 or BRCA-2 mutation carriers. Br J Cancer 2005; 93: 287–292.
7) Chadab TM, Bernstein J, Lifrieri A, et al. Is it worth the risk? Contralateral prophylactic mastectomy with immediate bilateral breast reconstruction. Ann Plast Surg 2021; 87: (Suppl 1) S2–S6.
8) Faverley DR, Burgers L, Bult P, et al. Three-dimensional imaging of mammary ductal carcinoma in situ: clinical implications. Sem Diag Pathol 1994; 11(3): 193–198.
9) Dunne C, Burke JP, Morrow M, et al. Effect of margin status on local recurrence after breast conservation and radiation therapy for ductal carcinoma in situ. J Clin Oncol 2009; 27(10): 1615–1620.
10) Marinovich ML, Azizi L, Macaskill P, et al. The association of surgical margins and local recurrence in women with ductal carcinoma in situ treated with breast conserving surgery: a meta-analysis. Ann Surg Oncol 2016; 23: 3811–3821.
11) Fisher B, Dignam J, Wolmark N, et al. Lumpectomy and radiation therapy for the treatment of intraductal breast cancer: findings from National Surgical Adjuvant Breast and Bowel Project B-17. J Clin Oncol 1998; 16: 441–452.
12) Bijker N, Meijnen P, Peterse JL, et al. Breast conserving treatment with or without radiotherapy in ductal carcinoma in situ: ten-year results of European Organisation for Research and Treatment of Cancer Randomised Phase III Trial 10853—a study by the EORTC Breast Cancer Cooperative Group and EORTC Radiotherapy Group. J Clin Oncol 2006; 24: 1–8.
13) Wapnir I, Dignam JJ, Fisher B, et al. Long term outcomes of invasive ipsilateral breast tumour recurrences after lumpectomy in NSABP B-17 and B-24 randomised clinical trials for DCIS. J Natl Cancer Inst 2011; 103: 478–488.
14) Killelea BK, Yang VQ, Mougalian S, et al. Neoadjuvant chemotherapy for breast cancer increases the rate of breast conservation: results from the national cancer database. J Am Coll Surg 2015; 220(6): 1063–1069.

15) Asselain B, Barlow W, Bartlett J, et al. Articles long-term outcomes for neoadjuvant versus adjuvant chemotherapy in early breast cancer: meta-analysis of individual patient data from ten randomised trials. Lancet Oncol 2018; 19: 27–39.
16) Fisher B, Brown A, Mamounas E, et al. Effect of preoperative chemotherapy on local-regional disease in women with operable breast cancer: findings from national surgical adjuvant breast and bowel project b-18. J Clin Oncol 1997; 15(7): 2483–2493.
17) Karakatsanis A, Tasoulis MK, Wärnberg F, et al. Metaanalysis of neoadjuvant therapy and its impact in facilitating breast conservation in operable breast cancer. Br J Surg 2018; 105(5): 469–81.
18) Cortazar P, Geyer CE Jr. Pathological complete response in neoadjuvant treatment of breast cancer. Ann Surg Oncol 2015; 22(5): 14441–14446.
19) Sikov WM, Berry DA, Perou CM, et al. Impact of the addition of carboplatin and/or bevaccizumab to neoadjuvant once-per-week paclitaxel followed by dose-dense doxorubicin and cyclophosphamide on pathologic complete response rates in stage II to III triple negative breast cancer: CALGB 40603 (Alliance). J Clin Oncol 2015; 33(1): 13–21.
20) Warren RML, Bobrow LG, Earl HM, et al. Can breast MRI help in the management of women with breast cancer treated by neoadjuvant chemotherapy? Br J Cancer 2004; 90: 1349–1360.
21) Heil J, Kuerer H, Pfob A, et al. Eliminating the breast cancer surgery paradigm after neoadjuvant systemic therapy: current evidence and future challenges. Ann Oncol 2020; 31(1): 61–71.
22) Mamounas EP. Optimizing surgical management of the axilla after neoadjuvant chemotherapy: an evolving story. Ann Surg Oncol 2018; 25: 2124–2126.
23) El Hage Chehade H, HeadonH, El Tokhy O, et al. Is sentinel lymph node biopsy a viable alternative to complete axillary dissection following neoadjuvant chemotherapy in women with node positive breast cancer at diagnosis? An updated meta-analysis involving 3,398 patients. Am J Surg 2016; 212(5): 969–981.
24) Boughey JC, Sumen VJ, Mittendorf EA, et al. Sentinel lymph node surgery after neoadjuvant chemotherapy in patients with node positive breast cancer: the ACOSOG Z1071 (ALLIANCE) clinical trial. JAMA 2013; 310(14): 1455–1461.
25) Caudle AS, Yang WT, Krishnamurthy S, et al. Improved axillary evaluation following neoadjuvant therapy for patients with node-positive breast cancer using selective evaluation of clipped nodes: implementation of targeted axillary dissection. J Clin Oncol 2016; 34(10): 1072–1078.
26) Montagna G, Lee MK, Sevilimedu V, et al. Is nodal clipping beneficial for node-positive breast cancer patients receiving neoadjuvant chemotherapy? Ann Surg Oncol 2022; 29(10): 6133–6139.
27) Mamounas E, Bandos H, White J, et al. Abstract OT2-04-01: phase III trial to determine if chest wall and regional nodal radiotherapy (CWRNRT) post mastectomy (Mx) or the addition of RNRT to whole breast RT post breast-conserving surgery (BCS) reduces invasive breast cancer recurrence-free interval (IBCR-FI) in patients (pts) with pathologically positive axillary (PPAx) nodes who are ypN0 after neoadjuvant chemotherapy (NC): NRG Oncology/NSABP b-51/RTOG 1304. Cancer Res 2019; 79(4 Supplement): OT2-04-01-OT2-04-01.
28) Goyal A, Cramp S, Marshall A, et al. ATNEC: a multicenter randomised trial investigating whether axillary treatment can be avoided in patients with T1-3N1M0 breast cancer patients with no residual cancer in the lymph glands after neoadjuvant chemotherapy. J Clin Oncol 2022; 40: TPS615.
29) Giacomo Montagna et al., Nodal Burden and Oncologic Outcomes in Patients With Residual Isolated Tumor Cells After Neoadjuvant Chemotherapy (ypN0i+): The OPBC-05/ICARO Study. JCO 0, JCO.24.01052 DOI:10.1200/JCO.24.01052

16

Adjuvant Treatments for Breast Cancer

E. R. Gatfield and M. B. Mukesh

16.1 Introduction

Breast cancer is the most common malignancy affecting women in Europe, with more than 550,000 cases diagnosed in 2020. With more than half of cases occurring in women aged 64 years and younger, the disease significantly impacts upon a population who are working and/or raising children (1). Breast cancer represents a substantial burden of disease globally, accounting for 1 out of 6 cancer deaths worldwide (1). There have been notable advancements in treatment of breast cancer over the past few decades, and mortality rates are decreasing in the majority of European countries (2). The reasons for this progressive decline in mortality are multi-factorial and include breast cancer screening, improvements in surgical techniques, and pathological assessment of margins after breast-conserving surgery together with advances in systemic therapies. This chapter summarises adjuvant treatments in management of breast cancer including radiotherapy, chemotherapy, endocrine therapies, targeted therapies, and bone-modifying agents.

16.2 Radiotherapy

Radiotherapy plays a crucial role in the management of breast cancer and is often a complementary modality of treatment following surgical resection of the primary tumour or axillary lymph nodes. Brachytherapy employing radium needles has been used since the first quarter of the 19th century (3), with external beam radiotherapy (EBRT) being introduced in the 1940s for treatment of breast cancer (4). Ionising radiation destroys cancer cells by causing double-strand DNA breaks. Radiotherapy encompasses a variety of techniques, including EBRT, brachytherapy, and intraoperative radiotherapy.

16.2.1 External Beam Radiotherapy

EBRT is the most commonly applied radiotherapy technique for treatment of breast cancer patients undergoing either mastectomy (chest wall irradiation) or breast-conserving surgery (breast irradiation). It employs high-energy photons, electrons, protons, or other ions as an energy source. Photon beam radiotherapy delivered using a linear accelerator is the most widely used technique (as shown in Figure 16.1). A large meta-analysis based on individual patient data has confirmed that adjuvant radiotherapy after breast-conserving surgery reduces the risk of recurrence by half and also improves overall survival in the longer term (5).

High-risk patients with tumours ≥50 mm, skin or chest wall involvement (T4), or four or more positive lymph nodes, as well as male patients, derive significant benefit from post-mastectomy radiotherapy that can reduce the chance of chest wall recurrence by up to three-quarters (6). For patients with 1–3 positive lymph nodes, other factors, such as tumour size and grade, should be taken into consideration and factored

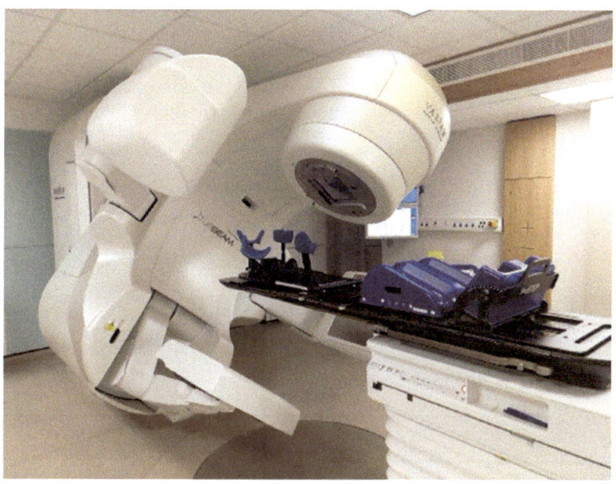

FIGURE 16.1
Linear accelerator.

DOI: 10.1201/9781003394785-16

into clinical decision-making for post-operative irradiation that may include the supraclavicular nodes (7). More recently, studies have demonstrated a modest improvement in overall survival from elective irradiation of regional lymph nodes in those patients with either four or more positive lymph nodes or 1–3 positive lymph nodes and a central or medial tumour (8, 9).

EBRT is generally well-tolerated and administered as outpatient treatment, although patients must attend daily for several visits. This fractionated regimen allows time for recovery of normal tissue between each treatment fraction. Early side effects include lethargy, skin erythema, itching and desquamation, breast discomfort, breast swelling, or change in breast texture. Radiation induces endarteritis obliterans and late side effects include skin colour changes, telangiectasia, changes in the appearance of the breast in terms of size, shape, or texture and breast pain. Rare long-term side effects may occur and include fibrosis of the underlying lung, rib fracture, and cardiac toxicity, such as myocardial infarction or cardiac failure. In addition, radiotherapy can induce secondary malignancy, such as angiosarcoma, that can be aggressive and associated with a worse prognosis than the original breast cancer.

16.2.2 Brachytherapy

Brachytherapy is a specific form of radiotherapy involving precise placement of radioactive sources directly into or adjacent to the tumour (primary radiotherapy) or tumour bed (adjuvant radiotherapy). There is rapid attenuation of radiation dose with increasing distance from the source and this serves to limit potentially harmful radiation exposure to surrounding tissues.

The majority of local recurrences after breast-conserving surgery are in close proximity to the tumour bed (10). This provided the rationale for use of brachytherapy to confine irradiation to the tissue immediately around the tumour bed and hence potentially reduce acute and long-term side effects associated with EBRT. A single-centre Hungarian trial revealed similar efficacy between brachytherapy and EBRT but more favourable cosmetic outcomes for brachytherapy amongst low-risk patients at 20 years follow-up (11). Both GEC-ESTRO and NSABP have approved this approach as an alternative form of irradiation in low-risk patient groups (12, 13). Patients deemed to be low-risk and suitable for brachytherapy based on guidelines from the American Brachytherapy Society (ABS), the American Society of Radiation Oncology (ASTRO), and the American Society of Breast Surgeons (ASBrS) are summarised in Table 16.1.

16.2.3 Intra-Operative Radiotherapy

Both EBRT and brachytherapy involve multiple visits to hospital for receipt of a treatment course, with brachytherapy often requiring two visits per day, six hours apart. Intra-operative radiotherapy (IORT) systems deliver a low dose of radiation to the tissue around the surgical cavity as a single session during or after surgery. This approach potentially reduces the toxic effects of radiation and has advantages from

TABLE 16.1

Low risk patient groups suitable for accelerated partial breast irradiation

Characteristic	ABS (2013)	ASTRO (2017)	ASBrS (2018)
Age	≥ 45 years	≥ 50 years	≥ 45 years
Histology	All invasive subtypes and ductal carcinoma in situ (DCIS)	Invasive ductal or favourable subtypes and low-risk DCIS (screen detected, grade 1 or 2)	All invasive subtypes and DCIS
Tumour size	≤ 30mm	≤ 20mm DCIS ≤ 25mm	≤ 30mm
Oestrogen receptor (ER)	Any	Positive	Any
Human epidermal growth factor receptor 2 (HER-2)	Negative (or will receive treatment with HER-2 targeted agents)	Negative	-
Surgical margins	Negative at inked margin for invasive disease ≥ 2mm for DCIS	≥ 2mm for invasive disease ≥ 3mm for DCIS	Negative at inked margin for invasive disease ≥ 2mm for DCIS
Extensive lymphovascular space invasion (LVSI)	Not present	Not present	Not present (focal acceptable)
Nodal status	Negative	Negative	Negative
Centricity	Unifocal	Unicentric, clinically unifocal	Multifocal acceptable if total span ≤ 30mm

the patient's perspective such as reduced travel time and subsequently the out-of-pocket expenses.

The TARGIT trial used an electron beam source with 50 kV X-rays to deliver IORT to lower-risk patients with tumours measuring up to 2.5 cm in size. This trial randomised patients to either EBRT or IORT with stratification into pre-pathology and post-pathology groups. Within the latter group, IORT was administered as a delayed procedure when final pathology results were known and patients with unexpectedly high-risk features received EBRT as a risk-adapted strategy. Higher rates of local (in-breast) recurrence were reported at 5 years for IORT compared to EBRT (14). By contrast, in the pre-pathology group, where IORT was delivered at the time of surgery, the five-year local recurrence rates were similar for the two arms, albeit with a relatively large non-inferiority margin. Moreover, 20% of patients in the IORT arm also received EBRT due to adverse histology (15). The long-term efficacy and toxicity data are awaited together with cosmetic outcomes, before this approach is considered to be a standard of care for early-stage breast cancer patients undergoing breast-conserving surgery.

The ELIOT trial employed 6–9 MeV beams for IORT in a largely unselected patient population. After 10 years, local recurrence rates were significantly higher in the IORT arm compared to EBRT (8.1% versus 1.1%) (16). These results highlighted the need for appropriate patient selection in the context of IORT (as was mandatory for brachytherapy studies).

16.2.4 Omission of Radiotherapy

The incidence of local recurrence is falling with better pre-operative imaging, rigorous pathology assessments and improvement in systemic therapies. This raises an important question on the need of adjuvant radiotherapy for all patients after breast-conserving surgery.

Hitherto, studies have failed to identify a group of patients for whom adjuvant radiotherapy can be safely omitted based on favourable factors relating to patient age, tumour size, nodal status, and endocrine sensitivity (17–19). Multiple biomarkers have been associated with risk of local and systemic cancer recurrence and biomarker-based studies are currently exploring this approach in randomised trials.

16.3 Adjuvant Systemic Therapies

Systemic anticancer therapy (SACT) includes chemotherapy, hormone therapy, immunotherapy, and targeted therapies, which all play a vital role in improving outcomes for breast cancer patients. We discuss each modality in detail in this section.

16.3.1 Chemotherapy

Chemotherapy agents exert lethal effects upon rapidly dividing cells by targeting different phases of the cell cycle. Cancer cells tend to multiply faster than the normal healthy cells, rendering them, more susceptible to the cytocidal action of chemotherapy drugs. Damaging healthy cells leads to adverse effects, but normal cells possess more efficient repair mechanisms compared to cancer cells, allowing for specific anti-cancer activity. Chemotherapy side effects include low blood cell counts with risk of neutropenic sepsis, anaemia, thrombocytopenia, lethargy, nausea, vomiting, diarrhoea, constipation, allergic reactions, mucositis, and alopecia. Specific side effects relating to anthracyclines include risk of cardiotoxicity, and there is a risk of peripheral neuropathy with taxanes.

Due to the aforementioned side effects, only patients at relatively high-risk of relapse are offered chemotherapy with a threshold of 5% for recommendation and 3–5% for discussion of chemotherapy. Historically, recurrence risk was calculated using parameters such as tumour size and grade along with axillary lymph node status that were incorporated into the Nottingham Prognostic Index (NPI) (20). Despite its clinical utility, the original NPI did not take account of biological features relating to expression of various cell surface receptors. These include oestrogen receptor (ER), progesterone receptor (PR), and human epidermal growth factor receptor 2 (HER2) whose expression is linked to risk of systemic (distant) recurrence. The online tool Predict Breast (access via https://breast.predict.nhs.uk) calculates the risk of death at 5 and 10 years and quantifies the benefit from systemic therapies (chemotherapy, hormonal therapy, trastuzumab, bisphosphonates) by integrating information on tumour size and grade, age at diagnosis, extent of lymph node involvement, and expression of markers—namely, ER, HER2, and Ki-67 (a proliferation index). The Predict Breast tool was developed with data from 5000 women with breast cancer, and its performance has been tested in another 23,000 women from around the world.

Most patients with ER-/PR-negative and/or HER2-positive disease benefit from adjuvant chemotherapy that is usually recommended for triple-negative breast cancers ≥1 cm and HER2-positive tumours ≥2 cm irrespective of nodal status. Over the last decade, several genomic assays, such as Oncotype DX, EndoPredict, and MammaPrint, have continued to be validated for clinical decision-making

TABLE 16.2

Genomic Assays to Help Predict Risk of Recurrence

Characteristic	Oncotype DX	MammaPrint	Endopredict
Oestrogen receptor (ER)	Positive	Positive	Positive
Human epidermal growth factor receptor 2 (HER-2)	Negative	Negative	Negative
Nodal status	Any (maximum three positive)	Any (maximum three positive)	Negative
Tumour size		≤50 mm	
Number of genes quantified in assay	21	70 (+BluePrint >150)	12
Reported outcome data	9 years	5 years	15 years
Chemotherapy benefit report	Recurrence score >26 = substantial benefit	High risk = substantial benefit	High risk = substantial benefit
Extended endocrine therapy report	No	No	5–15 year late recurrence

in ER-positive, HER2-negative patients. In particular, these assays can help identify those patients for whom absolute benefits from therapy are modest and omission of adjuvant chemotherapy is safe. The key features of these genomic assays are summarised in Table 16.2. Oncotype Dx assay is the most commonly used assay around the world and has been approved by NICE (National Institute for Health and Clinical Excellence). Moreover, this assay has recently been assessed in node-positive patients (1–3 nodes) and is the only genomic test that has been validated in large randomised studies (21, 22).

16.3.2 Endocrine Therapy

Endocrine therapy has a major role in management of hormone-receptor-positive breast cancer for both pre- and post-menopausal women, with proportionately greater effects in the latter. Tamoxifen is a selective oestrogen receptor modulator (SERM) with antagonist effects on breast cancers but agonist action in other tissues. All ER-positive patients derive benefit from adjuvant tamoxifen irrespective of tumour size, patient age, nodal status, or tumour differentiation. Within the breast tissue, tamoxifen blocks ER by competitive binding and inhibits growth of cells, whilst in bone, liver, and uterus it acts as an agonist leading to incidental effects such as uterine thickening. Apart from menopausal symptoms secondary to oestrogen deprivation, there is an increased risk of venous thromboembolism and a slightly increased risk of endometrial cancer and uterine sarcoma (23). The large Oxford overview with individual patient meta-analysis of 20 trials showed that five years of adjuvant tamoxifen reduced the risk of breast cancer recurrence and death with benefits of tamoxifen persisting at 15 years of follow-up (24).

Aromatase inhibitors such as letrozole or anastrozole represent another class of endocrine therapy whose principal action is to block the aromatase enzyme (oestrogen synthetase) in adipose tissue, preventing peripheral conversion of hormonal precursors into oestrogen. Aromatase inhibitors have clinical efficacy in post-menopausal women, where peripheral production of oestrogen is the main source of oestrogen in the absence of ovarian function. Apart from menopausal symptoms, this class of drugs can give rise to muscle and joint aches, which can be severe and troublesome to patients leading to poor compliance. Patients receiving aromatase inhibitors require a baseline DEXA scan and regular monitoring of bone health, especially when there is a family or personal history of osteoporosis. Dietary supplementation with vitamin D and calcium tablets is usually recommended and bisphosphonate therapy may be indicated for low bone density scores.

A meta-analysis from the Early Breast Cancer Trialists' Collaborative group (EBCTCG) evaluated individual patient data from several trials assessing aromatase inhibitors as adjuvant hormonal therapy. Comparison of five years of tamoxifen versus an aromatase inhibitor in post-menopausal women showed a reduction in ten-year breast cancer mortality with aromatase inhibitors (25). All-cause mortality favoured aromatase inhibitors that were associated with fewer endometrial cancers but more frequent bone fractures. Aromatase inhibitors are now the preferred choice of adjuvant endocrine agent for post-menopausal women but can be incorporated into a sequenced schedule with tamoxifen. For high-risk patients, extended endocrine therapy for up to ten years can be considered, although non-compliance due to side effects can be an issue. Patients should be evaluated after five years and continuation of therapy based on tolerance to date, risk of relapse, and sometimes cost.

In pre-menopausal women, the ovaries are the principal source of oestrogen and aromatase inhibitors alone do not suppress oestrogen activity and are therefore contraindicated. For high-risk pre-menopausal women, a gonadotrophin-releasing hormone (GnRH) agonist can be combined with endocrine therapy to achieve ovarian suppression and permit use of a more efficacious aromatase inhibitor. Combined results of two trials examining ovarian function suppression with either an aromatase inhibitor or tamoxifen for five years showed a small but significant improvement in disease free survival of 4.6% for the combination of a GnRH agonist with an aromatase inhibitor versus a GnRH agonist combined with tamoxifen (26). Improvement in overall survival was restricted to women aged 35 years or younger with tumours measuring >20 mm or grade 3 whose risk of recurrence is sufficiently high to recommend chemotherapy (26).

Cyclin-dependent kinase 4 and 6 (CDK 4/6) inhibitors act at the G1/S phase boundary of the cell cycle, leading to arrest of cell division and growth. Three approved CDK 4/6 inhibitors, abemaciclib, palbociclib, and ribociclib, are approved for use in hormone-receptor-positive, HER2-negative advanced breast cancer in combination with endocrine therapy. The MonarchE trial evaluated use of abemaciclib for two years alongside endocrine therapy in the adjuvant setting for patients with high-risk hormone-receptor-positive, HER2-negative early breast cancer. Patients were classed as high-risk if four or more axillary lymph nodes were positive, or between one and three axillary nodes contained metastases and the primary tumour was either grade 3, size ≥50 mm, or Ki-67 at least 20%. At four years, there was an absolute improvement of 6.4% in terms of invasive-disease-free survival compared to endocrine therapy alone with a trend towards an overall survival gain (27). The most common side effects within this trial included neutropenia (45%) and diarrhoea (84%) with discontinuation of therapy in almost one-fifth of patients receiving a CDK 4/6 inhibitor. Nonetheless, adjuvant abemaciclib is now approved in the adjuvant setting in both the United States and Europe for high-risk node-positive patients with hormone-receptor-positive, HER2-negative breast cancer.

16.3.3 Human Epidermal Growth Factor Receptor 2 (HER2) Directed Therapy

About 25% of invasive breast cancers have amplification or over-expression of the HER2 gene. These cancers are often more aggressive and historically carried a worse prognosis with a high risk of developing metastatic disease.

Over the last three decades, the availability of anti-HER2 targeted therapies has revolutionised the management of HER2-positive breast cancer. Trastuzumab is a humanised monoclonal chimeric antibody which binds to the extracellular domain of the HER2 receptor. This inhibits HER2 homo-dimerisation and in turn prevents HER2-mediated signalling. Pooled analysis of results from five large trials has confirmed that addition of trastuzumab to standard chemotherapy schedules reduces the risk of breast cancer recurrence and death (28). Cancer cells can develop resistance to trastuzumab by mechanisms that involve HER2 dimerisation with other members of the HER family of receptors, including HER1, HER3, and HER4. Trastuzumab and pertuzumab bind simultaneously to different epitopes of the HER2 receptor and interact synergistically by preventing both homo- and hetero-dimerisation of HER2. For patients with node-positive, HER2-positive breast cancer, the dual therapy with a combination of both trastuzumab and pertuzumab has been shown to improve invasive-disease-free survival by 5% at six years (29).

Neratinib is another targeted anti-HER2 agent that works by irreversibly binding to the intracellular tyrosine kinase domain of the HER2 receptor. Twelve months of neratanib treatment following trastuzumab modestly improves invasive-disease-free survival by 2–3% at five years, although patients often suffer troublesome diarrhoea and need prophylactic therapies (30).

Notable side effects of anti-HER2 targeted therapies include low blood counts, nausea, diarrhoea, constipation, joint aches, mucositis, palmer-plantar erythrodysesthesia, peripheral neuropathy, pneumonitis, and cardiotoxicity. The most concerning adverse effect of anti-HER2 treatment is cardiac failure and this may necessitate a break from treatment to allow recovery of left ventricular ejection fraction. Patients require regular monitoring of cardiac function with echocardiography prior to and during treatment.

16.3.4 Neoadjuvant and Tailored Adjuvant Therapy

Neoadjuvant therapy should be considered for HER2-positive and triple-negative breast cancer (TNBC) measuring ≥2 cm and ≥1 cm, respectively. Although the main advantage of upfront systemic therapy is to downsize the primary tumour to facilitate breast-conserving surgery, neoadjuvant therapy also provides prognostic information and allows tailoring of adjuvant therapy when there is residual disease after induction chemotherapy. Neoadjuvant chemotherapy ideally aims to achieve a complete pathological response with no viable cancer cells detected in the surgical resection specimen (breast and axillary lymph nodes). A complete pathological response rate has been shown to be associated with improved disease-free and overall survival for patients with HER2-positive or triple-negative disease (31).

For HER2-positive breast cancers, neoadjuvant therapy is considered for most patients with a tumour size ≥20 mm or node-positive disease. Treatment involves a combination of chemotherapy and dual HER2 blockade with trastuzumab and pertuzumab, which is associated with complete pathological response rates of approximately 65% (32). For patients who do not achieve a complete pathological response with neoadjuvant systemic therapy, the risk of disease recurrence is higher. For these patients, tailored adjuvant therapy can be employed to treat residual disease that is relatively resistant to systemic therapies. Treatment options include use of novel anti-HER2 therapies, especially antibody drug conjugates such as trastuzumab-emtansine (T-DM1). T-DM1 is an antibody-drug conjugate that accurately delivers a toxic payload (microtubule inhibitor) to cells expressing HER2. There is evidence from a randomised trial showing that use of adjuvant TDM-1 rather than trastuzumab in patients without a complete pathological response reduces risk of breast cancer recurrence or death by about half. However, these benefits were to some extent offset by a greater incidence of adverse effects including low blood cell counts and hypertension (33).

Neoadjuvant chemotherapy is considered for most TNBC patients with a tumour size ≥10 mm or node-positive disease. The most common chemotherapy regime is a combination of anthracycline and taxane, although addition of carboplatin has been shown to improve complete pathological response rates (34). It is now acknowledged that patients who achieve a complete pathological response have significantly improved disease-free and overall survival (35) and pathological response is to some extent a surrogate endpoint for long-term survival outcome.

Recent trials have confirmed that addition of immune checkpoint inhibitors to neoadjuvant chemotherapy schedules can further improve complete pathological response rates for triple-negative breast cancers (36). Administration of the immunotherapeutic agent pembrolizumab alongside standard neoadjuvant chemotherapy for 6 months with continuation as adjuvant therapy for a further 6 months can reduce the risk of recurrent disease. However, the addition of immune checkpoint inhibitors to a neoadjuvant schedule increases the risk of grade 3 or higher toxicities, including immune-mediated problems that can affect any organ and necessitate life-long treatment. For patients who do not achieve a complete response with neoadjuvant chemotherapy, the risk of cancer recurrence is high. The Create-X trial confirmed an overall survival benefit of 5% from use of adjuvant capecitabine in patients with TNBC and residual disease after neoadjuvant chemotherapy—albeit amongst a study population of oriental ethnicity with a 'mixed bag' of chemotherapy regimens (37). Interestingly, there is currently no data to support combined adjuvant treatment with capecitabine and pembrolizumab for these patients.

The high-risk predisposition genes BRCA1 and BRCA2 display tumour suppressor action and have an important role in homologous recombination and maintaining fidelity of DNA repair mechanisms. There is a clear association between germline mutations in these BRCA1 and BRCA2 genes and risk of developing breast cancer and/or ovarian cancer. BRCA-associated tumours often possess a defect in homologous recombination repair and this intrinsic weakness in DNA repair renders them vulnerable to the DNA-damaging effects of poly adenosine diphosphate-ribose polymerase (PARP) inhibitors. The PARP inhibitors olaparib and talazoparib have been approved in the United States for treatment of HER2-negative and metastatic triple negative breast cancer in high-risk BRCA1 and BRCA2 mutation carriers. Olaparib is not currently available for routine clinical used in the UK but can be obtained through a compassionate access scheme run by the relevant drug company. Olaparib has recently been evaluated as adjuvant therapy for TNBC patients with residual disease after neoadjuvant chemotherapy. Twelve months treatment with adjuvant olaparib significantly improved invasive-disease-free survival at three years compared with placebo with an absolute difference of almost 9% (86% versus 77%). Moreover, there was a trend towards improved overall survival (38).

16.4 Bisphosphonates and Other Bone-Modifying Agents

Bone is one of the common sites for breast cancer metastasis. Use of bone-modifying agents including bisphosphonates and denosumab can reduce the risk of skeletal-related events, including hypercalcemia, metastatic spinal cord compression, and pathological fractures. Bisphosphonates reduce the incidence of complications secondary to osteolytic bone lesions by limiting osteoclastic activity.

When these agents are used as a component of systemic therapy for early breast cancer, they can also reduce the risk of distant recurrence in bone and improve breast-cancer-specific survival (39). The EBCTCG meta-analysis involving more than 18,000 women included the two largest trials (AZURE and ABCSG-12) and also smaller trials without endpoints of breast cancer survival or recurrence. This meta-analysis found a reduction in bone recurrence (1.1%), a decrease in recurrence at all sites (1.4%) and a decrease in breast cancer mortality (1.7%) among post-menopausal women in receipt of adjuvant bisphosphonates compared to controls. A pre-specified subgroups analysis revealed no benefits among pre-menopausal women, but adjuvant bone-modifying agents can be beneficial with use of ovarian suppression therapy or oophorectomy in this group. Apart from menopausal status, no other clinical, patient, or pathological factors affect treatment efficacy. Notwithstanding these findings, all outcomes except bone recurrence were of borderline significance for post-menopausal patients.

It is common to develop flu-like reactions following treatment with bisphosphonates (zoledronic acid or denosumab). The major risk with bone-modifying agents is osteonecrosis of the jaw, although this is relatively uncommon with a pooled analysis suggesting an incidence of 1%. A dental assessment prior to treatment is mandatory for any patient with a history of dental problems—especially current ones. These should subsequently receive regular monitoring during treatment. These agents are also nephrotoxic and creatinine levels should be checked before commencing treatment. Bisphosphonates should be avoided if the creatinine levels are below 30 ml/min.

16.5 Unusual Situations

Male breast cancer is rare and represents between 0.5% and 1% of all breast cancers. This condition affects approximately 1 in 800 men over their lifetime. The majority of male patients have hormone-receptor-positive disease and are treated according to the same principles as female breast cancer. All male breast cancer patients should have BRCA2 gene mutation testing, and tamoxifen is used as the endocrine therapy (no robust data for benefit from aromatase inhibitors in male patients).

For cases of breast cancer occurring during pregnancy, it is important to consider the health of both the mother and the foetus—these may not be mutually exclusive. Radiotherapy is avoided during any stage of pregnancy due to teratogenic risks, but radioisotope may safely be used for sentinel lymph node biopsy. Mastectomy is preferred over breast-conserving surgery, but in the final trimester, wide tumour excision can be carried out with irradiation of the breast after delivery. Neoadjuvant or adjuvant chemotherapy can be considered from the second trimester onwards (when organogenesis is complete), and it is important to work in close collaboration with the obstetrician. HER2-directed therapy, endocrine therapy, and immunotherapy should all be avoided during pregnancy. It is important to liaise closely with obstetric services for pregnancy-associated breast cancer to promote patient-centred reproductive healthcare. There is now evidence from a large international trial that temporary interruption of endocrine therapy after 18–24 months to allow pregnancy to term does not adversely affect breast cancer outcomes with relatively short-term follow-up for hormone-receptor-positive disease.

16.6 Conclusion

The management of breast cancer has undergone significant advancements in recent years with much emphasis on a multidisciplinary approach and careful consideration of the sequencing of loco-regional and systemic therapies. With regard to the latter, a multitude of treatment options are now available in both the neoadjuvant and adjuvant settings. Collaborative working within the multidisciplinary team is essential to optimise personalised care, and ongoing research will ensure the continued evolution of breast cancer management.

References

1. Breast Cancer, [Internet] Europa Donna. Available from: https://www.europadonna.org/breast-cancer/.
2. Wojtyla C, Bertuccio P, Wojtyla A, Vecchia CL. European trends in breast cancer mortality, 1980–2017 and predictions to 2025. Eur J Cancer. 2021;152:4–17.
3. Keynes G. The radium treatment of carcinoma of the breast. Br J Surg. 1932;19(75):415–80.
4. McWhirter R. Simple mastectomy and radiotherapy in the treatment of breast cancer. Br J Radiol. 1955;28(327):128–39.
5. Early Breast Cancer Trialists' Collaborative Group (EBCTCG). Effect of radiotherapy after breast-conserving surgery on 10-year recurrence and 15-year breast cancer death: meta-analysis of individual patient data for 10 801 women in 17 randomised trials. Lancet. 2011;378(9804):1707–16.
6. Recht A, Edge SB, Solin LJ, et al. Postmastectomy radiotherapy: clinical practice guidelines of the American Society of Clinical Oncology. J Clin Oncol. 2001;19(5):1539–69.
7. Mukesh MB, Duke S, Parashar D, et al. The Cambridge post-mastectomy radiotherapy (C-PMRT) index: a practical tool for patient selection. Radiother Oncol. 2014;110(3):461–6.

8. Poortmans PM, Collette S, Kirkove C, et al. Internal mammary and medial supraclavicular irradiation in breast cancer. N Engl J Med. 2015;373(4):317–27.
9. Thorsen LBJ, Offersen BV, Danø H, et al. DBCG-IMN: a population-based cohort study on the effect of internal mammary node irradiation in early node-positive breast cancer. J Clin Oncol. 2016;34(4):314–20.
10. Salvadori B, Marubini E, Miceli R, et al. Reoperation for locally recurrent breast cancer in patients previously treated with conservative surgery. Br J Surg. 1999;86(1):84–7.
11. Polgár C, Major T, Takácsi-Nagy Z, Fodor J. Breast-conserving surgery followed by partial or whole breast irradiation: twenty-year results of a phase 3 clinical study. Int J Radiat Oncol Biol Phys. 2021;109(4):998–1006.
12. Strnad V, Polgár C, Ott OJ, et al. Accelerated partial breast irradiation using sole interstitial multicatheter brachytherapy compared with whole-breast irradiation with boost for early breast cancer: 10-Year results of a GEC-ESTRO randomised, phase 3, non-inferiority trial. Lancet Oncol. 2023;24(3):262–72.
13. Vicini FA, Cecchini RS, White JR, et al. Long-term primary results of accelerated partial breast irradiation after breast-conserving surgery for early-stage breast cancer: a randomised, phase 3, equivalence trial. Lancet. 2019;394(10215):2155–64.
14. Vaidya JS, Bulsara M, Saunders C, et al. Effect of delayed targeted intraoperative radiotherapy vs whole-breast radiotherapy on local recurrence and survival: long-term results from the TARGIT: a randomized clinical trial in early breast cancer. JAMA Oncol. 2020;6(7):e200249.
15. Vaidya JS, Bulsara M, Baum M, et al. Long term survival and local control outcomes from single dose targeted intraoperative radiotherapy during lumpectomy (TARGIT-IORT) for early breast cancer: TARGIT—a randomised clinical trial. BMJ. 2020;370:m2836.
16. Orecchia R, Veronesi U, Maisonneuve P, et al. Intraoperative irradiation for early breast cancer (ELIOT): long-term recurrence and survival outcomes from a single-centre, randomised, phase 3 equivalence trial. Lancet Oncol. 2021;22(5):597–608.
17. Hughes KS, Schnaper LA, Bellon JR, et al. Lumpectomy plus tamoxifen with or without irradiation in women age 70 years or older with early breast cancer: long-term follow-up of CALGB 9343. J Clin Oncol. 2013;31(19):2382–7.
18. Blamey RW, Bates T, Chetty U, et al. Radiotherapy or tamoxifen after conserving surgery for breast cancers of excellent prognosis: British Association of Surgical Oncology (BASO) II trial. Eur J Cancer. 2013;49(10):2294–302.
19. Kunkler IH, Williams LJ, Jack WJL, et al. Breast-conserving surgery with or without irradiation in early breast cancer. N Engl J Med. 2023;388(7):585–94.
20. Balslev I, Axelsson CK, Zedeler K, et al. The Nottingham Prognostic Index applied to 9,149 patients from the studies of the Danish Breast Cancer Cooperative Group (DBCG). Breast Cancer Res Treat. 1994;32(3):281–90.
21. Sparano JA, Gray RJ, Makower DF, et al. Adjuvant chemotherapy guided by a 21-gene expression assay in breast cancer. N Engl J Med. 2018;379(2):111–21.
22. Kalinsky K, Barlow WE, Gralow JR, et al. 21-Gene assay to inform chemotherapy benefit in node-positive breast cancer. N Engl J Med. 2021;385(25):2336–47.
23. Osborne CK. Tamoxifen in the treatment of breast cancer. N Engl J Med. 1998;339(22):1609–18.
24. Davies C, Godwin J, Gray R, et al. Relevance of breast cancer hormone receptors and other factors to the efficacy of adjuvant tamoxifen: patient-level meta-analysis of randomised trials. Lancet. 2011;378(9793):771–84.
25. (EBCTCG) EBCTCG. Aromatase inhibitors versus tamoxifen in early breast cancer: patient-level meta-analysis of the randomised trials. Lancet. 2015;386(10001):1341–52.
26. Pagani O, Walley BA, Fleming GF, et al. Adjuvant exemestane with ovarian suppression in premenopausal breast cancer: long-term follow-up of the combined TEXT and SOFT trials. J Clin Oncol. 2023;41(7):1376–82.
27. Johnston SRD, Toi M, O'Shaughnessy J, et al. Abemaciclib plus endocrine therapy for hormone receptor-positive, HER2-negative, node-positive, high-risk early breast cancer (monarchE): results from a preplanned interim analysis of a randomised, open-label, phase 3 trial. Lancet Oncol. 2023;24(1):77–90.
28. Viani GA, Afonso SL, Stefano EJ, et al. Adjuvant trastuzumab in the treatment of her-2-positive early breast cancer: a meta-analysis of published randomized trials. BMC Cancer. 2007;7(1):153.
29. Piccart M, Procter M, Fumagalli D, et al. Adjuvant pertuzumab and trastuzumab in early HER2-positive breast cancer in the APHINITY trial: 6 years' follow-up. J Clin Oncol. 2021;39(13):1448–57.
30. Martin M, Holmes FA, Ejlertsen B, et al. Neratinib after trastuzumab-based adjuvant therapy in HER2-positive breast cancer (ExteNET): 5-year analysis of a randomised, double-blind, placebo-controlled, phase 3 trial. Lancet Oncol. 2017;18(12):1688–700.
31. Cortazar P, Zhang L, Untch M, et al. Pathological complete response and long-term clinical benefit in breast cancer: the CTNeoBC pooled analysis. Lancet. 2014;384(9938):164–72.
32. Van Der Voort A, Liefaard MC, Van Ramshorst MS, et al. Efficacy of neoadjuvant treatment with or without pertuzumab in patients with stage II and III HER2-positive breast cancer: a nationwide cohort analysis of pathologic response and 5-year survival. Breast. 2022;65:110–5.
33. von Minckwitz G, Huang C-S, Mano MS, et al. Trastuzumab emtansine for residual invasive HER2-positive breast cancer. N Engl J Med. 2019;380(7):617–28.
34. Von Minckwitz G, Schneeweiss A, Loibl S, et al. Neoadjuvant carboplatin in patients with triple-negative and HER2-positive early breast cancer (GeparSixto; GBG 66): a randomised phase 2 trial. Lancet Oncol. 2014;15(7):747–56.
35. Shepherd JH, Ballman K, Polley MYC, et al. CALGB 40603 (alliance): long-term outcomes and genomic correlates of response and survival after neoadjuvant chemotherapy with or without carboplatin and bevacizumab in triple-negative breast cancer. J Clin Oncol. 2022;40(12):1323–34.
36. Schmid P, Cortes J, Pusztai L, et al. Pembrolizumab for early triple-negative breast cancer. N Engl J Med. 2020;382(9):810–21.
37. Masuda N, Lee S-J, Ohtani S, et al. Adjuvant capecitabine for breast cancer after preoperative chemotherapy. N Engl J Med. 2017;376(22):2147–59.
38. Tutt ANJ, Garber JE, Kaufman B, et al. Adjuvant olaparib for patients with BRCA1—or BRCA2—mutated breast cancer. N Engl J Med. 2021;384(25):2394–405.
39. Early Breast Cancer Trialists Collaborative Group. Adjuvant bisphosphonate treatment in early breast cancer: meta-analyses of individual patient data from randomised trials. Lancet. 2015;386(10001):1353–61.

Index

Note: Page numbers in *italics* indicate a figure and page numbers in **bold** indicate a table on the corresponding page.